IMMIGRATION AND ILLEGAL ALIENS

BURDEN OR BLESSING?

ISSN 1536-5263

IMMIGRATION AND ILLEGAL ALIENS

BURDEN OR BLESSING?

Cynthia S. Becker and David A. Becker

INFORMATION PLUS® REFERENCE SERIES
Formerly Published by Information Plus, Wylie, Texas

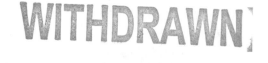

GALE
CENGAGE Learning

Detroit • New York • San Francisco • New Haven, Conn • Waterville, Maine • London

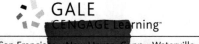

Immigration and Illegal Aliens: Burden or Blessing?

Cynthia S. Becker and David A. Becker

Paula Kepos, Series Editor

Project Editors: Kathleen J. Edgar, Elizabeth Manar

Rights Acquisition and Management: Jennifer Altschul, Barb McNeil

Composition: Evi Abou-El-Seoud, Mary Beth Trimper

Manufacturing: Cynde Lentz

For product information and technology assistance, contact us at
Gale Customer Support, 1-800-877-4253.
For permission to use material from this text or product,
submit all requests online at **www.cengage.com/permissions.**
Further permissions questions can be e-mailed to
permissionrequest@cengage.com

Cover photograph: Image copyright Jim Parkin, 2009. Used under license from Shutterstock.com.

Gale
27500 Drake Rd.
Farmington Hills, MI 48331-3535

ISBN-13: 978-0-7876-5103-9 (set)
ISBN-13: 978-1-4144-3379-0

ISBN-10: 0-7876-5103-6 (set)
ISBN-10: 1-4144-3379-4

ISSN 1536-5263

This title is also available as an e-book.
ISBN-13: 978-1-4144-5765-9 (set)
ISBN-10: 1-4144-5765-0 (set)
Contact your Gale sales representative for ordering information.

Printed in the United States of America
1 2 3 4 5 6 7 13 12 11 10 09

TABLE OF CONTENTS

PREFACE

Immigration and Illegal Aliens: Burden or Blessing? is part of the *Information Plus Reference Series.* The purpose of each volume of the series is to present the latest facts on a topic of pressing concern in modern American life. These topics include the most controversial and studied social issues in the twenty-first century: abortion, capital punishment, care of senior citizens, crime, the environment, health care, minorities, national security, social welfare, women, youth, and many more. Even though this series is written especially for high school and undergraduate students, it is an excellent resource for anyone in need of factual information on current affairs.

By presenting the facts, it is the intention of Gale, Cengage Learning to provide its readers with everything they need to reach an informed opinion on current issues. To that end, there is a particular emphasis in this series on the presentation of scientific studies, surveys, and statistics. These data are generally presented in the form of tables, charts, and other graphics placed within the text of each book. Every graphic is directly referred to and carefully explained in the text. The source of each graphic is presented within the graphic itself. The data used in these graphics are drawn from the most reputable and reliable sources, such as from the various branches of the U.S. government and from major independent polling organizations. Every effort has been made to secure the most recent information available. Readers should bear in mind that many major studies take years to conduct and that additional years often pass before the data from these studies are made available to the public. Therefore, in many cases the most recent information available in 2009 is dated from 2006 or 2007. Older statistics are sometimes presented as well, if they are of particular interest and no more-recent information exists.

Even though statistics are a major focus of the *Information Plus Reference Series*, they are by no means its only content. Each book also presents the widely held positions and important ideas that shape how the book's subject is discussed in the United States. These positions are explained in detail and, where possible, in the words of their proponents. Some of the other material to be found in these books includes historical background, descriptions of major events related to the subject, relevant laws and court cases, and examples of how these issues play out in American life. Some books also feature primary documents or have pro and con debate sections that provide the words and opinions of prominent Americans on both sides of a controversial topic. All material is presented in an even-handed and unbiased manner; readers will never be encouraged to accept one view of an issue over another.

HOW TO USE THIS BOOK

The United States is known as a melting pot, a place where people of different nationalities, cultures, ethnicities, and races have come together to form one nation. This process has been shaped by an influx of both legal immigrants and illegal aliens, and American attitudes toward both groups have varied over time. Legal immigrants have faced discrimination based on prevailing social and political trends; illegal aliens have been seen by some as undesirable, particularly after it became apparent that some or all of the terrorists behind the September 11, 2001, attacks had entered the United States legally but had overstayed their allotted time. This book discusses these and other legal, social, and political aspects of immigration and illegal aliens.

Immigration and Illegal Aliens: Burden or Blessing? consists of nine chapters and five appendixes. Each chapter is devoted to a particular aspect of immigration in the United States. For a summary of the information covered in each chapter, please see the synopses provided in the Table of Contents at the front of the book. Chapters generally begin with an overview of the basic facts and background information on the chapter's topic, then proceed to examine subtopics of particular interest. For example, Chapter 4, The

Worldwide Refugee Challenge, begins by explaining where refugees come from and how they were legally admitted before and after the Refugee Act of 1980. It then details how many refugees are admitted, annual refugee admissions limits, material support denials, the processing priority system, and the profile of admitted refugees. This is followed by an overview of asylum seekers, specifically their numbers, the claims they are required to file, affirmative and defensive asylum claims, legal challenges of immigration courts, and expedited removal. Two other groups of refugees are also discussed: victims of trafficking and violence and victims of torture. The chapter concludes by addressing the adjustment that refugees make to living in the United States, the benefits they receive to assist the transition, the support that is available for elderly and disabled refugees, and how unaccompanied children are handled. Readers can find their way through a chapter by looking for the section and subsection headings, which are clearly set off from the text. They can also refer to the book's extensive Index, if they already know what they are looking for.

Statistical Information

The tables and figures featured throughout *Immigration and Illegal Aliens: Burden or Blessing?* will be of particular use to readers in learning about this topic. These tables and figures represent an extensive collection of the most recent and valuable statistics on immigration and illegal aliens and related issues—for example, graphics cover the number of immigrant orphans adopted by U.S. citizens, the percentage of native-born and foreign-born workers employed in various industries, the living arrangements of native- and foreign-born children, and the use of welfare programs for native and immigrant households. Gale, Cengage Learning believes that making this information available to readers is the most important way to fulfill the goal of this book: to help readers understand the issues and controversies surrounding immigration and illegal aliens in the United States and to reach their own conclusions.

Each table or figure has a unique identifier appearing above it for ease of identification and reference. Titles for the tables and figures explain their purpose. At the end of each table or figure, the original source of the data is provided.

To help readers understand these often complicated statistics, all tables and figures are explained in the text. References in the text direct readers to the relevant statistics. Furthermore, the contents of all tables and figures are fully indexed. Please see the opening section of the Index at the back of this volume for a description of how to find tables and figures within it.

Appendixes

Besides the main body text and images, *Immigration and Illegal Aliens: Burden or Blessing?* has five appen-

dixes. The first is a reproduction of a pamphlet published by the U.S. Department of Justice titled *Federal Protections against National Origin Discrimination—U.S. Department of Justice: Potential Discrimination against Immigrants Based on National Origin*. The second appendix features maps of the world to assist readers in pinpointing the places of birth of the United States' immigrant population. The third is the Important Names and Addresses directory. Here, readers will find contact information for a number of government and private organizations that can provide further information on aspects of immigration and illegal aliens. The fourth appendix is the Resources section, which can also assist readers in conducting their own research. In this section the author and editors of *Immigration and Illegal Aliens: Burden or Blessing?* describe some of the sources that were most useful during the compilation of this book. The final appendix is the Index.

ADVISORY BOARD CONTRIBUTIONS

The staff of Information Plus would like to extend its heartfelt appreciation to the Information Plus Advisory Board. This dedicated group of media professionals provides feedback on the series on an ongoing basis. Their comments allow the editorial staff who work on the project to make the series better and more user-friendly. The staff's top priority is to produce the highest-quality and most useful books possible, and the Advisory Board's contributions to this process are invaluable.

The members of the Information Plus Advisory Board are:

- Kathleen R. Bonn, Librarian, Newbury Park High School, Newbury Park, California

- Madelyn Garner, Librarian, San Jacinto College, North Campus, Houston, Texas

- Anne Oxenrider, Media Specialist, Dundee High School, Dundee, Michigan

- Charles R. Rodgers, Director of Libraries, Pasco-Hernando Community College, Dade City, Florida

- James N. Zitzelsberger, Library Media Department Chairman, Oshkosh West High School, Oshkosh, Wisconsin

COMMENTS AND SUGGESTIONS

The editors of the *Information Plus Reference Series* welcome your feedback on *Immigration and Illegal Aliens: Burden or Blessing?* Please direct all correspondence to:

Editors
Information Plus Reference Series
27500 Drake Rd.
Farmington Hills, MI 48331-3535

CHAPTER 1
IMMIGRATION IN U.S. HISTORY

From its beginning, the United States has been a land of immigrants. People have come from all nations seeking free choice of worship, escape from cruel governments, and relief from war, famine, or poverty. All came with dreams of a better life for themselves and their families. The United States has accommodated people of diverse backgrounds, customs, and beliefs, although not without considerable friction along the way.

On the eastern shore of the peninsula that is now Florida, Spanish conquistadors established a settlement in 1565. The city of St. Augustine survived to become the oldest continuously occupied settlement of European origin in North America. However, it was the northern colonies that expanded rapidly and became central to the development of the nation. In *Immigration: From the Founding of Virginia to the Closing of Ellis Island* (2002), Dennis Wepman chronicles the immigrants who shaped the United States. Not long after English settlers established the first permanent colony on the James River in Virginia in 1607, the French developed a settlement on the St. Lawrence River in what is now Quebec, Canada. Dutch explorers soon built a fur trading post, Fort Nassau, on the Hudson River at what is now Albany, New York. Swedes settled on the Delaware River near present-day Wilmington. German Quakers and Mennonites joined William Penn's (1644–1718) experimental Pennsylvania colony. Jews from Brazil, Protestant Huguenots from France, and Puritans and Catholics from England all came to escape persecution of their religious beliefs and practices.

During the colonial period many immigrants came as indentured servants—meaning that they were required to work for four to seven years to earn back the cost of their passage. To the great aggravation of the colonists, some were convicts who accepted being shipped across the ocean as an alternative to imprisonment or death. Wepman estimates that as many as 50,000 British felons were sent to the colonies. The first Africans arrived in Jamestown in 1619 as indentured servants, but other Africans were soon brought in chains to be slaves.

A continual flow of immigrants provided settlers to develop communities along the Atlantic coast, pioneers to push the United States westward, builders for the Erie Canal and the transcontinental railways, pickers for cotton in the South and vegetables in the Southwest, laborers for U.S. industrialization, and intellectuals in all fields. Together, these immigrants have built, in the opinion of many people, the most diverse nation in the world.

According to Campbell Gibson and Kay Jung of the U.S. Census Bureau, in *Historical Census Statistics on Population Totals by Race, 1790 to 1990, and by Hispanic Origin, 1790 to 1990, for the United States, Regions, Divisions, and States* (September 2002, http://www.census.gov/population/www/documentation/twps0056/twps0056.html), the 1790 census in the United States showed a population of 3.2 million white people and 757,000 black people, of whom about 60,000 were free and the rest slaves. The U.S. population was predominantly English but also included people of German, Irish, Scottish, Dutch, French, and Spanish descent. Native Americans were not counted.

ATTITUDES TOWARD IMMIGRANTS

Even though immigration was the way of life in the country's first century, negative attitudes began to appear among the already settled English population. Officially, with the major exception of the Alien and Sedition Acts of 1798, the United States encouraged immigration. The Articles of Confederation, drafted in 1777, made citizens of each state citizens of every other state. The U.S. Constitution (written in 1787) made only one direct reference to immigration. Article 1, Section 9, Clause 1 provided that the "migration or importation of such persons as any of the states now existing shall think proper to admit, shall not be prohibited by the Congress prior to the year one thousand eight hundred and eight, but a tax or duty may be imposed on such importation, not exceeding ten dollars for each person." Article 1 also gave Congress power to establish "a uniform rule of naturalization" to grant U.S. citizenship.

Alien and Sedition Acts of 1798

Early federal legislation established basic criteria for naturalization: five years' residence in the United States, good moral character, and loyalty to the U.S. Constitution. These requirements were based on state naturalization laws. In 1798 the Federalist-controlled Congress proposed four laws, collectively called the Alien and Sedition Acts:

- The Naturalization Act lengthened the residence requirement for naturalization from 5 to 14 years.

- The Alien Act authorized the president to arrest and/ or expel allegedly dangerous aliens.

- The Alien Enemies Act allowed the imprisonment or deportation of aliens who were subjects of an enemy nation during wartime.

- The Sedition Act authorized fines and imprisonment for acts of treason including "any false, scandalous and malicious writing."

The Sedition Act was used by the Federalist administration of President John Adams (1735–1826) to arrest and silence a number of newspaper editors who publicly opposed the new laws. The strong public outcry against the Alien and Sedition Acts was partly responsible for the election of Thomas Jefferson (1743–1826), the Democratic-Republican presidential candidate, in the election of 1800. Jefferson pardoned the individuals convicted under the Sedition Act. The Naturalization Act was repealed by Congress, and the other three laws were allowed to lapse.

FIRST CENTURY OF IMMIGRATION

During the early 1800s U.S. territory more than doubled in size with the addition of 828,000 square miles (2.1 million square km) of land, which came to be known as the Louisiana Purchase. Reports of rich farmland and virgin forests provided by such explorers as Meriwether Lewis (1774–1809) and William Clark (1770–1838) enticed struggling farmers and skilled craftsmen, merchants and miners, laborers, and wealthy investors to leave Europe for the land of opportunity. The U.S. Department of Homeland Security's (DHS) Office of Immigration Statistics reports in *Yearbook of Immigration Statistics: 2008* (2008, http://www.dhs.gov/xlibrary/assets/statistics/yearbook/2008/table01.xls) that in 1820, the year when immigration records were first kept, only 8,385 immigrants were granted legal permanent residence in the United States. During the 1820s the number began to rise slowly to more than 22,000 in 1829.

Wave of Irish and German Immigration

Europe experienced a population explosion in the 1800s. As land in Europe became more and more scarce,

tenant farmers were pushed off their farms into poverty. Some immigrated to the United States to start a new life. This situation was made worse in Ireland, when a fungus that caused potato crops to rot struck in 1845. Many of the Irish were poor farmers who depended on potatoes for food. They suffered greatly from famine when their crops rotted, and epidemics of cholera and typhoid spread from village to village. The potato famine in Ireland forced people to choose between starving to death and leaving their country. In the 10-year period between 1830 and 1839, 170,672 Irish people arrived in the Unites States. (See Table 1.1.) Driven by the potato famine, between 1840 and 1849 the number of Irish immigrants rose more than 284% to 656,145. The flow of immigrants from Ireland to the United States peaked at 1,029,486 during the 1850s.

Increasing numbers of German immigrants, who were also affected by a potato famine as well as by failed political revolutions, paralleled that of the Irish. Between 1850 and 1859 the number of German immigrants (976,072) was not far behind the Irish (1,029,486). (See Table 1.1.) The influx of Germans peaked at 1,445,181 immigrants between 1880 and 1889.

Immigration, Politics, and the Civil War

This new wave of immigration led to intense anti-Irish, anti-German, and anti-Catholic sentiments among Americans, many of whom had been in the United States for only a few generations. It also triggered the creation of secret nativist societies (groups professing to protect the interests of the native-born against immigrants). Out of these groups grew a new political party, the Know Nothing movement (later known as the American Party), which claimed to support the rights of Protestant, American-born voters (and by implication, men, as women were not allowed to vote in federal elections until ratification of the 19th Amendment in 1920). The American Party managed to win 75 seats in Congress and 6 governorships in 1855 before it dissolved.

In contrast to the nativists, the 1864 Republican Party platform, written in part by Abraham Lincoln (1809–1865), stated, "Resolved, That foreign immigration, which in the past has added so much to the wealth, development of resources, and increase of power to the nation, the asylum of the oppressed of all nations, shall be fostered and encouraged by a liberal and just policy" (http://teachingamerican history.org/library/index.asp?document=1472).

In 1862 Lincoln had signed the Homestead Law, which offered 160 acres (65 ha) of free land to any adult citizen or prospective citizen who agreed to occupy and improve the land for 5 years. Wepman notes that between 1862 and 1904 over 147 million acres (59.5 million ha) of western land were claimed by adventurous citizens and eager new immigrants. In addition, efforts to complete a transcontinental railroad during the 1860s provided work for predominantly Irish and Chinese laborers.

TABLE 1.1

Immigration by region and selected country of last residence, fiscal years 1820–2007

Region and country of last residence[a]	1820 to 1829	1830 to 1839	1840 to 1849	1850 to 1859	1860 to 1869	1870 to 1879	1880 to 1889	1890 to 1899	1900 to 1909	1910 to 1919	1920 to 1929	1930 to 1939	1940 to 1949
Total	128,502	538,381	1,427,337	2,814,554	2,081,261	2,742,137	5,248,568	3,694,294	8,202,388	6,347,380	4,295,510	699,375	856,608
Europe	99,272	422,771	1,369,259	2,619,680	1,877,726	2,251,878	4,638,677	3,576,411	7,572,569	4,985,411	2,560,340	444,399	472,524
Austria-Hungary[b, c, d]	—	—	—	—	3,375	60,127	314,787	534,059	2,001,376	1,154,727	60,891	12,531	13,574
Austria[b, d]	—	—	—	—	2,700	54,529	204,805	268,218	532,416	589,174	31,392	5,307	8,393
Hungary[b]	—	—	—	—	483	5,598	109,982	203,350	685,567	565,553	29,499	7,224	5,181
Belgium	28	20	3,996	5,765	5,785	6,991	18,738	19,642	37,429	32,574	21,511	4,013	12,473
Bulgaria[e]	—	—	—	—	—	—	—	52	34,651	27,180	2,824	1,062	449
Czechoslovakia[f]	—	—	—	—	—	—	—	—	—	—	101,182	17,757	8,475
Denmark	173	927	671	3,227	13,553	29,278	85,342	56,671	61,227	45,830	34,406	3,470	4,549
Finland	—	—	—	—	—	—	—	—	—	—	16,922	2,438	2,230
France[g]	7,694	39,330	75,300	81,778	35,938	71,901	48,193	35,616	67,735	60,335	54,842	13,761	36,954
Germany[c, d]	5,753	124,726	385,434	976,072	723,734	751,769	1,445,181	579,072	328,722	174,227	386,634	119,107	119,506
Greece	17	49	17	32	51	209	1,807	12,732	145,402	198,108	60,774	10,599	8,605
Ireland[h]	51,617	170,672	656,145	1,029,486	427,419	422,264	674,061	405,710	344,940	166,445	202,854	28,195	15,701
Italy	430	2,225	1,476	8,643	9,853	46,296	267,660	603,761	1,930,475	1,229,916	528,133	85,053	50,509
Netherlands	1,105	1,377	7,624	11,122	8,387	14,267	52,715	29,349	42,463	46,065	29,397	7,791	13,877
Norway-Sweden[l]	91	1,149	12,389	22,202	82,937	178,823	586,441	334,058	426,981	192,445	170,329	13,452	17,326
Norway[l]	—	—	—	—	16,068	88,644	185,111	96,810	182,542	79,488	70,327	6,901	8,326
Sweden[l]	—	—	—	—	24,224	90,179	401,330	237,248	244,439	112,957	100,002	6,551	9,000
Poland[c]	19	366	105	1,087	1,886	11,016	42,910	107,793	—	—	223,316	25,555	7,577
Portugal	177	820	196	1,299	2,083	13,971	15,186	25,874	65,154	82,489	44,829	3,518	6,765
Romania	—	—	—	—	—	—	5,842	6,808	57,322	13,566	67,810	5,264	1,254
Russia[c, k]	86	280	520	423	1,670	35,177	182,698	450,101	1,501,301	1,106,998	61,604	2,463	605
Spain	2,595	2,010	1,916	8,795	6,966	5,540	3,995	9,189	24,818	53,262	47,109	3,669	2,774
Switzerland	3,148	4,430	4,819	24,423	21,124	25,212	81,151	37,020	32,541	22,839	31,772	5,990	9,904
United Kingdom[h, m]	26,336	74,350	218,572	445,322	532,956	578,447	810,900	328,759	469,518	371,878	341,552	61,813	131,794
Yugoslavia[n]	—	—	—	—	—	—	—	—	—	—	49,215	6,920	2,039
Other Europe	3	40	79	4	9	590	1,070	145	514	6,527	22,434	9,978	5,584
Asia	34	55	121	36,080	54,408	134,128	71,151	61,285	299,836	269,736	126,740	19,231	34,532
China	3	8	32	35,933	54,028	133,139	65,797	15,268	19,884	20,916	30,648	5,874	16,072
Hong Kong	—	—	—	—	—	—	—	—	—	—	—	—	—
India	9	38	33	42	50	166	247	102	3,026	3,478	2,076	554	1,692
Iran	—	—	—	—	—	—	—	—	—	—	208	198	1,144
Israel	—	—	—	—	—	—	—	—	—	—	—	—	98
Japan	—	—	—	—	138	193	1,583	13,998	139,712	77,125	42,057	2,683	1,557
Jordan	—	—	—	—	—	—	—	—	—	—	—	—	—
Korea	—	—	—	—	—	—	—	—	—	—	—	—	83
Philippines	—	—	—	—	—	—	—	—	—	—	—	391	4,099
Syria	—	—	—	—	—	—	—	—	—	—	5,307	2,188	1,179
Taiwan	—	—	—	—	—	—	—	—	—	—	—	—	—
Turkey	19	8	45	94	129	382	2,478	27,510	127,999	160,717	40,450	1,327	754
Vietnam	—	—	—	—	—	—	—	—	—	—	—	—	—
Other Asia	3	1	11	11	63	248	1,046	4,407	9,215	7,500	5,994	6,016	7,854
America	9,655	31,905	50,516	84,145	130,292	345,010	524,826	37,350	277,809	1,070,539	1,591,278	230,319	328,435
Canada and Newfoundland[o, p]	2,297	11,875	34,285	64,171	117,978	324,310	492,865	3,098	123,067	708,715	949,286	162,703	160,911
Mexico[o, q]	3,835	7,187	3,069	3,446	1,957	5,133	2,405	734	31,188	185,334	498,945	32,709	56,158
Caribbean	3,061	11,792	11,803	12,447	8,751	14,285	27,323	31,480	100,960	120,860	83,482	18,052	46,194
Cuba	—	—	—	—	—	—	—	—	—	—	12,769	10,641	25,976
Dominican Republic	—	—	—	—	—	—	—	—	—	—	—	1,026	4,802
Haiti	—	—	—	—	—	—	—	—	—	—	—	156	823
Jamaica[r]	—	—	—	—	—	—	—	—	—	—	—	—	—

TABLE 1.1

Immigration by region and selected country of last residence, fiscal years 1820–2007 [CONTINUED]

Region and country of last residence[a]	1820 to 1829	1830 to 1839	1840 to 1849	1850 to 1859	1860 to 1869	1870 to 1879	1880 to 1889	1890 to 1899	1900 to 1909	1910 to 1919	1920 to 1929	1930 to 1939	1940 to 1949	1950 to 1959	1960 to 1969	1970 to 1979	1980 to 1989	1990 to 1999	2000	2001	2002	2003	2004	2005	2006	2007
Other Caribbean[f]	3,061	11,792	11,803	12,447	8,751	14,285	27,323	31,480	100,960	120,860	70,713	6,229	14,593													
Central America	57	94	297	512	70	173	279	649	7,341	15,692	16,511	6,840	20,135													
Belize	—	—	—	—	—	—	—	—	77	40	285	193	433													
Costa Rica	—	—	—	—	—	—	—	—	—	—	—	431	1,965													
El Salvador	—	—	—	—	—	—	—	—	—	—	—	597	4,885													
Guatemala	—	—	—	—	—	—	—	—	—	—	—	423	1,303													
Honduras	—	—	—	—	—	—	—	—	—	—	—	679	1,874													
Nicaragua	—	—	—	—	—	—	—	—	—	—	—	405	4,393													
Panama[g]	—	—	—	—	—	—	—	—	—	—	—	1,452	5,282													
Other Central America	57	94	297	512	70	173	279	649	7,264	15,652	16,226	2,660	—													
South America	405	957	1,062	3,569	1,536	1,109	1,954	1,389	15,253	39,938	43,025	9,990	19,662													
Argentina	—	—	—	—	—	—	—	—	—	—	—	1,067	3,108													
Bolivia	—	—	—	—	—	—	—	—	—	—	—	50	893													
Brazil	—	—	—	—	—	—	—	—	—	—	4,627	1,468	3,653													
Chile	—	—	—	—	—	—	—	—	—	—	—	347	1,320													
Colombia	—	—	—	—	—	—	—	—	—	—	—	1,027	3,454													
Ecuador	—	—	—	—	—	—	—	—	—	—	—	244	2,207													
Guyana	—	—	—	—	—	—	—	—	—	—	—	131	596													
Paraguay	—	—	—	—	—	—	—	—	—	—	—	33	85													
Peru	—	—	—	—	—	—	—	—	—	—	—	321	1,273													
Suriname	—	—	—	—	—	—	—	—	—	—	—	25	130													
Uruguay	—	—	—	—	—	—	—	—	—	—	—	112	754													
Venezuela	—	—	—	—	—	—	—	—	—	—	—	1,155	2,182													
Other South America	405	957	1,062	3,569	1,536	1,109	1,954	1,389	15,253	39,938	38,398	4,010	7													
Other America[f]	—	—	—	—	—	—	—	—	—	—	29	25	25,375													
Africa	15	50	61	84	407	371	763	432	6,326	8,867	6,362	2,120	6,720													
Egypt	—	—	—	—	4	29	145	51	—	—	1,063	781	1,613													
Ethiopia	—	—	—	—	—	—	—	—	—	—	—	10	28													
Liberia	1	8	5	7	43	52	21	9	—	—	—	35	37													
Morocco	—	—	—	—	—	—	—	—	—	—	—	73	879													
South Africa	14	42	56	77	35	48	23	9	—	—	—	312	1,022													
Other Africa	—	—	—	—	325	242	574	363	6,326	8,867	5,299	909	3,141													
Oceania	3	7	14	166	187	9,996	12,361	4,704	12,355	12,339	9,860	3,306	14,262													
Australia	2	1	2	15	—	8,930	7,250	3,098	11,191	11,280	8,404	2,260	11,201													
New Zealand	—	—	—	—	—	39	21	12	—	—	935	790	2,351													
Other Oceania	1	6	12	151	187	1,027	5,090	1,594	1,164	1,059	521	256	710													
Not specified[t, u]	19,523	83,593	7,366	74,399	18,241	754	790	14,112	33,493	488	930	—	135													
Total														2,499,268	3,213,749	4,248,203	6,244,379	9,775,398	841,002	1,058,902	1,059,356	703,542	957,883	1,122,257	1,266,129	1,052,415
Europe														1,404,973	1,133,443	825,590	668,866	1,348,612	131,920	176,892	177,059	102,546	135,663	180,396	169,156	120,759
Austria-Hungary[b, c, d]														113,015	27,590	20,387	20,437	27,529	2,009	2,303	4,004	2,176	3,689	4,569	2,991	2,057
Austria[b, d]														81,354	17,571	14,239	15,374	18,234	986	996	2,650	1,160	2,442	3,002	1,301	849
Hungary[b]														31,661	10,019	6,148	5,063	9,295	1,023	1,307	1,354	1,016	1,247	1,567	1,690	1,208
Belgium														18,885	9,647	5,413	7,028	7,077	817	997	834	515	746	1,031	891	733
Bulgaria[e]														97	598	1,011	1,124	16,948	4,779	4,273	3,476	3,706	4,042	5,451	4,690	3,766
Czechoslovakia[f]														1,624	2,758	5,654	5,678	8,970	1,407	1,911	1,854	1,472	1,871	2,182	2,844	1,851
Denmark														10,918	9,797	4,405	4,847	6,189	549	732	651	435	568	714	738	505
Finland														4,923	4,310	2,829	2,569	3,970	377	497	365	230	346	549	513	385
France[g]														50,113	46,975	26,281	32,066	35,945	4,063	5,379	4,567	2,926	4,209	5,035	4,945	3,680
Germany[c, d]														576,905	209,616	77,142	85,752	92,207	12,230	21,992	20,977	8,061	10,270	12,864	10,271	8,640
Greece														45,153	74,173	102,370	37,729	25,403	5,113	1,941	1,486	900	1,213	1,473	1,544	1,152

TABLE 1.1

Immigration by region and selected country of last residence, fiscal years 1820–2007 [CONTINUED]

Region and country of last residence[a]	1950 to 1959	1960 to 1969	1970 to 1979	1980 to 1989	1990 to 1999	2000	2001	2002	2003	2004	2005	2006	2007
Ireland[h]	47,189	37,788	11,461	22,210	65,384	1,264	1,531	1,400	1,002	1,518	2,083	2,038	1,599
Italy	184,576	200,111	150,031	55,562	75,992	2,652	3,332	2,812	1,890	2,495	3,179	3,406	2,682
Netherlands	46,703	37,918	10,373	11,234	13,345	1,455	1,888	2,296	1,321	1,713	2,150	1,928	1,482
Norway-Sweden[l]	44,224	36,150	10,298	13,941	17,825	1,967	2,544	2,082	1,516	2,011	2,264	2,111	1,604
Norway[l]	22,806	17,371	3,927	3,835	5,211	508	582	460	385	457	472	532	388
Sweden[l]	21,418	18,779	6,371	10,106	12,614	1,459	1,962	1,622	1,131	1,554	1,792	1,579	1,216
Poland[c]	6,465	55,742	33,696	63,483	172,249	9,750	12,308	13,274	11,004	14,048	14,836	16,704	9,717
Portugal[l]	13,928	70,568	104,754	42,685	25,497	1,373	1,611	1,301	808	1,062	1,084	1,439	1,054
Romania	914	2,339	10,774	24,753	48,136	6,506	6,206	4,515	3,305	4,078	6,431	6,753	5,240
Russia[c, k]	453	2,329	28,132	33,311	433,427	43,156	54,838	55,370	33,513	41,959	60,344	59,720	41,593
Spain[l]	6,880	40,793	41,718	22,783	18,443	1,390	1,875	1,588	1,102	1,453	2,002	2,387	1,810
Switzerland	17,577	19,193	8,536	8,316	11,768	1,339	1,786	1,493	862	1,193	1,465	1,199	885
United Kingdom[h, m]	195,709	220,213	133,218	153,644	156,182	14,427	20,118	17,940	11,155	16,680	21,956	19,984	16,113
Yugoslavia[n]	6,966	17,990	31,862	16,267	57,039	11,960	21,854	28,051	8,270	13,213	19,249	11,066	6,364
Other Europe	11,756	6,845	5,245	3,447	29,087	3,337	6,976	6,723	6,377	7,286	9,485	10,994	7,847
Asia	135,844	358,605	1,406,544	2,391,356	2,859,899	254,932	336,112	325,749	235,339	319,025	382,707	411,746	359,387
China	8,836	14,060	17,627	170,897	342,058	41,804	50,677	55,901	37,342	50,280	64,887	83,590	70,924
Hong Kong	13,781	67,047	117,350	112,132	116,894	7,181	10,282	7,938	5,015	5,421	5,004	4,514	4,450
India	1,850	18,638	147,997	231,649	352,528	38,938	65,673	66,644	47,032	65,507	79,139	58,072	55,371
Iran	3,195	9,059	33,763	98,141	76,899	6,481	8,003	7,684	4,696	5,898	7,306	9,829	8,098
Israel	21,376	30,911	36,306	43,669	41,340	3,871	4,892	4,907	3,686	5,206	6,963	6,667	4,999
Japan	40,651	40,956	49,392	44,150	66,582	7,688	10,424	9,106	6,702	8,655	9,929	9,107	7,213
Jordan	4,899	9,230	25,541	28,928	42,755	4,476	5,106	4,774	4,008	5,186	5,430	5,512	5,516
Korea	4,845	27,048	241,192	322,708	179,770	15,107	19,728	19,917	12,076	19,441	26,002	24,472	21,278
Philippines	17,245	70,660	337,726	502,056	534,338	40,465	50,644	48,493	43,133	54,651	57,654	71,133	68,792
Syria	1,091	2,432	8,086	14,534	22,906	2,255	3,542	3,350	2,046	2,549	3,350	3,080	2,550
Taiwan	721	15,657	83,155	119,051	132,647	9,457	12,457	9,932	7,168	9,314	9,389	8,545	9,053
Turkey	2,980	9,464	12,209	19,208	38,687	2,702	3,463	3,914	3,318	4,491	6,449	6,433	4,728
Vietnam	290	2,949	121,716	200,632	275,379	25,159	34,537	32,372	21,227	30,074	30,832	29,701	27,510
Other Asia	14,084	40,494	174,484	483,601	637,116	49,348	56,684	50,817	37,890	52,352	70,373	91,091	68,905
America	921,610	1,674,172	1,904,355	2,695,329	5,137,743	392,461	470,794	477,363	305,936	408,972	432,726	548,812	434,272
Canada and Newfoundland[o, p]	353,169	433,128	179,267	156,313	194,788	21,289	29,991	27,142	16,447	22,439	29,930	23,913	20,324
Mexico[p, q]	273,847	441,824	621,218	1,009,586	2,757,418	171,445	204,032	216,924	114,758	173,711	157,992	170,042	143,180
Caribbean	115,661	427,235	708,850	790,109	1,004,687	84,250	96,384	93,914	67,498	82,116	91,371	144,477	114,318
Cuba	73,221	202,030	256,497	132,552	159,037	17,897	25,832	27,435	8,685	15,385	20,651	44,248	25,441
Dominican Republic	10,219	83,552	139,249	221,552	359,818	17,893	21,139	22,386	26,112	30,063	27,365	37,997	27,875
Haiti	3,787	28,992	55,166	121,406	177,446	21,977	22,470	19,151	11,924	13,695	13,491	21,625	29,978
Jamaica[r]	7,397	62,218	130,226	193,874	177,143	15,603	15,031	14,507	13,045	13,581	17,774	24,538	18,873
Other Caribbean[r]	21,037	50,443	127,712	120,725	131,243	11,400	11,912	10,435	7,732	9,392	12,090	16,069	12,151
Central America	40,201	98,560	120,374	339,376	610,189	60,331	72,504	66,298	53,283	61,253	52,629	74,244	53,834
Belize	1,133	4,185	6,747	14,964	12,600	774	982	983	616	888	901	1,263	1,089
Costa Rica	4,044	17,975	12,405	25,017	17,054	1,390	1,863	1,686	1,322	1,811	2,479	3,459	2,722
El Salvador	5,094	14,405	29,428	137,418	273,017	22,301	30,876	30,472	27,854	29,297	20,891	31,258	20,009
Guatemala	4,197	14,357	23,837	58,847	126,043	9,861	13,399	15,870	14,195	18,655	16,468	23,674	17,198
Honduras	5,320	15,078	15,651	39,071	72,880	5,851	6,546	6,355	4,582	5,339	6,825	8,036	7,300
Nicaragua	7,812	10,383	10,911	31,102	80,446	18,258	16,908	9,171	3,503	3,842	3,196	4,035	3,587
Panama[s]	12,601	22,177	21,395	32,957	28,149	1,896	1,930	1,761	1,211	1,421	1,869	2,519	1,929
Other Central America	—	—	—	—	—	—	—	—	—	—	—	—	—
South America	78,418	250,754	273,608	399,862	570,624	55,143	67,880	73,082	53,946	69,452	100,803	136,134	102,616
Argentina	16,346	49,384	30,303	23,442	30,065	2,472	3,426	3,791	3,193	4,672	6,945	7,239	5,375
Bolivia	2,759	6,205	5,635	9,798	18,111	1,744	1,804	1,660	1,365	1,719	2,164	4,000	2,326
Brazil	11,547	29,238	18,600	22,944	50,744	6,767	9,391	9,034	6,108	10,247	16,329	17,741	13,546

TABLE 1.1

Immigration by region and selected country of last residence, fiscal years 1820–2007 [CONTINUED]

Region and country of last residence[a]	1950 to 1959	1960 to 1969	1970 to 1979	1980 to 1989	1990 to 1999	2000	2001	2002	2003	2004	2005	2006	2007
Chile	4,669	12,384	15,032	19,749	18,200	1,660	1,881	1,766	1,255	1,719	2,354	2,727	2,202
Colombia	15,567	68,371	71,265	105,494	137,985	14,125	16,234	18,409	14,400	18,055	24,705	42,017	32,055
Ecuador	8,574	34,107	47,464	48,015	81,358	7,624	9,654	10,524	7,022	8,366	11,528	17,624	12,011
Guyana	1,131	4,546	38,278	85,886	74,407	5,255	7,835	9,492	6,373	5,721	8,771	9,010	5,288
Paraguay	576	1,249	1,486	3,518	6,082	394	464	413	222	324	523	725	518
Peru	5,980	19,783	25,311	49,958	110,117	9,361	10,838	11,737	9,169	11,369	15,205	21,300	17,056
Suriname	299	612	714	1,357	2,285	281	254	223	175	170	287	341	193
Uruguay	1,026	4,089	8,416	7,235	6,062	396	516	499	470	750	1,110	1,639	1,340
Venezuela	9,927	20,758	11,007	22,405	35,180	5,052	5,576	5,529	4,190	6,335	10,870	11,758	10,696
Other South America	17	28	97	61	28	12	7	5	4	5	12	13	10
Other America[t]	60,314	22,671	1,038	83	37	3	3	3	4	1	1	2	—
Africa	13,016	23,780	71,408	141,990	346,416	40,790	50,009	56,002	45,559	62,623	79,697	112,100	89,277
Egypt	1,996	5,581	23,543	26,744	44,604	4,323	5,333	6,215	3,928	6,590	10,296	13,163	10,178
Ethiopia	302	804	2,588	12,927	40,097	3,645	4,620	6,308	5,969	7,180	8,378	13,390	11,340
Liberia	289	841	2,391	6,420	13,587	1,225	1,477	1,467	1,081	1,540	1,846	3,736	3,771
Morocco	2,703	2,880	1,967	3,471	15,768	3,423	4,752	3,188	2,969	3,910	4,165	4,704	4,311
South Africa	2,278	4,360	10,002	15,505	21,964	2,814	4,046	3,685	2,088	3,335	4,425	3,173	2,842
Other Africa	5,448	9,314	30,917	76,923	210,396	25,360	29,781	35,139	29,524	40,068	50,587	73,934	56,835
Oceania	11,353	23,630	39,980	41,432	56,800	5,928	7,201	6,495	5,076	6,954	7,432	8,000	6,639
Australia	8,275	14,986	18,708	16,901	24,288	2,694	3,714	3,420	2,488	3,397	4,090	3,770	3,026
New Zealand	1,799	3,775	5,018	6,129	8,600	1,080	1,347	1,364	1,030	1,420	1,457	1,344	1,234
Other Oceania	1,279	4,869	16,254	18,402	23,912	2,154	2,140	1,711	1,558	2,137	1,885	2,886	2,379
Not specified[t,u]	12,472	119	326	305,406	25,928	14,971	17,894	16,688	9,086	24,646	39,299	16,315	42,081

—Represents zero or not available.

[a]Data for years prior to 1906 refer to country of origin; data from 1906 to 2007 refer to country of last residence.

[b]Data for Austria and Hungary not reported separately for all years during 1860 to 1869, 1890 to 1899, 1900 to 1909.

[c]From 1899 to 1919, data for Poland included in Austria-Hungary, Germany, and the Soviet Union.

[d]From 1938 to 1945, data for Austria included in Germany.

[e]From 1899 to 1910, included Serbia and Montenegro.

[f]Currently includes Czech Republic and Slovak Republic.

[g]From 1820 to 1910, included Corsica.

[h]Prior to 1926, data for Northern Ireland included in Ireland.

[i]Data for Norway and Sweden not reported separately until 1869.

[j]From 1820 to 1910, included Cape Verde and Azores Islands.

[k]From 1820 to 1920, data refer to the Russian Empire. Between 1920 and 1990 data refer to the Soviet Union. From 1991 to present, the data refer to the Russian Federation, Armenia, Azerbaijan, Belarus, Georgia, Kazakhstan, Kyrgyzstan, Moldova, Russia, Tajikistan, Ukraine, and Uzbekistan.

[l]From 1820 to 1910, included the Canary Islands and Balearic Islands.

[m]Since 1925, data for United Kingdom refer to England, Scotland, Wales and Northern Ireland.

[n]Currently includes Bosnia-Herzegovina, Croatia, Macedonia, Slovenia, and Serbia and Montenegro.

[o]Prior to 1911, data refer to British North America. From 1911, data includes Newfoundland.

[p]Land arrivals not completely enumerated until 1908.

[q]No data available for Mexico from 1886 to 1893.

[r]Data for Jamaica not reported separately until 1953. Prior to 1953, Jamaica was included in British West Indies.

[s]From 1932 to 1972, data for the Panama Canal Zone included in Panama.

[t]Included in 'Not specified' until 1925.

[u]Includes 32,897 persons returning in 1906 to their homes in the United States.

Note: From 1820 to 1867, figures represent alien passenger arrivals at seaports; from 1868 to 1891 and 1895 to 1897, immigrant aliens admitted for permanent residence; from 1892 to 1894 and 1898 to 2007, immigrant alien arrivals; from 1892 to 1903, aliens entering by cabin class were not counted as immigrants. Land arrivals were not completely enumerated until 1908. For this table, fiscal year 1843 covers 9 months ending September, 1843; fiscal years 1832 and 1850 cover 15 months ending December 31 of the respective years; and fiscal year 1868 covers 6 months ending June 30, 1868.

SOURCE: "Table 2. Persons Obtaining Legal Permanent Resident Status by Region and Selected Country of Last Residence: Fiscal Years 1820–2007," in Yearbook of Immigration Statistics: 2007, U.S. Department of Homeland Security, Office of Immigration Statistics, 2008, http://www.dhs.gov/xlibrary/assets/statistics/yearbook/2007/table02.xls (accessed October 16, 2008)

The Civil War (1861–1865) seemed to have little impact on immigration. The Office of Immigration Statistics reports in *Yearbook of Immigration Statistics: 2008* that even though the number of immigrants dropped from 153,640 in 1860 to just under 92,000 in both 1861 and 1862, there were 176,282 new arrivals in 1863, and the numbers continued to grow.

Post–Civil War Growth in Immigration

Post–Civil War America was characterized by the rapid growth of the Industrial Revolution, which fueled the need for workers in the nation's flourishing factories. The number of arriving immigrants continued to grow during the 1870s, dominated by people from Canada, Germany, Ireland, and the United Kingdom. (See Table 1.1.) Opposition to immigration continued among some factions of established citizens. Secret societies of white supremacists, such as the Ku Klux Klan, formed throughout the South to oppose not only African-American suffrage but also the influence of the Roman Catholic Church and rapid naturalization of foreign immigrants.

East European Influx during the 1880s

The decade from 1880 to 1889 marked a new era in immigration to the United States. The volume of immigrants nearly doubled from 2,742,137 in the 1870s to 5,248,568 in the 1880s. (See Table 1.1.) German arrivals peaked at 1,445,181, and the number arriving from Norway, Sweden, and the United Kingdom also reached their highest levels. A new wave of immigrants began to arrive from Russia (including a significant number of Jews fleeing massacres called pogroms), Poland, Austria-Hungary, and Italy. The mass exodus from eastern Europe foretold events that would result in World War I (1914–1918). These newcomers were different. They came from countries with limited public education and no sense of social equality. They were often unskilled and illiterate. They tended to form tight ethnic communities within the large cities, where they clung to their own language and customs, which further limited their ability to assimilate into U.S. culture.

A Developing Federal Role in Immigration

The increasing numbers of immigrants prompted a belief that there should be some type of administrative order to the ever-growing influx. In 1864 Congress created the Commission of Immigration under the U.S. Department of State. A one-person office was set up in New York City to oversee immigration.

The 1870s witnessed a national debate over the importation of contract labor and limiting immigration for such purposes. In 1875, after considerable debate, Congress passed the Page Law. The first major piece of restrictive immigration legislation, it prohibited alien convicts and prostitutes from entering the country.

With the creation of the Commission of Immigration, the federal government began to play a central role in immigration, which had previously been handled by the individual states. Beginning in 1849, court decisions strengthened the federal government's role and limited the states' role in regulating immigration. In 1875 the U.S. Supreme Court ultimately ruled in *Henderson v. Mayor of the City of New York* (92 U.S. 259) and *Chy Lung v. Freeman* (92 U.S. 275) that the immigration laws of New York, California, and Louisiana were unconstitutional. This ended the rights of states to regulate immigration and exclude undesirable aliens. From then on Congress and the federal government had complete responsibility for immigration.

In 1882 Congress passed the first general immigration law. The Immigration Act of 1882 established a centralized immigration administration under the U.S. secretary of the treasury. The law also allowed the exclusion of "undesirables," such as paupers, criminals, and the insane. A head tax was added at $0.50 per arriving immigrant to defray the expenses of immigration regulation and caring for the immigrants after their arrival in the United States.

Influx of Immigrants from Asia

Before the discovery of gold in California in 1848, few Asians (only 121 between 1840 and 1849) came to the United States. (See Table 1.1.) Between 1849 and 1852 large numbers of Asian immigrants began arriving in the United States. These early arrivals came mostly from southern China, spurred on by economic depression, famine, war, and flooding. Thousands of Chinese immigrants were recruited to build railroads and work in mines, construction, or manufacturing. Many became domestic servants. Former mining-camp cooks who had saved some of their income opened restaurants. Others invested small amounts in equipment to operate laundries, performing a service few other people wanted to tackle. Between 1850 and 1879, 223,100 immigrants from China arrived in the United States, whereas only a few thousand arrived from other Asian countries.

Some people became alarmed by this increase in Chinese immigration. Their fears were fueled by a combination of racism and concerns among American-born workers that employers were bringing over foreign workers to replace them and keep unskilled wages low. The public began to call for restrictions on Chinese immigration.

Chinese Exclusion Act

In 1882 Congress passed the Chinese Exclusion Act, which prohibited further immigration of Chinese laborers to the United States for 10 years. Exceptions included teachers, diplomats, students, merchants, and tourists. This act marked the first time the United States barred immigration of a national group. The law also prohibited Chinese immigrants in the United States from becoming naturalized U.S. citizens. Between 1890 and 1899 only 15,268 Chinese arrived. (See Table 1.1.)

Four other laws that prohibited the immigration of Chinese laborers followed the Chinese Exclusion Act. The Geary Act of 1892 extended the Chinese Exclusion Act for 10 more years. In cases brought before the U.S. Supreme Court, the court upheld the constitutionality of these two laws. The Immigration Act of 1904 made the Chinese exclusion laws permanent. Under the Immigration Act of 1917 the United States suspended the immigration of laborers from almost all Asian countries.

During World War II (1939–1945) the United States and China became allies against the Japanese in Asia. As a gesture of goodwill, on December 17, 1943, President Franklin D. Roosevelt (1882–1945) signed the Act to Repeal the Chinese Exclusion Acts, to Establish Quotas, and for Other Purposes. The new law lifted the ban on the naturalization of Chinese nationals but established a quota (a prescribed number) of 105 Chinese immigrants to be admitted per year.

Beginning of Japanese Immigration

Until the passage of the Chinese Exclusion Act, Japanese immigration was hardly noticeable, with the total flow at 331 between 1860 and 1879. (See Table 1.1.) Because Japanese immigrants were not covered by the Chinese Exclusion Act, Japanese laborers were brought in to replace Chinese workers. Consequently, Japanese immigration increased from 1,583 during the 1880s to 139,712 during the first decade of the 20th century. According to Marianne K. G. Tanabe of the University of Hawaii in *Health and Health Care of Japanese-American Elders* (2001, http://www.stanford.edu/group/ethnoger/japanese.html), the booming Hawaiian sugar industry offered so many jobs that by 1910 "Hawaii had four times as many Japanese as the U.S. mainland."

The same anti-Asian attitudes that had led to the Chinese Exclusion Act culminated in President Theodore Roosevelt's (1858–1919) Gentlemen's Agreement of 1907, an informal arrangement between the United States and Japan that cut the flow of Japanese immigration to a trickle. This anti-Asian attitude resurfaced a generation later in the National Origins Act of 1924. The immigration quota for any nationality group had been based on the number of people of that nationality that were residents in the United States during the 1910 census. The new law reduced quotas from 3% to 2% and shifted the base for quota calculations from 1910 back to 1890. Because few Asians lived in the United States in 1890, the 1924 reduction in Asian immigration was particularly dramatic. Asian immigration was not permitted to increase until after World War II.

Greater Government Control

In "U.S. Immigration and Naturalization Service—Populating a Nation: A History of Immigration and Naturalization" (September 10, 2008, http://www.cbp.gov/xp/cgov/about/history/ins_history.xml) the Department of Homeland Security provides an overview of the development of the implementation of immigration policy in the United States. In 1891 the federal government assumed total control over immigration issues. The Immigration Act of 1891 authorized the establishment of the U.S. Office of Immigration under the U.S. Department of the Treasury. This first comprehensive immigration law added to the list of inadmissible people those suffering from certain contagious diseases, polygamists (married people who had more than one spouse at the same time), and aliens convicted of minor crimes. The law also prohibited using advertisements to encourage immigration.

On January 1, 1892, a new federal immigration station began operating on Ellis Island in New York City. During its years of operation (1892–1954), more than 12 million immigrants were processed through Ellis Island. This figure represents about half of the more than 23 million total immigrants tallied by Table 1.1 during that period.

In 1895 the Office of Immigration became the Bureau of Immigration under the commissioner-general of immigration. In 1903 the Bureau of Immigration was transferred to the U.S. Department of Commerce and Labor. The Basic Naturalization Act of 1906 consolidated the immigration and naturalization functions of the federal government under the Bureau of Immigration and Naturalization. When the Department of Commerce and Labor was separated into two cabinet departments in 1913, two bureaus were formed: the Bureau of Immigration and the Bureau of Naturalization. In 1933 the two bureaus were reunited as the U.S. Immigration and Naturalization Service (INS).

A MILLION IMMIGRANTS PER YEAR BY 1905

By the 1890s the origins of those arriving in the United States had changed. Fewer immigrants came from northern Europe, whereas immigrants from southern, central, and eastern Europe increased every year. Of the 7.5 million European immigrants who arrived between 1900 and 1909, 5.4 million (72%) came from Italy, Russia, and Austria-Hungary. (See Table 1.1.) The exodus of Jews from eastern Europe was particularly significant. The American Immigration Law Foundation (December 6, 2004, http://www.ailf.org/exhibits/jewish2004/jewish_history.shtml) notes that many of these Jewish immigrants were merchants, shopkeepers, craftsmen, and professionals, contrary to the stereotype of poor, uneducated immigrants coming out of eastern Europe.

In *Yearbook of Immigration Statistics: 2008*, the Office of Immigration Statistics reports that the nation's already high immigration rate at the turn of the 20th century nearly doubled between 1902 and 1907. Immigration reached a million per year in 1905, 1906, 1907, 1910, 1913, and 1914, but declined to less than 325,000 per year from 1915 through 1919 because of World War I. Many Americans worried about the growing influx of immigrants, whose customs were unfamiliar to most of the native population.

Anti-Catholic sentiments, distrust of political radicalism (usually expressed as antisocialism), and racist movements gained prevalence along with a resurgence of nativism.

The Immigration Act of 1907 barred the immigration of "feeble-minded" people (those with physical or mental defects that might prevent them from earning a living) and people with tuberculosis. Increasing the head tax on each arriving immigrant to $5, the 1907 law also officially classified the arriving aliens as immigrants (people planning to take up residence in the United States) and nonimmigrants (people visiting for a short period to attend school, conduct business, or travel as tourists). All arrivals were required to declare their intentions for permanent or temporary stays in the United States. The law further authorized the president to refuse admission to people he considered harmful to the labor conditions in the nation.

Reflecting national concerns about conflicts between old and new immigrant groups, the Bureau of Immigration proposed in annual reports that the immigrants should be more widely dispersed throughout the rest of the country, instead of being concentrated mostly in the northeastern urban areas of the United States. Not only would such a distribution of aliens help relieve the nation's urban problems but also the bureau thought it might promote greater racial and cultural assimilation.

Immigration Act of 1917

The mounting negative feelings toward immigrants resulted in the Immigration Act of 1917, which was passed despite President Woodrow Wilson's (1856–1924) veto. Besides codifying previous immigration legislation, the 1917 act required that immigrants over age 16 be able to pass a literacy test, which proved to be a controversial clause. The new act also cited the following groups to the inadmissible classes of immigrants:

> All idiots, imbeciles, feeble-minded persons, epileptics, insane persons . . . persons with chronic alcoholism; paupers; professional beggars; vagrants; persons afflicted with tuberculosis in any form or a loathsome or dangerous contagious disease; persons not comprehended within any of the foregoing excluded classes who are found to be and are certified by the examining surgeon as being mentally or physically defective, such physical defect being of a nature which may affect the ability of such alien to earn a living; persons who have been convicted . . . of a felony or other crime or misdemeanor involving moral turpitude; polygamists, or persons who practice polygamy or believe in and advocate the practice of polygamy; anarchists, or persons who advocate the overthrow by force or violence of the Government of the United States, or of all forms of law . . . or who advocate the assassination of public officials, or who advocate and teach the unlawful destruction of property . . . ; prostitutes, or persons coming to the United States for the purpose of prostitution or immoral purposes.

The act also specifically disqualified those coming from the designated Asiatic "barred zone," which encompassed mostly Asia and the Pacific Islands. This provision was a continuation of the Chinese Exclusion Act and the Gentlemen's Agreement of 1907, in which the Japanese government had agreed to stop the flow of workers to the United States. In 1918 passports were required by presidential proclamation for all entries into the United States.

Denied Entry

Despite the restrictive immigration legislation, only a small percentage of those attempting to immigrate to the United States were turned away. Between 1892 and 1990, 650,252 people were denied entry for a variety of reasons. (See Table 1.2.) Aside from those attempting to enter without proper papers, the largest excluded group consisted of 219,399 people who were considered "likely to become public charges." The 30-year period from 1901 to 1930 was the peak era for exclusion of immigrants deemed likely to become public charges, mentally or physically defective, or immoral. The 1917 ban on illiterate immigrants excluded 13,679 aliens over the next 50 years.

Restrictions on Immigration Tighten

World War I temporarily stopped the influx of immigrants. According to the Office of Immigration Statistics, in *Yearbook of Immigration Statistics: 2008*, in 1914, 1,218,480 immigrants arrived; a year later the number dropped to 326,700. By 1918, the final year of the war, 110,618 immigrants ventured to the United States. However, the heavy flow of immigration started again after the war as people fled the war-ravaged European continent. In 1921, 805,228 immigrants arrived in the United States.

The new wave of immigrants flocked to major cities where they hoped to find relatives or other immigrants from their native country as well as jobs. According to the Census Bureau's *Increase of Population in the United States, 1910– 1920* (1922, http://www2.census.gov/prod2/decennial/documents/00476515n1_TOC.pdf), the 1920 census reported that for the first time in U.S. history the population living in cities exceeded that living in rural areas.

First Quota Law

Concern over whether the United States could continue to absorb such huge numbers of immigrants led Congress to introduce a major change in U.S. immigration policy. Other factors influencing Congress included racial fears about the new immigrants and apprehension over many of the immigrants' politically radical ideas.

The Quota Law of 1921 was the first quantitative immigration law. Congress limited the number of aliens of any nationality who could enter the United States to 3% of the number of foreign-born people of that nationality who lived in the United States in 1910 (based on the U.S. census). By

TABLE 1.2

Aliens excluded, by administrative reason for exclusion, fiscal years 1892–1990

Year	Total	Subversive or anarchist	Criminal or narcotics violations	Immoral	Mental or physical defect	Likely to become public charge	Stowaway	Attemped entry without inspection or without proper documents	Contract laborer	Unable to read (over 16 years of age)	Other
1892–1990	650,252	1,369	17,465	8,209	82,590	219,399	16,240	204,943	41,941	13,679	44,417
1892–1900	22,515	—	65	89	1,309	15,070	—	—	5,792	—	190
1901–10	108,211	10	1,681	1,277	24,425	63,311	—	—	12,991	—	4,516
1911–20	178,109	27	4,353	4,824	42,129	90,045	1,904	—	15,417	5,083	14,327
1921–30	189,307	9	2,082	1,281	11,044	37,175	8,447	94,084	6,274	8,202	20,709
1931–40	68,217	5	1,261	253	1,530	12,519	2,126	47,858	1,235	258	1,172
1941–50	30,263	60	1,134	80	1,021	1,072	3,182	22,441	219	108	946
1951–60	20,585	1,098	2,017	361	956	149	376	14,657	13	26	932
1961–70	4,831	128	383	24	145	27	175	3,706	—	2	241
1971–80	8,455	32	814	20	31	31	30	7,237	—	—	260
1981–90	19,759	NA	3,675	NA	NA	NA	NA	14,960	—	—	1,124

Note: From 1941–53, statistics represent all exclusions at sea and air ports and exclusions of aliens seeking entry for 30 days or longer at land ports. After 1953, includes aliens excluded after formal hearings.
— Represents zero.
NA Not available.

SOURCE: Adapted from "Table 44. Aliens Excluded by Administrative Reason for Exclusion: Fiscal Years 1892–1990," in *Yearbook of Immigration Statistics: 2004*, U.S. Department of Homeland Security, Office of Immigration Statistics, 2004, http://www.dhs.gov/xlibrary/assets/statistics/yearbook/2003/2003ENF.pdf (accessed April 1, 2009)

1910, however, many south and east Europeans had already entered the country, a fact legislators had overlooked. Consequently, to restructure the makeup of the immigrant population, Congress approved the National Origins Act of 1924. This act set the first permanent limitation on immigration, called the national origins quota system. The law immediately limited the number of people of each nationality to 2% of the population of that nationality who lived in the United States in 1890.

The 1924 law provided that after July 1, 1927, an overall cap would allow a total of 150,000 immigrants per year. Quotas for each national origin group were to be developed based on the 1920 census. Exempted from the quota limitation were spouses or dependents of U.S. citizens, returning alien residents, or natives of Western Hemisphere countries not subject to quotas (natives of Mexico, Canada, or other independent countries of Central or South America). The 1924 law further required that all arriving nonimmigrants present visas (government authorizations permitting entry into a country) obtained from a U.S. consulate abroad. U.S. immigration law consisted of the 1917 and 1924 acts until 1952.

Impact of Quotas

The new laws also barred all Asian immigration, which soon led to a shortage of farm and sugar plantation workers. Filipinos filled the gap because the Philippines was a U.S. territory and did not come under the immigration quota laws. In addition, large numbers of Caribbean immigrants arrived, peaking during the 1910 to 1919 period, when 120,860 Caribbean immigrants entered the United States. (See Table 1.1.)

Before World War I, Caribbean workers had moved among the islands and to parts of South and Central America. Following the war many went north in search of work. Similarly, after World War II, when agricultural changes in the Caribbean forced many people off farms and into cities, many traveled on to the United States or the United Kingdom in search of work.

With the new quota laws, the problem of illegal aliens arose for the first time. Previously, only a few who had failed the immigration standards tried to sneak in, usually across the U.S.-Mexican or U.S.-Canadian land borders. With the new laws, the number of illegal aliens began to increase. Subsequently, Congress created the U.S. Border Patrol in 1924 (under the Labor Appropriation Act) to oversee the nation's borders and prevent illegal aliens from coming into the United States. This in turn resulted in a system of appeals and deportation actions.

IMMIGRATION DURING WORLD WAR II

Immigration dropped well below 100,000 arrivals per year during the Great Depression because the United States offered no escape from the unemployment that was rampant throughout most of the world. However, in the latter half of the 1930s Nazi persecution caused a new round of immigrants to flee Europe. In 1940 the INS was transferred from the U.S. Department of Labor to the U.S. Department of Justice. This move reflected the growing fear of war, making the surveillance of aliens a question of national security rather than of how many to admit. The job of the INS shifted from the exclusion of aliens to combating alien criminal and subversive elements. This required closer cooperation with the U.S. attorney general's office and the Federal Bureau of Investigation.

Alien Registration

World War II began with the German invasion of Poland in September 1939. Growing concern about an increase in refugees that might result from the war in Europe led Congress to pass the Alien Registration Act of 1940 (also known as the Smith Act). Among its provisions, this act required all aliens to register. Those over 14 years old also had to be fingerprinted. All registration and fingerprinting took place at local post offices between August 27 and December 26, 1940. Each alien was identified by an alien registration number, known as an A-number. For the first time, the government had a means of identifying individual immigrants. The law has been challenged by the courts, but the A-number system is still in use in the 21st century. Following registration, each alien received by mail an Alien Registration Receipt Card, which he or she was required to keep to prove registration. Each alien was also required to report any change of address within five days. Managing such a vast number of registrants and documents in a short time created a monumental challenge for the federal government. The ranks of employees in the Alien Registration Division of the INS increased dramatically in late 1940 and early 1941.

The United States officially entered World War II on December 8, 1941, the day after the Japanese attack on Pearl Harbor, Hawaii. President Roosevelt immediately proclaimed all "nationals and subjects" of nations with which the country was at war to be enemy aliens. According to the INS, on January 14, 1942, the president issued a proclamation requiring further registration of aliens from enemy nations (primarily Germany, Italy, and Japan). All such aliens aged 14 and older were directed to apply for a Certificate of Identification during the month of February 1942.

Alien registrations were used by a variety of government agencies and private industry to locate possible enemy subversives, such as aliens working for defense contractors, aliens with radio operator licenses, and aliens trained to pilot aircraft. According to the INS, one out of every 23 workers in U.S. industry at that time was a noncitizen.

Japanese Internment

Following the recommendation of military advisers, President Roosevelt issued Executive Order 9066 on February 19, 1942, which authorized the forcible internment of people of Japanese ancestry. Lieutenant General John L. DeWitt (1880–1962) was placed in charge of removal of the Japanese to internment camps, which were located in remote areas in western states, including Arizona, California, Colorado, Idaho, Utah, and Wyoming. Two camps were also established in Arkansas. In *Final Report: Japanese Evacuation from the West Coast 1942* (1943), DeWitt stated that during a period of less than 90 days 110,442 people of Japanese ancestry were evacuated from the West Coast. More than two-thirds were U.S. citizens. Relocation began in April 1942. The last camp was vacated in March 1946.

Executive Order 9066 was never formally terminated after the war ended. Over the years many Japanese-Americans expressed concern that it could be implemented again. On February 19, 1976, President Gerald Ford (1913–2006) issued a proclamation officially terminating the provisions of Executive Order 9066 retroactive to December 31, 1946. In 1988 President Ronald Reagan (1911–2004) signed a bill into law providing restitution ($20,000) to each of the surviving internees.

POSTWAR IMMIGRATION LAW

A growing fear of communist infiltration arose during the post–World War II period. One result was the passage of the Internal Security Act of 1950, which made membership in communist or totalitarian organizations cause for exclusion (denial of an alien's entry into the United States), deportation, or denial of naturalization. The law also required resident aliens to report their addresses annually and made reading, writing, and speaking English prerequisites for naturalization.

The Immigration and Nationality Act of 1952 added preferences for relatives and skilled aliens, gave immigrants and aliens certain legal protections, made all races eligible for immigration and naturalization, and absorbed most of the Internal Security Act of 1950. The act changed the national origin quotas to only one-sixth of 1% of the number of people in the United States in 1920 whose ancestry or national origin was attributable to a specific area of the world. It also excluded aliens on ideological grounds, homosexuality, health restrictions, criminal records, narcotics addiction, and involvement in terrorism.

Once again, countries within the Western Hemisphere were not included in the quota system. President Harry S. Truman (1884–1972) vetoed the legislation, but Congress overrode his veto. Even though there were major amendments, the Immigration and Nationality Act remained the basic statute governing who could gain entry into the United States until the passage of new laws following the September 11, 2001, terrorist attacks.

During the 1950s a half-dozen special laws allowed the entrance of additional refugees. Many of the laws resulted from World War II, but some stemmed from new developments, including laws relaxing the quotas for refugees fleeing the failed 1956 Hungarian revolution and those seeking asylum following the Cuban revolution in 1959.

A TWO-HEMISPHERE SYSTEM

In 1963 President John F. Kennedy (1917–1963) submitted a plan to change the quota system. Two years later

Congress passed the Immigration and Nationality Act Amendments of 1965. Since 1924 sources of immigration had changed. During the 1950s immigration from Asia to the United States nearly quadrupled from 34,532 (between 1940 and 1949) to 135,844 (between 1950 and 1959). (See Table 1.1.) In the same period immigrants to the United States from North, Central, and South America increased dramatically.

The 1965 legislation canceled the national origins quota system and made visas available on a first-come, first-served basis. A seven-category preference system was implemented for families of U.S. citizens and permanent resident aliens for the purpose of family reunification. In addition, the law set visa allocations for people with special occupational skills, abilities, or training needed in the United States. It also established an annual ceiling of 170,000 Eastern Hemisphere immigrants with a 20,000 per-country limit, and an annual limit of 120,000 for the Western Hemisphere without a per-country limit or preference system.

The Immigration and Nationality Act Amendments of 1976 extended the 20,000 per-country limit to Western Hemisphere countries. Some legislators were concerned that the 20,000-person limit for Mexico was inadequate, but their objections were overruled. The Immigration and Nationality Act Amendments of 1978 combined the separate ceilings for the Eastern and Western Hemispheres into a single worldwide ceiling of 290,000.

PROGRAMS FOR REFUGEES

Official U.S. refugee programs began in response to the devastation of World War II, which created millions of refugees and displaced people (DPs). (A displaced person was a person living in a foreign country as a result of having been driven from his or her home country because of war or political unrest.) This was the first time the United States formulated policy to admit people fleeing persecution. The Presidential Directive of December 22, 1945, gave priority in issuing visas to about 40,000 DPs. The directive was followed by the Displaced Persons Act of 1948, which authorized the admission of 202,000 people from eastern Europe, and the Refugee Relief Act of 1953, which approved entry of another 209,000 defectors from communist countries over a three-year period. The Displaced Persons Act counted the refugees in the existing immigration quotas, whereas the Refugee Relief Act admitted them outside the quota system.

Parole Authority—A Temporary Admission Policy

In 1956 the U.S. attorney general used the parole authority (temporary admission) under section 212(d) (15) of the Immigration and Nationality Act of 1952 for the first time on a large scale. This section authorized the attorney general to temporarily admit any alien to the United States. Even though parole was not admission for permanent residence, it could lead to permanent resident or immigrant status. Aliens already in the United States on a temporary basis

could apply for asylum (to stay in the United States) on the grounds they were likely to suffer persecution if returned to their native land. The attorney general was authorized to withhold deportation on the same grounds.

In *Americans at the Gate: The United States and Refugees during the Cold War* (2008), Carl J. Bon Tempo estimates that this parole authority was used to admit approximately 32,000 of the 38,000 Hungarians who fled the failed Hungarian revolution in 1956. The other 6,000 entered under the Refugee Relief Act of 1953 and were automatically admitted as permanent residents. Similarly, in *Defining America through Immigration Policy* (2004), Bill Ong Hing notes that the parole provision had been used to accommodate 15,000 refugees leaving China following the communist revolution there in 1949, and was used again in 1962 to admit several thousand Chinese refugees from Hong Kong to the United States.

Refugees as Conditional Entrants

In 1965, under the Immigration and Nationality Act Amendments, Congress added section 203(a) (7) to the Immigration and Nationality Act of 1952, creating a group of conditional entrant refugees from communist or Middle Eastern countries, with status similar to the refugee parolees. Sections 203(a) (7) and 212(d) (15) were used to admit thousands of refugees, including Czechoslovakians escaping their failed revolution in 1968, Ugandans fleeing their dictatorship in the 1970s, and Lebanese avoiding the civil war in their country in the 1980s.

The United States did not have a general policy governing the admission of refugees until the Refugee Act of 1980. This act eliminated refugees as a category in the preference system and set a worldwide ceiling on immigration of 270,000, not counting refugees. It also removed the requirement that refugees had to originate from a communist or Middle Eastern nation.

ILLEGAL IMMIGRATION LEADS TO REFORM

In *Temporary Migration to the United States: Nonimmigrant Admissions under U.S. Immigration Law* (January 2006, http://www.uscis.gov/files/nativedocuments/Nonimmigrants_2006.pdf), the U.S. Citizenship and Immigration Services explains that the U.S. attorney general "authorized the temporary admission of agricultural workers under the Ninth Proviso of Section 3 of the Immigration Act of 1917, and later legislation provided for the temporary admission of seasonal farm labor in what would become known as the Bracero Program. Between 1942 and 1964, the United States welcomed more than 4.5 million nonimmigrant workers from Mexico known as braceros (Spanish for the strong-armed). The Bracero Program was developed in response to labor shortages during World War II." In 1964 the United States ended the program following an agreement with Mexico that allowed migrant workers to enter the United States to supply seasonal agricultural labor. However, ending the program did not stop migrants from crossing the border for work they had come to rely on. Those who could get visas often overstayed their time limit. Others simply crossed the border illegally and found jobs. A population of illegal immigrants began to grow.

During the 1970s the Vietnam War (1955–1975) divided the nation, oil prices skyrocketed, and gasoline shortages caused long waiting lines at the pumps. Price controls were implemented and removed to control rampant inflation. In this period of political, social, and economic uncertainty many people saw immigrants as straining the already limited welfare and educational systems. States with growing immigrant populations, such as California, Florida, Illinois, New York, and Texas, pushed Congress for immigration reform.

A surge of refugees from Vietnam and Cambodia as well as Cubans escaping the Fidel Castro (1926–) regime in the mid-1970s added to Americans' concerns. The major source of immigrants had changed from Europe to Latin America and Asia. Many people were uncomfortable with the faces and cultures of these new arrivals.

President Ford established a cabinet-level Domestic Council Committee on Illegal Aliens. Its December 1976 report recommended sanctions against employers who knowingly hired undocumented workers, increased border enforcement, and called for legalization for certain illegal aliens who arrived in the United States before July 1, 1968. In 1979 Congress established the Select Commission on Immigration and Refugee Policy. The commission spent the next two years evaluating the problem. Its 1981 *Final Report* fostered ideas that would become part of major new immigration reform legislation in 1986. More than 20 years later, however, Congress and the nation were still debating such issues as employers hiring undocumented workers, border enforcement, and legalization of long-term illegals.

CHAPTER 2
IMMIGRATION LAWS AND POLICIES SINCE THE 1980s

In "Immigration: Shaping and Reshaping America" (*Population Bulletin*, vol. 61, no. 4, December 2006), Philip Martin and Elizabeth Midgley point out that before the 1980s U.S. immigration laws might have changed once in a generation, but the quickening pace of global change after 1980 brought major new immigration legislation in 1986, 1990, and 1996. The September 11, 2001 (9/11), terrorist attacks led to antiterrorism laws that had considerable impact on immigration policies and procedures and that effected changes to immigration legislation. This chapter covers the most significant immigration laws from the 1980s through 2008.

IMMIGRATION REFORM AND CONTROL ACT OF 1986

On November 6, 1986, after 34 years with no new major immigration legislation and a 6-year effort to send an acceptable bill through both houses of Congress, the Immigration Reform and Control Act (IRCA) of 1986 was signed into law by President Ronald Reagan (1911–2004).

To control illegal immigration, the IRCA adopted three major strategies:

- Legalization of a portion of the undocumented population (aliens in the country without legal papers), thereby reducing the number of aliens illegally resident in the United States

- Sanctions against employers who knowingly hired illegal aliens

- Additional border enforcement to impede further unlawful entries

Arrivals before 1982

Two groups of immigrants became eligible to apply for legalization under the IRCA. The largest group consisted of those who could prove they had continuously resided in the United States without authorization since January 1, 1982. This large group of aliens had entered the United States in one of two ways: they arrived as illegal aliens before January 1, 1982, or they arrived on temporary visas (government authorizations permitting entry into a country) that expired before January 1, 1982.

To adjust to the legal status of permanent resident, aliens were required to prove eligibility for admission as immigrants and have at least a minimal understanding and knowledge of the English language, U.S. history, and the U.S. government. They could apply for citizenship five years from the date permanent resident status was granted.

Special Agricultural Workers

The second group of immigrants that became eligible to apply for legalization under the IRCA were referred to as special agricultural workers (SAWs). This category was created because many fruit and vegetable farmers feared they would lose their workers, many of whom were illegal aliens, if the IRCA provisions regarding length of continuous residence were applied to seasonal laborers. Most of these workers were migrants who returned home to live in Mexico when there was no work available in the fields. The SAW program permitted aliens who had performed labor in perishable agricultural commodities for a minimum of 90 days between May 1985 and May 1986 to apply for legalization.

HOW MANY WERE LEGALIZED? Nancy Rytina of the U.S. Citizenship and Immigration Services (USCIS) estimates in *IRCA Legalization Effects: Lawful Permanent Residence and Naturalization through 2001* (October 25, 2002, http://www.dhs.gov/xlibrary/assets/statistics/publications/irca0114int.pdf) that 3 million to 5 million illegal aliens were living in the United States in 1986. More than 3 million aliens applied for temporary residence status under the IRCA. Nearly 2.7 million (88%) of these applicants were eventually approved for permanent residence. By 2001 one-third (889,033) of these residents had become naturalized citizens. Rytina notes that a majority (75%) of applicants under the IRCA provisions were born in Mexico.

The IRCA barred newly legalized aliens from receiving most federally funded public assistance for five years. Exceptions included access to Medicaid for children, pregnant women, the elderly, the handicapped, and for emergency care. The State Legalization Impact Assistance Grant program reimbursed state and local governments the costs for providing public assistance, education, and public health services to the legalized aliens. In *Measuring the Fallout: The Cost of IRCA Amnesty after 10 Years* (May 1997, http://www.cis.org/articles/1997/back197.htm), David Simcox of the Center for Immigration Studies reports that the program reimbursed states $3.5 billion, averaging $1,167 per eligible legalized alien, during its seven years of operation.

Employer Sanctions

The employer sanctions provision of the IRCA was intended to correct a double standard that prohibited unauthorized aliens from working in the United States but permitted employers to hire them. The IRCA prohibited employers from hiring, recruiting, or referring for a fee aliens known to be unauthorized to work in the United States. Employers who violated the law were subject to a series of civil fines or criminal penalties when a pattern or practice of violations was found.

DOCUMENTING ELIGIBILITY FOR EMPLOYMENT. The burden of proof was on employers to demonstrate that their employees had valid proof of identity and were authorized to work. The IRCA required employers to complete the Employment Eligibility Verification form, known as Form I-9, for each employee hired. In completing the form the employer certified that the employee had presented valid proof of identity and eligibility for employment and that these documents appeared genuine. The IRCA also required employers to retain the completed I-9 forms and produce them in response to an official government request.

In February 2009 the USCIS revised Form I-9 and the list of documents acceptable to prove work eligibility. The new form applied only to employees hired after the form was implemented. (See Figure 2.1.) Even though Form I-9 is available in English and Spanish, only employers in Puerto Rico may have employees complete the Spanish version for their records. Employers in the 50 states and other U.S. territories may use the Spanish version as a translation guide for Spanish-speaking employees, but must complete the English version for company records. Employees may also use or ask for a translator/preparer to assist them in completing the form.

The most significant change was the new requirement that all documents presented during the Form I-9 completion process must be unexpired. Removed from List A (documents that establish both identity and employment authorization) were Temporary Resident Cards and the outdated Employment Authorization Cards I-688A and I-688B. Two documents were added to List A: a machine-readable immigrant visa with a temporary I-551 printed notation

along with a foreign passport with a temporary I-551 stamp, and a passport from the Federated States of Micronesia (FSM) or the Republic of the Marshall Islands (RMI) along with a Form I-94 or I-94A indicating nonimmigrant admission under the Compact of Free Association between the FSM or RMI. Under these agreements, most citizens of the FSM or RMI are eligible for nonimmigrant admission and have the privilege of residing and working in the United States. The new Form I-9 also allows an employee to attest to being either a citizen or noncitizen national of the United States. According to the USCIS, in "Questions and Answers: USCIS Revises Employment Eligibility Verification Form" (February 12, 2009, http://www.uscis.gov/), noncitizen nationals are people born in American Samoa, certain citizens of the former Trust Territory of the Pacific Islands, and certain children of nationals born abroad.

Undocumented Workers and Identity Theft

Many job seekers who lacked proof of eligibility to work in the United States bought false identity documents. The Federal Trade Commission (FTC) reports in its *Consumer Sentinel Network Data Book for January–December 2008* (February 2009, http://www.ftc.gov/ sentinel/reports/ sentinel-annual-reports/sentinel-cy2008.pdf) that in 2008 there were 313,982 nationwide complaints of identity theft. Border states and states with large immigrant populations in 2008 had the highest rates of identity theft complaints per 100,000 population, including Arizona (149 per 100,000 population), California (139.1), Florida (133.3), Texas (130.3), and Nevada (126). By comparison, South Dakota (33.8) registered the lowest number of complaints per 100,000 population in 2008.

The FTC also reported that 15% of victims' identities had been used to fraudulently obtain government documents or benefits, including tax refunds, and 15% had been used to secure employment. In the press release "3 Sentenced for Possessing, Selling Counterfeit Identification Documents" (October 24, 2008, http://www.ice.gov/pi/nr/ 0810/081024houston.htm), U.S. Immigration and Customs Enforcement (ICE) states that in 2008 the U.S. District Court in Houston, Texas, found three men guilty of conspiracy and fraud in connection with the possession with intent to transfer counterfeit identification documents. One of the men possessed 13 counterfeit Texas Identification cards, 21 Social Security cards, 4 resident alien cards, and 16 Permanent Resident Alien cards. Because all three were illegally in the United States, they will be subject to deportation after their release from prison.

Verifying Employee Eligibility for Work

To assist employers in complying with the Illegal Immigration Reform and Immigrant Responsibility Act of 1996 (IIRIRA; see below) and the IRCA, the Social Security Administration began the Basic Pilot Program, a computerized system that allowed employers to check the validity

FIGURE 2.1

Form I-9, Employment Eligibility Verification

Department of Homeland Security
U.S. Citizenship and Immigration Services

Read instructions carefully before completing this form. The instructions must be available during completion of this form.

ANTI-DISCRIMINATION NOTICE: It is illegal to discriminate against work-authorized individuals. Employers CANNOT specify which document(s) they will accept from an employee. The refusal to hire an individual because the documents have a future expiration date may also constitute illegal discrimination.

Section 1. Employee Information and Verification. *(To be completed and signed by employee at the time employment begins.)*

Print Name: Last	First	Middle Initial	Maiden Name

Address *(Street Name and Number)*		Apt. #	Date of Birth *(month/day/year)*

City	State	Zip Code	Social Security #

I am aware that federal law provides for imprisonment and/or fines for false statements or use of false documents in connection with the completion of this form.

I attest, under penalty of perjury, that I am (check one of the following):

☐ A citizen of the United States
☐ A noncitizen national of the United States (see instructions)
☐ A lawful permanent resident (Alien #) _____
☐ An alien authorized to work (Alien # or Admission #) _____
untill (expiration date, if applicable-*month/day/year*)

Employee's Signature

Date *(month/day/year)*

Preparer and/or Translator Certification *(To be completed and signed if Section 1 is prepared by a person other than the employee.)* I attest, under penalty of perjury, that I have assisted in the completion of this form and that to the best of my knowledge the information is true and correct.

Preparer's/Translator's Signature	Print Name

Address *(Street Name and Number, City, State, Zip Code)*	Date *(month/day/year)*

Section 2. Employer Review and Verification *(To be completed and signed by employer. Examine one document from List A OR examine one document from List B and one from List C, as listed on the reverse of this form, and record the title, number and expiration date, if any, of the document(s).)*

List A	OR	List B	AND	List C
Document title:				
Issuing authority:				
Document #:				
Expiration Date *(if any)*:				
Document #:				
Expiration Date *(if any)*:				

CERTIFICATION: I attest, under penalty of perjury, that I have examined the document(s) presented by the above-named employee, that the above-listed document(s) appear to be genuine and to relate to the employee named, that the employee began employment on *(month/day/year)* _____ and that to the best of my knowledge the employee is authorized to work in the United States. (State employment agencies may omit the date the employee began employment.)

Signature of Employer or Authorized Representative	Print Name	Title

Business or Organization Name and Address *(Street Name and Number, City, State, Zip Code)*	Date *(month/day/year)*

Section 3. Updating and Reverification *(To be completed and signed by employer.)*

A. New Name *(if applicable)*	B. Date of Rehire *(month/day/year) (if applicable)*

C. If employee's previous grant of work authorization has expired, provide the information below for the document that establishes current employment authorization.

Document Title: _____	Document #: _____	Expiration Date *(if any)*: _____

I attest, under penalty of perjury, that to the best of my knowledge, this employee is authorized to work in the United States, and if the employee presented document(s), the document(s) I have examined appear to be genuine and to relate to the individual.

Signature of Employer or Authorized Representative	Date *(month/day/year)*

FIGURE 2.1

Form I-9, Employment Eligibility Verification [CONTINUED]

LISTS OF ACCEPTABLE DOCUMENTS
All documents must be unexpired

LIST A	LIST B	LIST C
Documents that Establish Both Identity and Employment Authorization	Documents that Establish Identity	Documents that Establish Employment Authorization
	OR	AND
1. U.S. Passport or U.S. Passport Card	1. Driver's license or ID card issued by a State or outlying possession of the United States provided it contains a photograph or information such as name, date of birth, gender, height, eye color, and address	1. Social Security Account Number card other than one that specifies on the face that the issuance of the card does not authorize employment in the United States
2. Permanent Resident Card or Alien Registration Receipt Card (Form I-551)		
		2. Certification of Birth Abroad issued by the Department of State (Form FS-545)
3. Foreign passport that contains a temporary I-551 stamp or temporary I-551 printed notation on a machine-readable immigrant visa	2. ID card issued by federal, state or local government agencies or entities, provided it contains a photograph or information such as name, date of birth, gender, height, eye color, and address	
		3. Certification of Report of Birth issued by the Department of State (Form DS-1350)
4. Employment Authorization Document that contains a photograph (Form I-766)	3. School ID card with a photograph	
	4. Voter's registration card	4. Original or certified copy of birth certificate issued by a State, county, municipal authority, or territory of the United States bearing an official seal
5. In the case of a nonimmigrant alien authorized to work for a specific employer incident to status, a foreign passport with Form I-94 or Form I-94A bearing the same name as the passport and containing an endorsement of the alien's nonimmigrant status, as long as the period of endorsement has not yet expired and the proposed employment is not in conflict with any restrictions or limitations identified on the form	5. U.S. Military card or draft record	
	6. Military dependent's ID card	
	7. U.S. Coast Guard Merchant Mariner Card	5. Native American tribal document
	8. Native American tribal document	
	9. Driver's license issued by a Canadian government authority	6. U.S Citizen ID Card (Form I-197)
	For persons under age 18 who are unable to present a document listed above:	7. Identification Card for Use of Resident Citizen in the United States (Form I-179)
6. Passport from the Federated States of Micronesia (FSM) or the Republic of the Marshall Islands (RMI) with Form I-94 or I-94A indicating nonimmigrant admission under the Compact of Free Association Between the United States and the FSM or RMI	10. School record or report card	8. Employment authorization document issued by the Department of Homeland Security
	11. Clinic, doctor, or hospital record	
	12. Day-care or nursery school record	

Illustrations of many of these documents appear in Part 8 of the Handbook for Employers (M-274)

SOURCE: "Form I-9, Employment Eligibility Verification," U.S. Department of Homeland Security, U.S. Citizenship and Immigration Services, February 2, 2009, http://www.uscis.gov/files/form/I-9.pdf (accessed April 28, 2009)

of Social Security numbers (SSNs) presented by new hires. It was tested with employers in California, Florida, Illinois, and Texas before being expanded on December 1, 2004, to voluntary employers in all states. The program returned a tentative non-confirmation (known as a TNC) if the name, date of birth, or gender of the new hire did not match Social Security records; if the SSN had never been issued; or if records indicated the person issued that SSN was deceased. The new hire had a set time limit for resolving the problem with the Social Security Administration before the employer could terminate the individual.

In "Illegal Immigrants at Center of New Identity Theft Crackdown" (*New York Times*, December 14, 2006), Rachel L. Swarns reports that in December 2006 the U.S. Department of Homeland Security (DHS) raided six Swift & Company meat processing plants. It detained 1,282 illegal aliens and charged 65 people with identity theft. Swift & Company had participated in the Basic Pilot Program for several years, but the raids showed that the system did not recognize identity theft. Basic Pilot confirmed the validity of the SSN but did not check to see how many times and in what locations the number had been used for employment. Thus, several people could be using the same number on fraudulent identification (IDs). Even though the Swift raids left employers feeling threatened, they were assured that by using the tools provided by the government, they would be hiring legally eligible workers.

The Basic Pilot Program was renamed E-Verify in 2007 and expanded to include a feature that would allow employers to scan a new hire's photo identification to be compared against the 14.8 million images stored in DHS immigration databases. In "E-Verify: Frequently Asked Questions" (January 12, 2009, http://www.ncsl.org/programs/immig/EVerifyFAQ.htm), the National Conference of State Legislatures (NCSL) indicates that in fiscal year (FY) 2007, E-Verify had 3.6 million queries, up from 1.7 million in FY 2006, and that 100,000 employers were registered with E-Verify as of January 2009. Comparing E-Verify queries to NCSL's estimate of 7 million employers in the United States with 60 million new hires per year suggests that use of E-Verify is limited. According to the NCSL, in January 2009 a dozen states required the use of E-Verify for public and/or private employers—nine through legislation and three through executive orders.

IMMIGRATION MARRIAGE FRAUD AMENDMENTS OF 1986

Before 1986 the U.S. Immigration and Naturalization Service (INS) granted permanent residence fairly quickly to the foreign spouses of U.S. citizens or lawful permanent residents (LPRs). However, a number of marriages between Americans and foreigners occurred purely to attain U.S. permanent residence status for the foreigner. Some U.S. citizens or LPRs agreed to marry aliens for money. After

the alien gained permanent residence, the marriage was dissolved. Other cases involved aliens entering into marriages by deceiving U.S. citizens or LPRs with declarations of love.

The Immigration Marriage Fraud Amendments of 1986 specified that aliens basing their immigrant status on a marriage of less than two years were considered conditional immigrants. To remove the conditional immigrant status, the alien had to apply for permanent residence within 90 days after the second-year anniversary of receiving conditional status. The alien and his or her spouse were required to show that the marriage was and continued to be a valid one; otherwise, conditional immigrant status was terminated and the alien could be deported.

Wendy Koch notes in "Va. Case Highlights Fraudulent Marriages" (*USA Today*, November 8, 2006) that between FYs 2004 and 2006 ICE investigated 700 cases of marriage fraud. ICE found that marriage fraud organizations typically charged $2,500 to $6,000 to arrange a marriage for immigration purposes. Marriage fraud took on more serious implications after 9/11. Koch reports that according to the Center for Immigration Studies, half of the 36 suspected 9/11 terrorists gained legal status by marrying Americans, 10 through sham marriages.

In "Hello, I Love You, Won't You Tell Me Your Name: Inside the Green Card Marriage Phenomenon" (November 2008, http://www.cis.org/marriagefraud), David Seminara of the Center for Immigration Studies points out that marriage to an American citizen accounted for the highest number of immigrants who successfully gained legal permanent residency (often called "green card" status) in the United States in 2007. Seminara found that based on DHS data, more than 2.3 million foreigners gained LPR status in the United States based on marriage to an American between 1998 and 2007. The Department of Homeland Security reports in its *Yearbook of Immigration Statistics: 2008* (March 24, 2009, http://www.dhs.gov/xlibrary/assets/statistics/yearbook/2008/table06d.xls) that in 2008 more than a quarter-million people (265,671) gained permanent legal residence in the United States through marriage to a U.S. citizen.

Although Seminara notes that many marriages are legitimate, he also discusses the ways in which people use sham marriages to abuse provisions in the immigration laws that are intended to benefit American citizens and their immediate families. Among the most common types of marriage fraud, Seminara lists:

Mail-order brides

Arranged marriages

Financial arrangements in which a foreigner pays a fee to obtain an American spouse

Relatives or friends who marry someone as a gesture of kindness

Foreign nationals who feign attachment and trick an American into marriage

Other types of trafficking or exploitation by Americans taking advantage of foreigners seeking status in the United States

In addition, he terms some marriages "I do, I don't, I do" arrangements, in which a married noncitizen divorces a spouse in his or her home country, then marries an American to gain LPR status, then divorces the American and reunites with the original spouse.

Battered Brides

Spousal abuse sometimes results during the two-year period of conditional immigrant status. Particularly in cases of mail-order brides and brides from countries where women have few, if any, rights, some husbands take advantage of the power they have as the wife's sponsor. The new wives are dependent on their husbands to obtain permanent U.S. residence. The U.S. Department of Justice finds cases of alien wives who are virtual prisoners, afraid they will be deported if they defy their husband or report abuse. In addition, some of the women come from cultures in which divorced women are outcasts with no place in society.

The Violence against Women Act of 1994—which is part of the Violent Crime Control and Law Enforcement Act of 1994—and the Victims of Trafficking and Violence Prevention Act of 2000 were enacted to address the plight of such abused women and their children. The 1994 law allows the women and/or children to self-petition for immigrant status without the abuser's participation or consent. Abused males can also file a self-petition under this law. The 2000 law created a new nonimmigrant U-visa for victims of serious crimes. Recipients of the U-visa, including victims of crimes against women, can adjust to lawful permanent resident status based on humanitarian grounds as determined by the U.S. attorney general.

IMMIGRATION ACT OF 1990

Shortly after the IRCA was passed, Senators Edward M. Kennedy (1932–; D-MA) and Alan K. Simpson (1931–; R-WY) began work to change the Immigration and Nationality Act Amendments of 1965, which determined legal immigration into the United States. The senators asserted that the family-oriented system allowed one legal immigrant to bring too many relatives into the country. They proposed to cut the number of dependents admitted and replace them with individuals who had the skills or money to immediately benefit the U.S. economy. The result of their efforts was the Immigration Act (IMMACT) of 1990.

Enacted on November 29, 1990, IMMACT represented a major overhaul of immigration law. The focus of the new law was to raise the annual number of immigrants allowed from 500,000 to 700,000 and give greater priority to employment-based immigration. A diversity program encouraged applications from countries with low immigration history by allotting 50,000 visas per year in this category.

Diversity Visa Program

IMMACT made new provisions for the admission of immigrants from countries with low rates of immigration to the United States. The program was introduced as a transitional measure from 1992 to 1994. Ruth Ellen Wasem and Karma Ester explain in "Immigration: Diversity Visa Lottery" (April 22, 2004, http://www.ilw.com/immigdaily/news/ 2005,0809-crs.pdf) that under the permanent program, which began in 1995, no country was permitted more than 7% (3,850) of the total 55,000 visas, and Northern Ireland was treated as a separate state rather than included within the United Kingdom. To be eligible, aliens were required to have at least a high school education or equivalent, or at least two years of work experience in an occupation that required a minimum of two years' training or two years' experience within the past five years. An alien selected under the lottery program could apply for permanent residence and, if granted, was authorized to work in the United States. The alien's spouse and unmarried children under age 21 were also allowed to enter the United States.

Beginning in FY 1999, 5,000 visas were reserved for participants in the 1997 Nicaraguan Adjustment and Central American Relief Act. This law provided various immigration benefits and relief from deportation to certain Nicaraguans, Cubans, Salvadorans, Guatemalans, nationals of former Soviet-bloc countries, and their dependents.

RESULTS OF THE 2009 DIVERSITY LOTTERY. According to the U.S. Department of State, in "Diversity Visa Lottery 2009 (DV-2009) Results" (March 30, 2009, http://travel.state.gov/visa/immigrants/types/types_4317.html), more than 9.1 million qualified entries for DV-2009 were received during the 60-day application period that ran from noon on October 3, 2007, until noon on December 2, 2007. Even though only 50,000 permanent resident visas are available through the lottery, the State Department contacts a larger number of applicants to ensure that none of the 50,000 visas go unused. The countries with the highest representation among the 99,600 potential immigrants in DV-2009 included Ghana (7,322), Nigeria (6,041), Bangladesh (6,023), Ukraine (5,502), and Ethiopia (5,200).

Changing Grounds for Entry

IMMACT changed the political and ideological grounds for exclusion and deportation. The law repealed the ban against the admission of communists and representatives of other totalitarian regimes that had been in place since 1950. In addition, immigration applicants who had been excluded previously because of associations with communism were provided exceptions if the applicants had been involuntary members of the communist party, had terminated membership, or merely had close family relationships with people affiliated with communism.

Temporary Protected Status

IMMACT authorized the U.S. attorney general to grant temporary protected status (TPS) to undocumented aliens present in the United States when a natural disaster, ongoing armed conflict, or other extraordinary occurrence in their country posed a danger to their personal safety.

TPS lasts for 6 to 18 months unless conditions in the alien national's country warrant an extension of stay. TPS does not lead to permanent resident status, although such aliens can obtain work authorization. Once the TPS designation ends, the foreign nationals resume the same immigrant status they had before TPS (unless that status has expired) or any new status obtained while in TPS. According to the USCIS, in "Temporary Protected Status" (April 13, 2009, http://www.uscis.gov/), applicants from Burundi, Somalia, and Sudan were eligible for TPS in 2009.

WELFARE REFORM LAW OF 1996

Under Title IV of the Personal Responsibility and Work Opportunity Reconciliation Act of 1996, federal welfare benefits for legal immigrants were cut substantially and the responsibility for public assistance was shifted from the federal government to the states. (Illegal immigrants were already ineligible for most major welfare programs.) The law was designed to ensure that available welfare benefits did not serve as an incentive for immigration and that immigrants admitted to the United States would be self-reliant.

In the past legal immigrants had generally been eligible for the same welfare benefits as citizens. Under the new rules immigrants who had become naturalized citizens remained eligible for federal benefits, but most noncitizens were barred from participating in federal programs such as Temporary Assistance for Needy Families (TANF), food stamps, Supplemental Security Income (SSI), and Medicaid. (TANF is a federal block grant program for needy families with dependent children. Medicaid is a joint federal-state health insurance program for certain low-income and needy people. SSI is a federal income supplement program funded by general tax revenues—not Social Security taxes—that assists aged, blind, and disabled people who have little or no income.) States were given the option of using federal funds for TANF and Medicaid for immigrants who arrived before the act took effect. Immigrants who arrived legally after the law took effect were ineligible for any federal funds for five years; states then had the option of granting their applications for TANF and/or Medicaid. On August 15, 1997, the Balanced Budget Act restored SSI and Medicaid benefits to legal immigrants who had been receiving these benefits when the welfare reform law was passed.

Food Stamps

According to the U.S. General Accounting Office (now the U.S. Government Accountability Office), in *Welfare Reform: Many States Continue Some Federal or State Benefits for Immigrants* (July 1998, http://www.gao.gov/archive/1998/he98132.pdf), when the food stamp restrictions went into effect in 1997, an estimated 940,000 of the 1.4 million legal immigrants receiving food stamps lost their eligibility. Nearly one-fifth were immigrant children. During 1997 and 1998, 14 states created food stamp programs that served about a quarter of this immigrant group nationwide. Most recipients were children, the elderly, and the disabled. Some states continued to provide food assistance to ineligible legal immigrants. In "State-Funded Food Programs for Legal Immigrants" (February 17, 2009, http://www.fns.usda.gov/FSP/rules/Memo/PRWORA/StatePrograms.htm), the Food and Nutrition Service indicates that in 2008 only four states—California, Nebraska, New York, and Wisconsin—had food programs in place to assist some immigrants who were not eligible for the federal food stamps.

ILLEGAL IMMIGRATION REFORM AND IMMIGRANT RESPONSIBILITY ACT OF 1996

On September 30, 1996, the Illegal Immigration Reform and Immigrant Responsibility Act (IIRIRA) became law. In an effort to reduce illegal immigration, the IIRIRA included the following among its many provisions:

- Required doubling the number of U.S. Border Patrol agents to 5,000 by 2001 and increasing equipment and technology at air and land ports of entry

- Authorized improvements of southwestern border barriers

- Toughened penalties for immigrant smuggling (up to 10 years in prison, 15 years for third and subsequent offenses) and document fraud (up to 15 years in prison)

- Increased the number of INS investigators for worksite enforcement, tracking aliens who overstayed visas, and investigating alien smuggling

- Instituted a new "expedited removal" proceeding (denial of an alien's entry into the United States without a hearing) to speed deportation of aliens with no documents or with fraudulent documents

- Authorized three voluntary pilot programs to enable employers to verify the immigrant status of job applicants and to reduce the number and types of documents needed for identification and employment eligibility

- Instituted a bar on admissibility for aliens seeking to reenter the United States after having been unlawfully present in the country—a bar of 3 years for aliens unlawfully present from 6 months to a year and a bar of 10 years for those unlawfully present for more than a year

GREEN CARD

The USCIS states in "Lawful Permanent Residence ('Green Card')" (2008, http://www.uscis.gov/greencard) that "a 'green card' gives you official immigration status (Lawful Permanent Residency) in the United States." An LPR carries this document as proof of legal status in the country. Yet, the card is not green. What is known as a green card came in a variety of different colors at different times in history. The card, formally known as the Alien Registration Receipt Card, Form I-151 or I-551, entitles an alien to certain benefits, and those benefits originated at a time when the card was actually green. The USCIS provides a history of this important document in "Q: Green Card Not Green?" (2008, http://www.uscis.gov/).

The first receipt card, Form AR-3, resulted from the Alien Registration Act of 1940, a national defense measure enacted during World War II (1939–1945). The act required all non-U.S. citizens (legal or illegal) to register at post offices. From there the registration forms were forwarded to the INS. The receipt card was mailed to each alien as proof of his or her compliance with the law. These receipts were printed on white paper.

When the war ended, alien registration became part of the regular immigration procedure. Aliens registered at ports of entry and the INS issued different types of Alien Registration Receipt Cards based on each alien's admission status. For example, temporary foreign laborers received an I-100a card and visitors received an I-94c. Permanent residents received the I-151. The cards were different colors to make it easy to identify the immigration status of each alien. The permanent resident card was green and was necessary to get a job.

The Internal Security Act of 1950 made the I-151 even more valuable. Effective April 17, 1951, any alien holding an AR-3 card (the type issued to all aliens during the war) had to apply to have it replaced with the green I-151 card. Anyone who could not prove his or her legal admission to the United States did not qualify for a green card and could be subject to prosecution for violation of immigration laws.

By 1951 the green card represented security for an alien, because it indicated the right to permanently live and work in the United States. The Alien Registration Receipt Card, Form I-151, became commonly known to aliens, immigration attorneys, enforcement officers, and employers by its color. The term *green card* designated not only the document but also the official status so desired by many legal nonimmigrants (students, tourists, and temporary workers) and by illegal aliens.

The green card was so desirable that counterfeiting became a problem. In response to this counterfeiting, the INS issued 19 different designs of the card between 1940 and 1977. The 1964 version was pale blue, and in 1965 the card became dark blue. In January 1977 the INS introduced the new style, machine-readable Alien Registration Receipt Card, Form I-551, which has since been issued in a variety of colors, including pink and a pink and blue combination. Form I-151 and its successor, Form I-551, have such vital meaning to immigrants that despite changes in form number, design, and color, it will probably always be known as a green card.

PATRIOT ACT OF 2001

Following 9/11 it became apparent that some, if not all, of the perpetrators had entered the United States legally, and many had overstayed their visas with no notice taken by the INS or any other enforcement agency. As a result, several laws were enacted to address immigration concerns related to terrorism. The first such law was the Uniting and Strengthening America by Providing Appropriate Tools Required to Intercept and Obstruct Terrorism Act (also known as the Patriot Act), which was signed into law in October 2001. With reference to immigration, the act:

- Mandated that the number of personnel at the northern border be tripled, appropriated funds for technology improvements, and gave the INS access to the Federal Bureau of Investigation's (FBI) criminal databases. The INS was to begin the task of locating hundreds of thousands of foreigners who had been ordered deported and entering their names into the FBI database.

- Amended the Immigration and Nationality Act to clarify that an alien who solicited funds or membership or provided material support to a certified terrorist organization could be detained or removed from the country.

- Directed the U.S. attorney general to implement an entry-exit system, with particular focus on biometric information gathered during the visa application process, and develop tamper-resistant documents. The new system would require certain nonimmigrants to register with the INS and submit fingerprints and photographs on arrival in the United States; report to the INS in person within 30 days of arrival and annually thereafter; and notify an INS agent of their departure. Those who failed to comply could face criminal prosecution.

- Appropriated $36.8 million to implement a foreign-student monitoring system with mandatory participation by all institutions of higher education that enrolled foreign students or exchange visitors. The act expanded the list of participating institutions to include air flight schools, language training schools, and vocational schools.

- Established provisions to ensure that the immigration status of 9/11 victims and their families was not adversely affected as a result of the attacks. The family members of some victims were facing deportation.

HOMELAND SECURITY ACT OF 2002

On November 25, 2002, President George W. Bush (1946–) signed into law the Homeland Security Act of 2002, which implemented the largest restructuring of the government in several decades. This act created the cabinet-level U.S. Department of Homeland Security and consolidated the functions of more than 20 federal agencies into one department that employs over 170,000 people. One of the affected agencies was the INS.

INS Reorganization

Title IV, Section 402 of the Homeland Security Act transferred the responsibilities of the INS from the Justice Department to the DHS. With the goal of separating immigration services from immigration law enforcement, the INS became on March 1, 2003, the U.S. Citizenship and Immigration Service, responsible for processing visas and petitions for naturalization, asylum, and refugee status. Immigration enforcement became the responsibility of the U.S. Immigration and Customs Enforcement.

Border Security

Section 402 of the Homeland Security Act outlined the responsibilities of the undersecretary for border and transportation security. These included:

- Preventing the entry of terrorists and the instruments of terrorism into the United States

- Securing the borders, territorial waters, ports, terminals, waterways, and air, land, and sea transportation systems of the United States

- Administering the immigration and naturalization laws of the United States, including the establishment of rules governing the granting of visas and other forms of permission to enter the United States to individuals who are not citizens or lawful permanent residents

- Administering the customs laws of the United States

- Ensuring the speedy, orderly, and efficient flow of lawful traffic and commerce in carrying out these responsibilities

OTHER POST-9/11 CHANGES

Since 9/11 hundreds of policy changes have been inaugurated by the Justice Department, the State Department, the DHS, and the INS/USCIS. In November 2001 the State Department mandated background checks on all male visa applicants between the ages of 16 and 45 from 26 mostly Muslim countries. The Enhanced Border Security and Visa Entry Reform Act of 2002 prohibited issuing nonimmigrant visas to nationals of seven countries (Cuba, Iran, Iraq, Libya, North Korea, Sudan, and Syria) unless it was determined after a thorough background check that the individuals were not security threats. The list of prohibited countries could change as directed by the attorney general.

Increased Visa Restrictions for Foreign Students

The IIRIRA had mandated the creation of a database that stored information about international students, but the system had not yet been launched when 9/11 occurred. In May 2002 the INS launched the Student and Exchange Visitor Information System (SEVIS) to track foreigners who enter the country on student visas. New rules required that foreign students present a confirmation of acceptance from an American school before a visa would be issued, and colleges were required to report enrollment information and dates of students' arrivals or failure to arrive.

Reporting Change of Address

The INS took steps to enforce the long-standing but essentially ignored requirement that all noncitizens in the country for more than 30 days must report any change of address within 10 days of moving. Failure to report could be grounds for fines, penalties, or deportation.

Police Participation in Immigration Enforcement

The Justice Department ruled that effective August 2002 local police could detain individuals for immigration violations, a right formerly reserved for federal agents. The measure was part of the IIRIRA but had not previously been finalized. Florida became the test state, initiating a Memorandum of Understanding with the Justice Department, which authorized specially trained local police officers to assist federal agents in locating and detaining wanted aliens.

INTELLIGENCE REFORM AND TERRORISM PREVENTION ACT AND REAL ID ACT

On December 17, 2004, President Bush signed the Intelligence Reform and Terrorism Prevention Act of 2004. This act set national standards for driver's licenses, Social Security cards, and birth certificates.

The REAL ID Act of 2005 furthered the effort to improve identification standards. Preceding it, the National Commission on Terrorist Attacks on the United States (also known as the 9/11 Commission) was created in late 2002 by Congress and the president to prepare a complete account of the circumstances surrounding the 9/11 terrorist attacks and the nation's response. The commission was also mandated to provide recommendations designed to guard against future attacks.

One recommendation by the 9/11 Commission was improved, secure identification for all Americans. The Intelligence Reform and Terrorism Prevention Act of 2004 had established a committee of federal and state officials to set new security and verification standards for driver's licenses. On May 11, 2005, President Bush signed the REAL ID Act, which mandated federal standards for state-issued driver's licenses. The new act transferred responsibility for driver's license security from the U.S. Department of Transportation to the DHS.

The new law required states to develop security upgrades and security clearances for Department of Motor Vehicles (DMV) personnel; verify all documents with the original issuing agency and verify U.S. citizenship or lawful immigration status before issuing a driver's license or non-driver's identification card; and establish new data management, storage, and sharing protocols. States were prohibited from accepting any foreign documents other than an official passport for identity purposes. States were required to be certified by May 11, 2008, in compliance with the DHS and the Transportation Department. According to the DHS, in "REAL ID: States Granted Extensions" (November 10, 2008, http://www.dhs.gov/xprevprot/programs/gc_1204567770971.shtm), all 50 states applied for extensions of the original May 11, 2008, compliance deadline or received unsolicited extensions, meaning that the REAL ID Act would not become an issue at federal facilities and airports until December 31, 2009. After this date, licenses and ID cards issued by noncertified states would not be accepted for federal purposes, including boarding an airplane, receiving federal benefits such as Social Security, or filing an employment eligibility verification form (the I-9).

Cost Projections for the REAL ID Act

The REAL ID Act: National Impact Analysis (September 2006, http://www.nga.org/Files/pdf/0609REALID.PDF), the result of a survey jointly sponsored by the National Governors Association, the NCSL, and the National Association of Motor Vehicle Administrators, projects that implementation of the act will cost more than $11 billion over five years. Besides new applicants, all 245 million current holders of state driver's licenses or ID cards will be required to make a personal visit to a DMV office to present original documents verifying identity and be reenrolled in the state's computer system. The cost of additional staff and work hours necessary to reenroll that number of people within the five-year deadline was projected at $8.5 billion. Upgrading state and national systems to facilitate verification of each document presented by a driver's license applicant or reenrollee was estimated to cost $1.4 billion. The price tag for license redesign to comply with required security features was projected at $1.1 billion. Other items, such as security clearances and fraudulent document training for employees processing license applications, added an additional $40 million.

SUSPICIONS OF GOVERNMENT INVASION OF PRIVACY. Following on the heels of the Patriot Act, the REAL ID Act was viewed by civil libertarians as one more example of the erosion of privacy rights allowed by Congress under the guise of fighting terrorism. Angela French of Citizens against Government Waste states in *REAL ID: Big Brother Could Cost Big Money* (October 17, 2005, http://www.cagw.org/site/DocServer/Real_ID_FINAL_with_cover.pdf?docID=1281):

> Some view the implementation of the REAL ID Act as a chance to convince the government that the best way

to secure licenses is to embed them with a tiny little chip, creating a "smartcard," which has the potential to track every movement and decision made by the cardholder.... The Orwellian plot seems far-fetched, but the government already made the mistake of mandating that U.S. passports will be updated using this technology.... If the government opts to use these brittle chips,... U.S. drivers will be forced to carry a license that has the memory to store every detail about the person, including health records, family history, bank and credit card transactions, as well as a wealth of other information.

REBELLION IN THE STATES. Reports on the impact of the REAL ID Act generated a stir in state legislatures, and several introduced legislation prohibiting its implementation, either by directing state agencies not to implement it or by denying the funding necessary for its implementation. By 2009 the American Association of Motor Vehicle Administrators reported in "2008 Year End Real ID Status Report" (http://www.aamva.org/) that 11 states had enacted anti–REAL ID legislation, including Alaska, Arizona, Georgia, Idaho, Louisiana, Maine, Montana, New Hampshire, Oklahoma, South Carolina, and Washington, and 7 more had introduced such bills.

LEGISLATION IN THE STATES

California's Efforts to Legislate against Illegal Aliens

In November 1994 increasing concern about the effects of a large population of illegal aliens culminated in California voters approving Proposition 187. The ballot initiative prohibited illegal aliens and their children from receiving any welfare services, education, or emergency health care. It further required local law enforcement authorities, educators, medical professionals, and social service workers to report suspected illegal aliens to state and federal authorities. It also considered the manufacture, distribution, and sale of fraudulent documents to be a state felony punishable by up to five years in prison.

The day after California voters approved Proposition 187, civil rights groups filed suit in federal district court to block implementation of the ballot initiative. One week later a temporary restraining order was issued. In November 1995 the U.S. district judge Mariana R. Pfaelzer (1926–) ruled unconstitutional Proposition 187's provision denying elementary and secondary education for undocumented children. Pfaelzer cited the U.S. Supreme Court decision in *Plyler v. Doe* (457 U.S. 202 [1982]), which held that the equal protection clause of the 14th Amendment prohibited states from denying education to illegal immigrants. Civil rights and education groups had argued that states had no legal rights to regulate immigration, which was a federal responsibility.

In March 1998 Pfaelzer permanently barred Proposition 187's restrictions on benefits for aliens and declared much of the legislation unconstitutional. Pfaelzer did allow, however, the criminal provision to consider as a felony the manufacture, distribution, and use of false documents.

Arizona Succeeds Where California Failed

In November 2004, Arizona voters approved Proposition 200, which required proof of citizenship when registering to vote and applying for public benefits. It also required state, county, and municipal employees to report suspected undocumented immigrants to immigration authorities. The Mexican American Legal Defense and Educational Fund filed suit to block implementation of Proposition 200. In December 2004, the U.S. district judge David C. Bury (1942–) lifted a temporary order barring implementation of Proposition 200, which allowed it to become law in Arizona.

Immigration Legislation in States in 2008

The apparent success of Arizona's Proposition 200 sparked interest in similar laws in other states. According to the NCSL, 300 immigration-related bills were introduced in state legislatures in 2005; new immigration laws reached a peak of 1,562 in 2007 and dropped slightly to 1,305 in 2008. (See Table 2.1.) By the end of November 2008, 41 states enacted a total of 205 new immigration laws.

The NCSL notes that employment, law enforcement, and IDs were key subjects of new legislation. (See Table 2.2.) Thirteen states enacted employment laws including employer sanctions for hiring unauthorized workers and employment eligibility verification requirements and penalties. Ten states dealt with immigrant detention processes, bail determinations, and law enforcement officer responsibilities. Sixteen states enacted new laws related to eligibility requirements for licenses, including 14 laws for driver's licenses, 12 laws covering professional licenses, and 6 laws pertaining to firearm and hunting/fishing licenses. Eight states addressed education issues such as in-state tuition eligibility, student loans, English language acquisition, and English as a second language programs. Eight states further defined eligibility for health care benefits and the licensing of health care professionals. Miscellaneous laws in 21 states provided for commissions and studies, including assessing the economic impact of immigration. For example, Virginia enacted a

voting law requiring that people found not to be U.S. citizens must receive notice and be allowed 14 days to submit a sworn statement of citizenship before their voter registration is canceled. The 64 resolutions passed by 19 state legislatures included requests for action by the governor, Congress, or the president. Other resolutions honored certain immigrants or institutions.

TABLE 2.1

Immigration-related activity in state legislatures, 2005–08

Fiscal year	2005	2006	2007	2008
Bills introduced	300	570	1,562	1,305
Laws enacted	38	84	240	205

SOURCE: Adapted from *State Laws Related to Immigrants and Immigration in 2008, January 1–November 30, 2008,* National Conference of State Legislatures, December 18, 2008, http://www.ncsl.org/print//immig/State%20Immigration%20Report%20December%2018%202008.pdf (accessed December 30, 2008)

TABLE 2.2

Immigration laws enacted by states, 2008

Main topics	Number of laws enacted	States
Education	12	8
Employment	19	13
Health	11	8
Human trafficking	5	5
ID/driver's licenses and other licenses	32	16
Law enforcement	12	10
Legal services	2	2
Miscellaneous	35	21
Omnibus/multi-issue measures	3	3
Public benefits	9	7
Voting	1	1
Resolutions	64	19
Total	**205**	**41**

SOURCE: "State Immigration Laws and Resolutions, by Policy Arena (As of November 28, 2008)," in *State Laws Related to Immigrants and Immigration in 2008, January 1–November 30, 2008*, National Conference of State Legislatures, December 18, 2008, http://www.ncsl.org/print//immig/State%20Immigration%20Report%20December%2018%202008.pdf (accessed December 30, 2008)

CHAPTER 3
CURRENT IMMIGRATION STATISTICS

The U.S. Census Bureau estimates in the press release "Census Bureau Projects Population of 305.5 Million on New Year's Day" (December 29, 2008, http://www.census.gov/Press-Release/www/releases/archives/population/013127.html) that the United States receives a new resident from another country every 36 seconds. Comparing this information with U.S. birth and death rates, and other data, the Census Bureau projects that immigrants will represent 13.3% of the population in 2050, then drop to 10.9% by 2100. (See Table 3.1.)

To understand the scope of the immigration issue in the United States, it is important to know the number of immigrants in the country, where they came from, why they came, and why some did not get to stay. Because immigrant statistics have been the basis for legislation and project funding, information about immigrants' ages, skills, ability to work, and location of settlement in the United States is collected in a variety of forms. The Census Bureau uses statistical methods to estimate the nation's population size and foreign-born component based on the most recent census counts and sampling surveys.

COUNTING IMMIGRANTS

Counting resident people spread across 2.3 billion acres (930.8 million ha) of land is a major challenge. Besides births, deaths, and people moving out of the country, the U.S. Customs and Border Protection (2008, http://cbp.gov/xp/cgov/travel) states that on a typical day more than 1.1 million international travelers enter the United States at land, air, and sea ports. Some of them stay beyond the time allowed by their visas (government authorizations permitting entry into a country for a specific purpose and for a finite amount of time). Other people cross the borders illegally. For this reason, population counts are reported as estimates.

In the press release "One in Five Speak Spanish in Five States" (September 23, 2008, http://www.census.gov/Press-Release/www/releases/archives/american_community_survey_acs/012634.html), the Census Bureau discusses its American Community Survey data. These estimates, based on interviews with population samples across the country, provide a profile of the nation's immigrant population in 2007:

• The foreign-born population reached an all-time high of 38.1 million, or 12.6% of the total population.

• About 12 million people, or 31% of all foreign born, were born in Mexico.

• The five states with the largest foreign-born populations were California (27.4%), New York (21.8%), New Jersey (19.9%), Nevada (19.4%), and Florida (18.9%).

• About 19.7% of the population aged five and older spoke a language other than English at home in 2007. That figure was 17.9% in 2000 and 13.8% in 1990.

• An estimated 35 million people, or about 12.3%, spoke Spanish at home.

THE U.S. FOREIGN-BORN POPULATION

In March 2007 the Census Bureau estimated the foreign-born population of the United States to be 37.3 million. (See Figure 3.1.) This represented an increase of 53% over the 1995 estimate of 24.3 million foreign born.

Steven A. Camarota of the Center for Immigration Studies calculates an even greater number of 37.9 million foreign born. In *Immigrants in the United States, 2007: A Profile of America's Foreign-Born Population* (November 2007, http://www.cis.org/articles/2007/back1007.pdf), Camarota notes that the Census Bureau's number did not include 613,000 immigrants living in group quarters (mostly prisons and nursing homes). The Census Bureau did, however, include an estimated 11.3 million illegal aliens and about 1 million students and guest workers with long-term temporary visas. According to Camarota, one out of eight people in the United States was an immigrant.

TABLE 3.1

Population projections for native and foreign-born, selected years 2006–2100

[Numbers in thousands]

	July 1, 2006	July 1, 2025	July 1, 2050	July 1, 2075	July 1, 2100
Total					
Population	290,152	337,814	403,686	480,504	570,954
Percent of total	100.0	100.0	100.0	100.0	100.0
Native population	258,917	296,999	349,890	420,957	508,694
Percent of total	89.2	87.9	86.7	87.6	89.1
Foreign-born population	31,235	40,814	53,796	59,546	62,259
Percent of total	10.8	12.1	13.3	12.4	10.9

SOURCE: Adapted from "Projections of the Resident Population by Race, Hispanic Origin, and Nativity: Middle Series, 1999–2100 (NP-T5-C; NP-T5-F; NP-T5-G; NP-T5-H)," U.S. Census Bureau, http://www.census.gov/population/projections/nation/summary/np-t5-c.txt (accessed December 15, 2008)

FIGURE 3.1

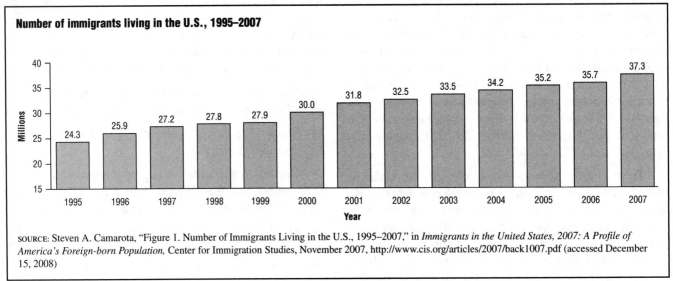

Number of immigrants living in the U.S., 1995–2007

SOURCE: Steven A. Camarota, "Figure 1. Number of Immigrants Living in the U.S., 1995–2007," in *Immigrants in the United States, 2007: A Profile of America's Foreign-born Population,* Center for Immigration Studies, November 2007, http://www.cis.org/articles/2007/back1007.pdf (accessed December 15, 2008)

Region of Birth

Half of the foreign-born population in the United States in 2007 came from nearby countries and regions: Mexico (32%), Central America (7%), the Caribbean (9%), and Canada (1.9%). In Figure 3.2, the Canadian-born population is counted among "Other" source countries. The second-largest foreign-born group came from Asia (23%). These numbers reflect a major shift in immigration patterns that occurred during the 20th century. The U.S. Department of Homeland Security's (DHS) Office of Immigration Statistics indicates in *Yearbook of Immigration Statistics: 2007* (2008, http://www.dhs.gov/xlibrary/assets/statistics/yearbook/2007/ois_2007_yearbook.pdf) that between 1900 and 1909 the vast majority (7.5 million, or 92%) of immigrants came from Europe. The 38,529 immigrants who came from Central America and Mexico represented only 0.5% of the 8.2 million immigrants who arrived in the United States during that time.

Where Foreign-Born Residents Live

California, with nearly 10 million foreign-born residents, had more than twice the number of the next highest state, New York (4.1 million). (See Table 3.2.) Camarota reports that in 2007 more than half of all immigrants resided in four states: California (27%), New York (11%), Florida (9.3%), and Texas (9.2%). Of the 37.3 million foreign-born people counted in 2007, 10.3 million (28%) arrived between 2000 and 2007. The impact of these new arrivals was much greater in some states. The 67,000 immigrants who settled in Kentucky between 2000 and 2007 represented 61% of the state's foreign-born population by 2007. More than half (52%; 99,000) of Alabama's immigrant population settled in the state between 2000 and 2007.

The Pew Research Center conducted a survey on Americans' mobility, and its findings were published by D'Vera Cohn and Rich Morin in *American Mobility: Who Moves?*

FIGURE 3.2

Nativity of all immigrants living in the United States, 2007

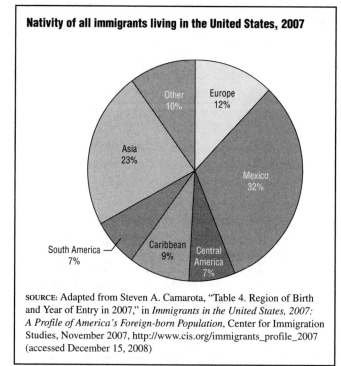

SOURCE: Adapted from Steven A. Camarota, "Table 4. Region of Birth and Year of Entry in 2007," in *Immigrants in the United States, 2007: A Profile of America's Foreign-born Population*, Center for Immigration Studies, November 2007, http://www.cis.org/immigrants_profile_2007 (accessed December 15, 2008)

TABLE 3.2

Immigrants by state, 2007

[In thousands]

		Number of immigrants	Immigrants who arrived 2000 to 2007*
1	California	9,980	2,022
2	New York	4,105	877
3	Florida	3,453	1,068
4	Texas	3,438	1,071
5	New Jersey	1,869	501
6	Illinois	1,702	491
7	Georgia	953	383
8	Massachusetts	897	203
9	Arizona	891	284
10	Virginia	856	276
11	Maryland	731	276
12	Washington	722	239
13	North Carolina	623	282
14	Pennsylvania	581	154
15	Michigan	493	113
16	Nevada	457	105
17	Connecticut	443	134
18	Colorado	435	124
19	Ohio	421	139
20	Minnesota	375	135
21	Oregon	357	107
22	Tennessee	286	144
23	Wisconsin	257	81
24	Utah	239	79
25	Indiana	236	93
26	Hawaii	226	47
27	Missouri	208	77
28	Alabama	190	99
29	New Mexico	179	68
30	Kansas	148	66
31	South Carolina	144	67
32	Rhode Island	140	21
33	Iowa	132	49
34	Louisiana	113	37
35	Nebraska	113	30
36	Arkansas	111	37
37	Oklahoma	111	26
38	Kentucky	110	67
39	New Hampshire	83	29
40	D.C.	78	30
41	Delaware	77	35
42	Idaho	72	17
43	Mississippi	66	26
44	Alaska	39	11
45	Maine	34	6
46	Vermont	30	10
47	South Dakota	19	8
48	Montana	15	4
49	West Virginia	15	1
50	Wyoming	14	7
51	North Dakota	13	2
	Nation	**37,280**	**10,258**

*Indicates the year that immigrants said they came to the United States. Included in totals are a tiny number of people who did not indicate a year of arrival.

SOURCE: Adapted from Steven A. Camarota, "Table 1. Immigrants by State, 2007," in *Immigrants in the United States, 2007: A Profile of America's Foreign-born Population*, Center for Immigration Studies, November 2007, http://www.cis.org/articles/2007/back1007.pdf (accessed December 15, 2008)

Who Stays Put? Where's Home? (October 2008, http://pewsocialtrends.org/assets/pdf/Movers-and-Stayers.pdf). When people were asked why they move from one community or state to another, according to Cohn and Morin, the most frequent response was for business or job opportunities (44%). Finding a good place to raise children was cited by 36% of respondents and to be near family was the reason given by 35%. These are the same reasons most immigrants come to the United States.

According to Cohn and Morin, people were also asked "Where's home?" Among U.S. natives who have moved to a different community at least once in their life, 60% said home is where they live now. The answer for foreign-born residents depends on how long they have lived in the United States. Survey results in Figure 3.3 reveal that nearly two-thirds (62%) of immigrants living in the United States for less than 20 years consider home to be the country where they were born. Among immigrants who have lived in the United States for 20 years or more, three-quarters (76%) call the United States home.

CONTACT WITH NATIVE COUNTRY. Pew also gathered information about how immigrants in the United States keep in touch with family and friends in their native countries. Cohn and Morin report that more than half of foreign-born Americans (56%) visit their home country at lease once every five years; about one-third (32%) visit their native country at least once a year. (See Table 3.3.) More men (38%) than women (26%) return home annually. This is likely due to the greater number of men who come to the United States to work while their wives and children remain

at home. Nearly half (48%) of immigrants surveyed keep in touch with people in their native country at least once per month through e-mail, text messaging, or Internet sites such as Facebook. Even though immigrants with higher family income were more likely to call home weekly or maintain

FIGURE 3.3

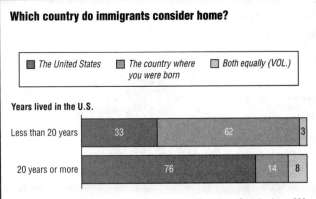

Which country do immigrants consider home?

Note: Based on those born in a foreign country or U.S. territory. Sample size = 229. Don't know/refused not shown.

SOURCE: D'Vera Cohn and Rich Morin, "Which Country Do Immigrants Consider Home?" in *American Mobility: Who Moves? Who Stays Put? Where's Home?* Pew Research Center, December 17, 2008, http://pewsocialtrends.org/assets/pdf/Movers-and-Stayers.pdf (accessed December 22, 2008)

FIGURE 3.4

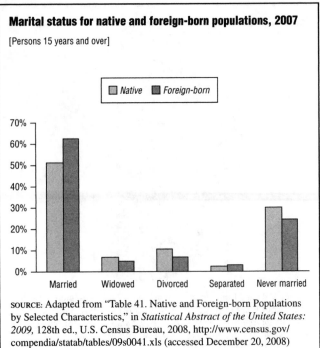

Marital status for native and foreign-born populations, 2007

[Persons 15 years and over]

SOURCE: Adapted from "Table 41. Native and Foreign-born Populations by Selected Characteristics," in *Statistical Abstract of the United States: 2009*, 128th ed., U.S. Census Bureau, 2008, http://www.census.gov/compendia/statab/tables/09s0041.xls (accessed December 20, 2008)

TABLE 3.3

How foreign-born residents maintain contact with their native country

QUESTION: ABOUT HOW OFTEN DO YOU HAVE CONTACT WITH FRIENDS OR FAMILY LIVING IN THE COUNTRY WHERE YOU WERE BORN THROUGH ELECTRONIC DEVICES SUCH AS EMAIL, TEXT MESSAGES OR INTERNET SITES LIKE FACEBOOK: EVERY DAY, ONCE A WEEK, ONCE A MONTH, SEVERAL TIMES A YEAR, ONCE A YEAR, OR LESS OFTEN THAN THAT?

	Call at least once a week	Send email, text msg., etc. at least once a month	Visit at least once a year
	%	%	%
Total	42	48	32
Gender			
Men	49	46	38
Women	36	50	26
Age			
18–40	51	57	32
41+	34	38	32
Education			
College grad	40	57	24
Not a grad	44	45	34
Family income			
$50,000+	47	58	28
LT $50k	39	42	34

Note: Based on those born in a foreign country or U.S. territory.

SOURCE: D'Vera Cohn and Rich Morin, "Staying in Touch When Home Is Another Country," in *American Mobility: Who Moves? Who Stays Put? Where's Home?* Pew Research Center, December 17, 2008, http://pewsocialtrends.org/assets/pdf/Movers-and-Stayers.pdf (accessed December 22, 2008)

Internet contact, income was not a factor in going home to visit at least once per year. Among individuals with family incomes less than $50,000, 34% returned to their native country at least once per year, compared with 28% of those with incomes more than $50,000.

Marriage and Families

The Census Bureau's *Statistical Abstract of the United States: 2009* (2008, http://www.census.gov/compendia/statab/2009edition.html) indicates that immigrants are more likely than native-born residents to be married. Figure 3.4 shows that 62% of foreign-born people were married, compared with 51% of natives. Smaller percentages of immigrants than natives are widowed, divorced, or never married. In 2007, 77% of foreign-born people lived in a family household, compared with 66% of native-born people. (See Figure 3.5.) Foreign-born households were also more likely than native households to be headed by a married couple.

Employment

During 2007 the increase in the number of foreign-born workers accounted for half of the total U.S. labor force growth, according to the Bureau of Labor Statistics (BLS). Among foreign-born workers, more than half (56%) were employed in the production, service, and construction sectors: 24% provided services such as food preparation and health-care support, 16% worked in construction, and 16% held production or transportation jobs. (See Figure 3.6.) These percentages stayed fairly constant in 2008, with 23% of foreign workers employed in service occupations, 15% employed in the construction sector, and 16% in production and transportation jobs. By contrast, 26% of U.S.-born workers in 2007 held office/sales positions, 21% professional positions, and 16% management positions. In 2008 the rates

FIGURE 3.5

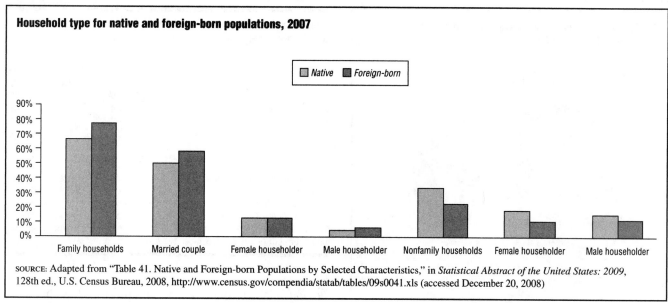

Household type for native and foreign-born populations, 2007

SOURCE: Adapted from "Table 41. Native and Foreign-born Populations by Selected Characteristics," in *Statistical Abstract of the United States: 2009*, 128th ed., U.S. Census Bureau, 2008, http://www.census.gov/compendia/statab/tables/09s0041.xls (accessed December 20, 2008)

were similar for native-born U.S. workers: office/sales (26%), professional (22%), and management (16%).

Education was a factor in the types of jobs workers held and their income. Table 3.4 compares the median (average) weekly incomes for foreign- and native-born workers by education level. Among foreign-born workers, 28% had less than a high school education, compared with 5% of native workers. These foreign-born workers took home a weekly average of $405 per week, which was less than the native workers with the same level of education. About one-third of both foreign-born (32%) and native-born workers (31%) held college degrees, but immigrant workers still averaged slightly lower earnings per week— $1,057, compared with $1,075 for workers born in the United States.

In *Foreign-Born Workers: Labor Force Characteristics in 2008* (March 26, 2009, http://www.bls.gov/news.release/pdf/forbrn.pdf), the Bureau of Labor Statistics estimates that 24.1 million foreign-born residents aged 16 and older were in the labor force in 2008, compared with 130.2 million native-born residents in the same age group. Included in the BLS estimates are documented and undocumented immigrants, including legal permanent residents, temporary workers, refugees, students, and illegal aliens; the BLS based its estimates on a survey of 60,000 households. The breakdown for foreign-born workers included 22.7 million who were employed, and 1.4 million who were unemployed but actively seeking work in 2008. The unemployment rate for both immigrant and native-born workers overall was 5.8% in 2008, but native-born men (6.2%) and foreign-born women (6%) were unemployed at higher rates than foreign-born men (5.7%) or native-born women (5.3%).

HOUSEHOLD INCOME. In 2007 the U.S. median annual family income was $59,894. (See Table 3.5.) The median income for foreign-born families was $44,706, about 27% less than the $61,565 median income of native-born families. However, for foreign-born families who had become naturalized citizens the median income was $60,733, or 1% less than the median income of native-born families. Immigrant households tend to be larger than native households and may be supported by multiple incomes. Figure 3.7 shows that 62% of native households contain only one or two people (28% one-person and 34% two-person), compared with 42% of foreign-born households (17% one-person and 25% two-person). Foreign-born residents are more likely to live in households of three or more people.

WORKING IMMIGRANTS AND POVERTY. Camarota reports that in 2007, 82% of immigrant households had at least one worker, compared with 73% of native households. Despite this higher percentage, a worker was present in 78% of immigrant households that use at least one welfare program. In 2007, 17% of foreign-born residents were in or near poverty, compared with 14% of native residents. (See Figure 3.8.) Naturalized citizens had the lowest poverty rate at 10%, whereas 27% of the most recent arrivals (between 2000 and 2007) lived below the poverty level.

Education

Camarota states that "there is no single better predictor of economic success in modern America than one's education level." In 2007, 29% of all immigrants over the age of 18 in the workforce and 35.5% of immigrants who arrived between 2000 and 2007 had less than a high school education. (See Table 3.6.) By contrast, just 7.5% of native-born workers had not completed high school. According to Camarota, "the fact that so many adult immigrants have little education means that their income, poverty rates, welfare use, and other measures of economic attainment lag far behind natives."

FIGURE 3.6

TABLE 3.4

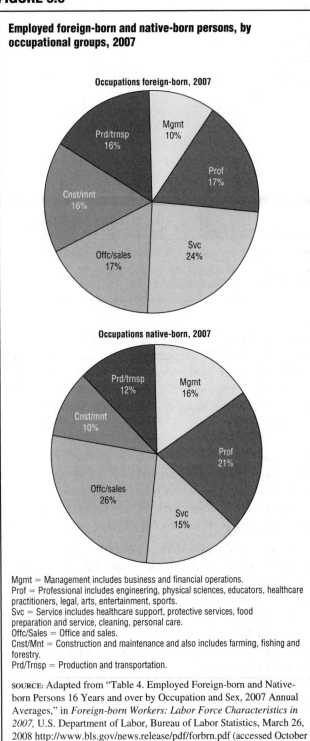

Employed foreign-born and native-born persons, by occupational groups, 2007

Occupations foreign-born, 2007

Occupations native-born, 2007

Mgmt = Management includes business and financial operations.
Prof = Professional includes engineering, physical sciences, educators, healthcare practitioners, legal, arts, entertainment, sports.
Svc = Service includes healthcare support, protective services, food preparation and service, cleaning, personal care.
Offc/Sales = Office and sales.
Cnst/Mnt = Construction and maintenance and also includes farming, fishing and forestry.
Prd/Trnsp = Production and transportation.

SOURCE: Adapted from "Table 4. Employed Foreign-born and Native-born Persons 16 Years and over by Occupation and Sex, 2007 Annual Averages," in *Foreign-born Workers: Labor Force Characteristics in 2007*, U.S. Department of Labor, Bureau of Labor Statistics, March 26, 2008 http://www.bls.gov/news.release/pdf/forbrn.pdf (accessed October 17, 2008)

Educational attainment by native-born and foreign-born workers age 25 and older, 2007

	Native	Median weekly earnings	Foreign-born	Median weekly earnings
Less than high school diploma	5%	$479	28%	$405
High school graduate	30%	$617	24%	$511
Some college or associate degree	30%	$714	16%	$617
Bachelor's degree or higher	31%	$1,075	32%	$1,057
Total number workers	**79,864**		**16,225**	

SOURCE: Adapted from "Table 5. Median Usual Weekly Earnings of Full-Time Wage and Salary Workers for the Foreign Born and Native Born by Selected Characteristics, 2006–07 Annual Averages," in *Foreign-born Workers: Labor Force Characteristics in 2007*, U.S. Department of Labor, Bureau of Labor Statistics, March 26, 2008 http://www.bls.gov/news.release/pdf/forbrn.pdf (accessed December 18, 2008)

ulation Survey (http://www.census.gov/cps/). Kochhar indicates that the median annual income of noncitizen immigrant households (52% of all immigrant households) fell 7.3% between 2006 and 2007. The median annual income of all U.S. households increased 1.3% during this same period. Kochhar describes the situation of these noncitizen immigrants: "Most arrived in the U.S. in recent years with only a high school education or less. Many are employed in blue-collar production and construction occupations or lower-rung occupations in the service sector. The majority (56%) of non-citizen households are Hispanic. And nearly half (45%) of non-citizen immigrant households are headed by an undocumented immigrant."

IMMIGRANT STATUS AND ADMISSIONS

U.S. immigration law defines an immigrant as a person legally admitted for permanent residence in the United States. Some arrive in the country with immigrant visas issued abroad by U.S. Department of State consular offices. Others who already reside in the United States become immigrants when they adjust their status from temporary to permanent residence. These include individuals who enter the country as foreign students, temporary workers, refugees and asylees (those seeking asylum), and some illegal immigrants.

There are various ways to qualify for immigration to the United States, but the U.S. Citizenship and Immigration Services (USCIS) generally classifies admissions into four major groups:

• Family-sponsored preference

• Employment-based preference

• Diversity Program

• Other—including Amerasians (typically children of Asian mothers and U.S. military or civilian personnel), parolees, refugees and asylees, individuals whose order for removal was canceled, and other legal provisions

In "Non-citizen Immigrant Households Suffer Sharp Decline in Income, 2006–2007" (October 2, 2008, http://pewresearch.org/pubs/979/non-citizen-immigrant-households), Rakesh Kochhar of the Pew Hispanic Center reports that "the current economic slowdown has taken a far greater toll on non-citizen immigrants than it has on the United States population as a whole." This observation is based on analysis of the Census Bureau's March 2008 *Current Pop-*

TABLE 3.5

Family income by native, foreign-born, and citizenship status, and 2000–07 arrival period, 2007

Income levels	All U.S. families	Native	Foreign-born	Foreign-born naturalized	Foreign-born not a citizen	Foreign-born arrived 2000–2007
$1 to $9,999 or less	4%	4%	5%	3%	6%	7%
$10,000 to $14,999	3%	3%	4%	3%	5%	5%
$15,000 to $19,999	4%	4%	6%	4%	7%	7%
$20,000 to $24,999	5%	4%	6%	5%	7%	7%
$25,000 to $34,999	10%	10%	13%	11%	14%	15%
$35,000 to $49,999	15%	14%	17%	14%	19%	18%
$50,000 to $74,999	20%	21%	18%	19%	17%	19%
$75,000 and over	39%	40%	31%	40%	23%	22%
Median income = $59,894	$59,894	$61,565	$44,706	$60,733	$41,650	$49,241

SOURCE: Adapted from "Table 41. Native and Foreign-born Populations by Selected Characteristics," in *Statistical Abstract of the United States: 2009*, 128th ed., U.S. Census Bureau, 2008, http://www.census.gov/compendia/statab/tables/09s0041.xls (accessed December 20, 2008)

FIGURE 3.7

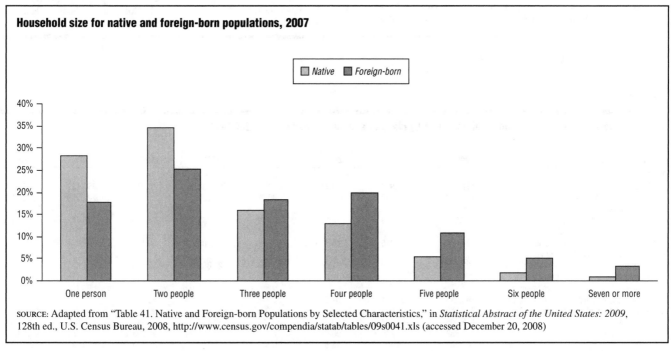

Household size for native and foreign-born populations, 2007

SOURCE: Adapted from "Table 41. Native and Foreign-born Populations by Selected Characteristics," in *Statistical Abstract of the United States: 2009*, 128th ed., U.S. Census Bureau, 2008, http://www.census.gov/compendia/statab/tables/09s0041.xls (accessed December 20, 2008)

With the passage of the Immigration Act (IMMACT) of 1990, the number of immigrants was limited to a total of 675,000 per year. However, the annual limit is flexible; it can exceed 675,000 if the maximum number of visas are not issued in the preceding year. Furthermore, the USCIS reports that some categories of immigrants are exempt from the annual limits. These include:

• Immediate relatives of U.S. citizens

• Refugee and asylee adjustments

• Certain parolees from Southeast Asia and the former Soviet Union

• Certain special agricultural workers

• Canceled removals

• Aliens who applied for adjustment of status after having unlawfully resided in the United States since January 1, 1982

New Arrivals

The United States offers two general methods for foreign-born people to attain immigrant status. In the first method an alien living abroad can apply for an immigrant visa and then become a legal resident when approved for admission at a U.S. port of entry. According to the Office of Immigration Statistics, in *Yearbook of Immigration Statistics: 2007*, nearly 1.1 million people obtained legal permanent resident (LPR) status in fiscal year (FY) 2007. (See Table 3.7.) This represented a 17% decrease from the 1.3 million people admitted to LPR status in FY 2006.

FIGURE 3.8

Percent of population below poverty level, by nativity, citizenship status, and 2000–07 arrival period, 2007

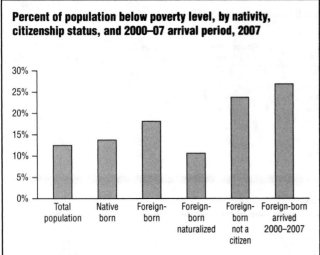

SOURCE: Adapted from "Table 41. Native and Foreign-born Populations by Selected Characteristics," in *Statistical Abstract of the United States: 2009,* 128th ed., U.S. Census Bureau, 2008, http://www.census.gov/compendia/statab/tables/09s0041.xls (accessed December 20, 2008)

TABLE 3.6

Selected characteristics of immigrants and natives, 2007

	Natives	All immigrants	Arrived 2000–07[a]
Less than high school	7.5%	29.0%	35.5%
High school only	30.9%	24.8%	24.6%
Some college	30.7%	17.7%	13.9%
Bachelor's	20.8%	17.4%	16.0%
Graduate or professional	10.1%	11.0%	10.0%
Median annual earnings[b]	$40,344	$31,074	$24,712
Median household income[c]	$49,201	$43,933	$39,691
Average household size[c]	2.43	3.11	3.06
Average age[d]	35.9	40.5	29.4

Note: Education figures are for persons 18 and older in the labor force.
[a]Indicates the year that immigrants said they came to the United States.
[b]Earnings are for full-time year-round workers.
[c]Immigrant and native households based on nativity of household head. Income is from all sources.
[d]All persons.

SOURCE: Steven A. Camarota, "Table 6. Selected Characteristics of Immigrants and Natives," in *Immigrants in the United States, 2007: A Profile of America's Foreign-born Population,* Center for Immigration Studies, November 2007, http://www.cis.org/articles/2007/back1007.pdf (accessed December 15, 2008)

TABLE 3.7

Persons obtaining legal permanent resident status by class of admission, fiscal years 2000–07

Type and class of admission	2000	2001	2002	2003	2004	2005	2006	2007
Total								
Total	841,002	1,058,902	1,059,356	703,542	957,883	1,122,257	1,266,129	1,052,415
Family-sponsored preferences	235,092	231,699	186,880	158,796	214,355	212,970	222,229	194,900
First: unmarried sons/daughters of U.S. citizens and their children	27,635	27,003	23,517	21,471	26,380	24,729	25,432	22,858
Second: spouses, children, and unmarried sons/daughters of alien residents	124,540	112,015	84,785	53,195	93,609	100,139	112,051	86,151
Third: married sons/daughters of U.S. citizens and their spouses and children	22,804	24,830	21,041	27,287	28,695	22,953	21,491	20,611
Fourth: brothers/sisters of U.S. citizens (at least 21 years of age) and their spouses and children	60,113	67,851	57,537	56,843	65,671	65,149	63,255	65,280
Immediate relatives of U.S. citizens	346,350	439,972	483,676	331,286	417,815	436,115	580,348	494,920
Spouses	196,405	268,294	293,219	183,796	252,193	259,144	339,843	274,358
Children*	82,638	91,275	96,941	77,948	88,088	94,858	120,064	103,828
Parents	67,307	80,403	93,516	69,542	77,534	82,113	120,441	116,734
Employment-based preferences	106,642	178,702	173,814	81,727	155,330	246,877	159,081	162,176
First: priority workers	27,566	41,672	34,168	14,453	31,291	64,731	36,960	26,697
Second: professionals with advanced degrees or aliens of exceptional ability	20,255	42,550	44,316	15,406	32,534	42,597	21,911	44,162
Third: skilled workers, professionals, and unskilled workers	49,589	85,847	88,002	46,415	85,969	129,070	89,922	85,030
Fourth: special immigrants	9,014	8,442	7,186	5,389	5,407	10,133	9,539	5,481
Fifth: employment creation (investors)	218	191	142	64	129	346	749	806
Diversity	50,920	41,989	42,820	46,335	50,084	46,234	44,471	42,127
Refugees	56,091	96,870	115,601	34,362	61,013	112,676	99,609	54,942
Asylees	6,837	11,111	10,197	10,402	10,217	30,286	116,845	81,183
Parolees	3,162	5,349	6,018	4,196	7,121	7,715	4,569	1,999
Children born abroad to alien residents	1,004	899	783	743	707	571	623	597
Nicaraguan Adjustment and Central American Relief Act (NACARA)	20,364	18,663	9,307	2,498	2,292	1,155	661	340
Cancellation of removal	12,154	22,188	23,642	28,990	32,702	20,785	29,516	14,927
Haitian Refugee Immigration Fairness Act (HRIFA)	435	10,064	5,345	1,406	2,451	2,820	3,375	2,448
Other	1,951	1,396	1,273	2,801	3,796	4,053	4,802	1,856

*Includes orphans.

SOURCE: Adapted from "Table 6. Persons Obtaining Legal Permanent Resident Status by Type and Major Class of Admission: Fiscal Years 1998 to 2007," in *Yearbook of Immigration Statistics: 2007,* U.S. Department of Homeland Security, Office of Immigration Statistics, 2008, http://www.dhs.gov/xlibrary/assets/statistics/yearbook/2007/ois_2007_yearbook.pdf (accessed December 27, 2008)

The second method of gaining immigrant status is by adjustment of status. This procedure allows certain aliens already in the United States to apply for immigrant status, including certain undocumented residents, temporary workers, foreign students, and refugees. The Office of Immigration Statistics states that in FY 2008 a total of 640,568 individuals had their status adjusted (March 2009, http://www.dhs.gov/xlibrary/assets/statistics/publications/lpr_fr_2008.pdf).

New Arrivals by Adoption

Included in the category of immediate relatives are orphans and other children adopted by U.S. citizens. In October 2000 Congress passed the Child Citizenship Act, granting automatic U.S. citizenship to foreign-born biological and adopted children of U.S. citizens.

The adoption of foreign-born children reached a peak in FY 2004 with a total of 22,884 children admitted as citizens. (See Figure 3.9.) By FY 2008 the number of foreign-born children admitted through adoption dropped 24% to 17,438. The largest share of international adoptions to the United States came from Asia (42%). (See Figure 3.10.)

ADOPTING CHILDREN FROM CHINA. In FY 2007 the People's Republic of China was the leading source of children adopted to the United States. Out of a total of 5,397 children adopted from China, 4,571 (85%) were female, reflecting parents' willingness to give up a female in hopes of having a male child in a country with a one-child-per-couple rule. (See Table 3.8.) Holt International Children's Services, a nonprofit adoption service, notes in "FAQs about the China Adoption Process" (2008, http://www.holtintl.org/china/chinafaq.shtml) that nearly all the children available for adoption from China were abandoned. Child abandonment is illegal, so children are usually left in public places with no identifying information.

In "China's One-Child Policy to Stay" (*Guardian* [Manchester, England], March 10, 2008), Tania Branigan reports that China's minister of the state population and family planning commission said the country is entering a birth peak. By 2018 an estimated 200 million Chinese women will reach the age of fertility. "The current rules, which in fact allow many rural couples to have two children but restrict most urban families to one, have slowed the growth of China's 1.3 [billion]-strong population and reduced the strain on the country's resources."

According to the State Department's Office of Children's Issues, in *Intercountry Adoption* (September 30, 2008, http://adoption.state.gov/news/total_chart.html), U.S. adoptions from China dropped from 7,906 in FY 2005 to 3,909 in FY 2008. This was the result of the Chinese government

FIGURE 3.9

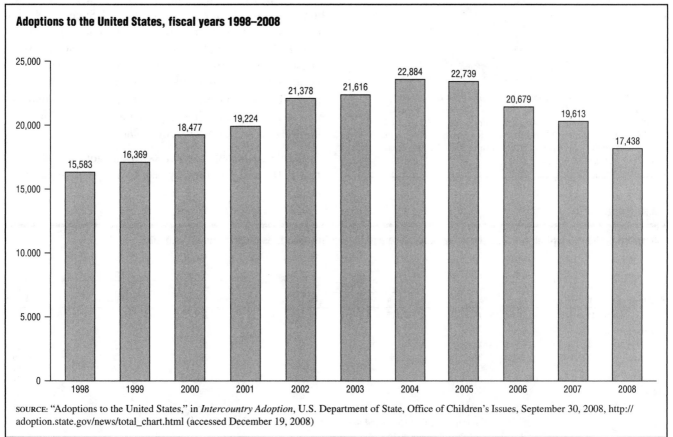

Adoptions to the United States, fiscal years 1998–2008

SOURCE: "Adoptions to the United States," in *Intercountry Adoption*, U.S. Department of State, Office of Children's Issues, September 30, 2008, http://adoption.state.gov/news/total_chart.html (accessed December 19, 2008)

implementing new rules for adopting Chinese orphans that went into effect in May 2007. Pam Belluck and Jim Yardley explain in "China Tightens Adoption Rules for Foreigners" (*New York Times*, December 20, 2006) that the new rules bar adoption by people who are single, obese, older than 50, or have criminal records. The couples applying to adopt Chinese orphans must be married at least two years and have no more than two divorces between them. If either is divorced, then five years are required in the current marriage. Health requirements include freedom from acquired immunodeficiency syndrome (AIDS), cancer, and certain mental health conditions. Financial minimums include a net worth of at least $80,000 and a household income equivalent to $30,000 per year plus $10,000 per child living in the home.

ADOPTING CHILDREN FROM GUATEMALA. As adoptions from China became more challenging, Guatemala became the top international adoption source for U.S. parents in 2008. In FY 2008, U.S. families adopted 4,123 Guatemalan children. However, the State Department (http://adoption.state.gov/news/guatemala.html) issued an "Adoption Alert" on September 12, 2008, advising potential adoptive parents not to initiate new adoptions from Guatemala. On April 1, 2008, the United Stated adopted the Hague Convention on Protection of Children and Co-operation in Respect of Intercountry Adoption, which requires any newly initiated international adoptions with other "convention countries" to comply with the Hague standards. The standards are designed to protect children. Guatemala adopted the Hague Convention in 2003 but failed to establish the regulations and infrastructure required.

LEGAL PERMANENT RESIDENTS

People who are granted admission to the United States with a so-called green card are considered to be LPRs. There are two ways to gain LPR status. Foreign nationals can apply for an immigrant visa through a State Department consular office in their country. When approved, they become an LPR when admitted at a U.S. port of entry. Foreign nationals already in the United States, including refugees, certain temporary workers, students, family members, and certain undocumented residents, can apply for adjustment of status through the USCIS. In 2007 over 1 million people became LPRs. (See Figure 3.11.) The peak in new LPRs occurred in 1990, when 2.7 million undocumented immigrants gained legal status under the Immigration Reform and Control Act of 1986.

Table 3.9 shows new LPRs by category of admission from 2005 to 2007. Employment-based preferences repre-

FIGURE 3.10

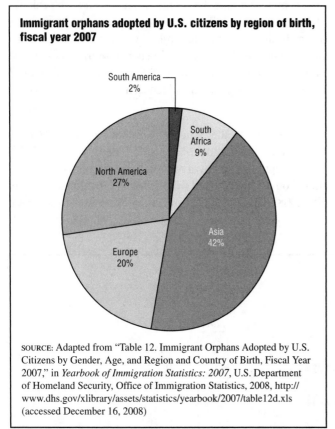

Immigrant orphans adopted by U.S. citizens by region of birth, fiscal year 2007

South America 2%
South Africa 9%
North America 27%
Asia 42%
Europe 20%

SOURCE: Adapted from "Table 12. Immigrant Orphans Adopted by U.S. Citizens by Gender, Age, and Region and Country of Birth, Fiscal Year 2007," in *Yearbook of Immigration Statistics: 2007*, U.S. Department of Homeland Security, Office of Immigration Statistics, 2008, http://www.dhs.gov/xlibrary/assets/statistics/yearbook/2007/table12d.xls (accessed December 16, 2008)

TABLE 3.8

Immigrant orphans adopted by U.S. citizens by gender and age for top five countries of birth, fiscal year 2007

Region and country of birth	Total	Gender		Age		
		Male	Female	Under 1 year	1 to 4 years	5 years and over
Total immigrants adopted	19,471	7,625	11,846	7,789	8,462	3,220
Country						
China, People's Republic	5,397	826	4,571	1,728	3,322	347
Guatemala	4,721	2,268	2,453	3,328	1,202	191
Russia	2,301	1,236	1,065	157	1,626	518
Ethiopia	1,203	544	659	396	430	377
Korea	945	543	402	849	89	7

SOURCE: Adapted from "Table 12. Immigrant Orphans Adopted by U.S. Citizens by Gender, Age, and Region and Country of Birth, Fiscal Year 2007," in *Yearbook of Immigration Statistics: 2007*, U.S. Department of Homeland Security, Office of Immigration Statistics, 2008, http://www.dhs.gov/xlibrary/assets/statistics/yearbook/2007/table12d.xls (accessed December 16, 2008)

FIGURE 3.11

Flow of legal permanent residents (LPRs) to the U.S., 1900–2007

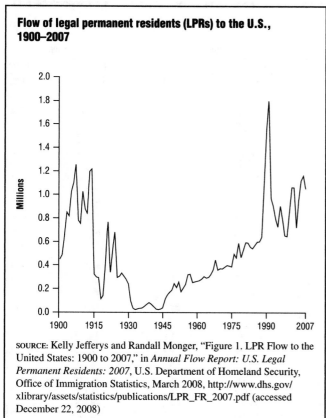

SOURCE: Kelly Jefferys and Randall Monger, "Figure 1. LPR Flow to the United States: 1900 to 2007," in *Annual Flow Report: U.S. Legal Permanent Residents: 2007*, U.S. Department of Homeland Security, Office of Immigration Statistics, March 2008, http://www.dhs.gov/xlibrary/assets/statistics/publications/LPR_FR_2007.pdf (accessed December 22, 2008)

sented 15.4% of all LPRs in 2007. Even though this was an increase over the 12.6% share of all LPRs in 2006, it was still far below the 22% share of all LPRs who were employment-based preferences in 2005. In *Annual Flow Report: U.S. Legal Permanent Residents, 2007* (March 2008, http://www.dhs.gov/xlibrary/assets/statistics/publications/LPR_FR_2007.pdf), Kelly Jefferys and Randall Monger of the Office of Immigration Statistics note that the historically high number of LPRs in 2005 resulted from the American Competitiveness in the 21st Century Act of 2000 and the REAL ID Act of 2005. These acts allowed the recapture of certain unused employment-based visas from 1999 to 2004. The 2007 employment-based LPRs included 10,849 recaptured REAL ID visas. These visas were available only after the 147,148 annual limit was reached.

Some preference categories have annual limits that are determined by the State Department's Bureau of Consular Affairs. For family-sponsored preferences, the annual limit is 480,000 minus the number of certain categories of aliens who adjusted to LPR status the previous year and certain categories of aliens paroled into the United States. Unused preferences from the previous year are then added to determine the final annual limit for the current year. The minimum number of family-sponsored preferences in any year is 226,000. The employment-preference annual limit is 140,000 plus unused family-sponsored preferences in the previous year. The employment-preference for 2007 was 140,000 plus 7,148 unused family-sponsored preferences from 2006 for a total of 147,148. (See Table 3.10.)

About two-thirds of LPRs between 2005 and 2007 came from North America and Asia. In 2007, 32.2% came from North America and 36.4% came from Asia. (See Table 3.11.) Between 2005 and 2007 China and the Philippines replaced India as the Asian leading countries of birth for LPRs. Mexico remained the leading country of birth for LPRs overall and from North America.

One-fourth (272,537) of the total 1,052,415 LPRs in 2007 were students or children. (See Table 3.12.) Among the 194,900 family-sponsored LPRs, 75,929 (39%) were students or children. Among the 136,125 refugees and asylees who became LPRs in 2007, 39,405 (29%) were students or children. The largest share of employment-based LPRs who worked (52,803) were in management and professional occupations. Among working refugees and asylees, the greatest share (12,258) worked in service occupations.

NATURALIZATION—BECOMING A CITIZEN

Naturalization refers to the conferring of U.S. citizenship on a person after birth. A naturalization court grants citizenship if the naturalization occurs within the United States, whereas a representative of the USCIS confers citizenship occurring outside the United States. Beginning in 1992 IMMACT also permitted people to naturalize through administrative hearings with the U.S. Immigration and Naturalization Service (now the USCIS). When individuals become U.S. citizens, they pledge allegiance to the United States and renounce allegiance to their former country.

On October 1, 2008, the USCIS implemented a revised naturalization test (http://www.uscis.gov/files/nativedocuments/New_Test_Fact_Sheet.pdf). "The content now follows a basic U.S. history and government curriculum. For the civics test, an applicant will be asked up to 10 questions from [a] list of 100 civics questions and answers. Applicants must answer correctly at least six of the 10 questions to pass the civics test." The applicant must also pass reading and writing tests in English. The content for these portions is also based on civics. To help applicants prepare for the test, beginning on October 1, 2008, applicants received the booklet *Learn about the United States* (http://www.uscis.gov/files/nativedocuments/M-638.pdf) at the time they were fingerprinted (a standard part of the naturalization process). The booklet contains short lessons based on each of the 100 civics questions and information to help applicants prepare for the English reading and writing portion of the new test.

General Requirements

To naturalize, most immigrants must meet certain general requirements. They must be at least 18 years old, have been legally admitted to the United States for permanent

TABLE 3.9

LPR flow by major category of admission, fiscal years 2005–07

Category of admission	2007		2006		2005	
	Number	Percent	Number	Percent	Number	Percent
Total	1,052,415	100.0	1,266,129	100.0	1,122,257	100.0
Family-sponsored immigrants	689,820	65.5	802,577	63.4	649,085	57.8
Family-sponsored preferences	194,900	18.5	222,229	17.6	212,970	19.0
Unmarried sons/daughters of U.S. citizens	22,858	2.2	25,432	2.0	24,729	2.2
Spouses and children of alien residents	86,151	8.2	112,051	8.8	100,139	8.9
Married sons/daughters of U.S. citizens	20,611	2.0	21,491	1.7	22,953	2.0
Siblings of U.S. citizens	65,280	6.2	63,255	5.0	65,149	5.8
Immediate relatives of U.S. citizens	494,920	47.0	580,348	45.8	436,115	38.9
Spouses	274,358	26.1	339,843	26.8	259,144	23.1
Parents	116,734	11.1	120,441	9.5	82,113	7.3
Children	103,828	9.9	120,064	9.5	94,858	8.5
Employment-based preferences	162,176	15.4	159,081	12.6	246,877	22.0
Priority workers	26,697	2.5	36,960	2.9	64,731	5.8
Professionals with advanced degrees	44,162	4.2	21,911	1.7	42,597	3.8
Skilled workers, professionals, unskilled workers	85,030	8.1	89,922	7.1	129,070	11.5
Special immigrants	5,481	0.5	9,539	0.8	10,133	0.9
Investors	806	0.1	749	0.1	346	0.0
Diversity programs	42,127	4.0	44,471	3.5	46,234	4.1
Refugees and asylees	136,125	12.9	216,454	17.1	142,962	12.7
Refugee adjustments	54,942	5.2	99,609	7.9	112,676	10.0
Asylee adjustments	81,183	7.7	116,845	9.2	30,286	2.7
Parolees	1,999	0.2	4,569	0.4	7,715	0.7
Other categories	20,168	1.9	38,977	3.1	29,384	2.6
Children born abroad to alien residents	597	0.1	623	0.0	571	0.1
NACARA* section 202	340	0.0	661	0.1	1,155	0.1
Cancellation of removal	14,927	1.4	29,516	2.3	20,785	1.9
Subject to annual limit	3,148	0.3	3,566	0.3	5,188	0.5
Not subject to limit (NACARA[1] section 203)	11,779	1.1	25,950	2.0	15,597	1.4
Haitian Refugee Immigrant Fairness Act	2,448	0.2	3,375	0.3	2,820	0.3
Other	1,856	0.2	4,802	0.4	4,053	0.4

*Nicaraguan Adjustment and Central American Relief Act of 1997.

SOURCE: Kelly Jefferys and Randall Monger, "Table 2. Legal Permanent Resident Flow by Major Category of Admission: Fiscal Years 2005 to 2007," in *Annual Flow Report: U.S. Legal Permanent Residents: 2007*, U.S. Department of Homeland Security, Office of Immigration Statistics, March 2008, http://www.dhs .gov/xlibrary/assets/statistics/publications/LPR_FR_2007.pdf (accessed December 22, 2008).

residence, and have lived in the country continuously for at least 5 years. They must also be able to speak, read, and write English; know how the U.S. government works; have a basic knowledge of U.S. history; and be of good moral character.

Special Provisions

A small share of people are naturalized under special provisions of the naturalization laws that exempt them from one or more of the general requirements. For example, spouses of U.S. citizens can become naturalized in three years instead of the normal five. Children who immigrated with their parents generally receive their U.S. citizenship through the naturalization of their parents. Aliens with LPR status who served honorably in the U.S. military are also entitled to certain exemptions from the naturalization requirements.

Expedited Naturalization of Active-Duty Military

In 2008 President George W. Bush (1946–) signed into law the Military Personnel Citizenship Processing Act, which was intended to speed up the naturalization process

for military personnel and veterans. He also authorized an increase in the number of Iraqi translators and contractors, employed for at least one year after March 20, 2003, who may be admitted as immigrants. Section 1244 of the Defense Authorization Act for FY 2008 authorized 5,000 special immigrant visas per year for Iraqi employees and contractors and their spouses and children from FYs 2008 to 2012.

In "Immigrants in the U.S. Armed Forces" (May 2008, http://www.migrationinformation.org/feature/display.cfm? ID=683), Jeanne Batalova of the Migration Policy Institute states that as of February 2008 the ranks of U.S. armed forces personnel included more than 65,000 immigrants. Batalova also notes that since September 2001, 37,250 foreign-born service members had been naturalized. Another 111 were granted posthumous citizenship. About 5% of all active-duty personnel in 2008 were foreign born.

Naturalization Rates

The longer immigrants live in the United States, the more likely they are to become naturalized citizens. Figure 3.12

TABLE 3.10

Annual limits for preference and diversity immigrants, fiscal year 2007

Preference/description	Limit
Family-sponsored preferences	**226,000**
First: unmarried sons and daughters of U.S. citizens and their children	23,400[a]
Second: spouses, children, and unmarried sons and daughters of permanent resident aliens	114,200[b]
Third: married sons and daughters of U.S. citizens	23,400[b]
Fourth: brothers and sisters of U.S. citizens (at least 21 years of age)	65,000[b]
Employment-based preferences	**147,148**
First: priority workers	42,084[c]
Second: professionals with advanced degrees or aliens of exceptional ability	42,084[b]
Third: skilled workers, professionals, and needed unskilled workers	42,084[b]
Fourth: special immigrants	10,448
Fifth: employment creation ("investors")	10,448
Diversity	**50,000**

[a]Plus unused family 4th preference visas.
[b]Visas not used in higher preferences may be used in these categories.
[c]Plus unused employment 4th and 5th preference visas.

SOURCE: Kelly Jefferys and Randall Monger, "Table A1. Annual Limits for Preference and Diversity Immigrants: Fiscal Year 2007," in *Annual Flow Report: U.S. Legal Permanent Residents: 2007*, U.S. Department of Homeland Security, Office of Immigration Statistics, March 2008, http://www.dhs.gov/xlibrary/assets/statistics/publications/LPR_FR_2007.pdf (accessed December 22, 2008

shows the changing patterns of naturalization by world region from which immigrants came. In the 1961–70 period, the majority (62.4%) of naturalizations were people from Europe. By the 1991–2000 period, Europe represented just 12% of naturalized U.S. citizens. Figure 3.13 reports naturalizations between 2001 and 2007, in which 40% of naturalized citizens were from Asia. Table 3.13 indicates that specific country of origin is also a factor in the choice for naturalization. Among the top 25 countries of birth for all immigrants in the United States in 2007, 76.3% of those who came from Italy had become U.S. citizens by 2007. Immigrants from Iran had the second-highest citizenship rate (75.8%), followed by immigrants from Vietnam (68.8%), Germany (62.6%), Jamaica (60.4%), and the Philippines (60.3%).

NONIMMIGRANTS

There are no restrictions on the number of nonimmigrants allowed to enter the United States. In fact, the United States, like most other countries, encourages tourism and tries to attract as many visitors as possible. Even though it is easy to get in, strict rules do apply to the conditions of the visit. For example, students can stay only long enough to complete their studies, and business people can stay only six months (although a six-month extension is available). Most nonimmigrants are not allowed to hold jobs while in the United States, although exceptions are made for students and the families of diplomats. An undetermined number of visitors, amounting to many tens of thousands, overstay their nonimmigrant visas and continue to live in the United States illegally.

Tourists, Students, and Others

Table 3.14 lists the nonimmigrant visa classifications and the numbers of nonimmigrant visas issued by the State Department between FYs 2003 and 2007. The impact of increased security following the September 11, 2001, terrorist attacks can be seen in the continuing drop in total visas issued from 180.5 million in 2003 to 171.4 million in 2007. Despite this downward trend in total nonimmigrant visas, foreign visitors traveling for pleasure, business, or passing through the United States to other places (nonresidents in Table 3.14) increased 35%, from 24.7 million in 2003 to 33.3 million in 2007.

Visas Processed by the State Department

In *Fiscal Year 2009 Budget in Brief* (February 2008, http://www.state.gov/documents/organization/100033.pdf), the State Department indicates that in FY 2007 over $2.1 billion in fees related to immigrant and nonimmigrant visa processing were collected. (See Table 3.15.) The State Department reports "major increases in the cost of providing consular services as a result of enhanced security measures implemented to strengthen U.S. homeland security." The budget report offers data on numbers of visas processed:

- Non-immigrant visa requests from foreign tourists, students, business people, investors, and government officials undergo a rigorous adjudication process at missions abroad. In FY 2007, the Department processed 8.56 million non-immigrant visa applications that generated Machine Readable Visa fee revenue.... The State Department expects that demand for non-immigrant visa services will grow to 9.64 million applications in FY 2008 and 10.1 million applications in FY 2009.

- Persons seeking immigrant visas to the United States also undergo comprehensive screening during the adjudication process by Consular Officials overseas. In FY 2007, the Department processed a total of 680,000 immigrant visa applications. This workload is expected to remain at the same level in FY 2008 and FY 2009.

- Routine and emergency assistance must be provided to American citizens in distress. In FY 2008 and FY 2009, the Department projects that it will respond to 2 million citizen services requests worldwide each year.

- In FY 2007, the Department processed 18.4 million passport applications. Workload is expected to grow to 29 million applications in FY 2008 and between 30 and 36 million in FY 2009.

Temporary Foreign Workers

A temporary worker is an alien coming to the United States to work for a limited period. Most legal temporary workers arrive with H-class visas, which include H-1B/H-1B1 and H-2/H-2A visas. According to the Bureau of Consular Affairs, in *Report of the Visa Office 2007* (2008, http://travel.state.gov/visa/frvi/statistics/statistics_4179.html#), among workers admitted to the United States on H-class visas in

TABLE 3.11

LPR flow by region and country of birth, fiscal years 2005–07

Region/country of birth	2007 Number	2007 Percent	2006 Number	2006 Percent	2005 Number	2005 Percent
Total	1,052,415	100.0	1,266,129	100.0	1,122,257	100.0
Region:						
Africa	94,711	9.0	117,422	9.3	85,098	7.6
Asia	383,508	36.4	422,284	33.4	400,098	35.7
Europe	120,821	11.5	164,244	13.0	176,516	15.7
North America	339,355	32.2	414,075	32.7	345,561	30.8
Caribbean	119,123	11.3	146,768	11.6	108,591	9.7
Central America	55,926	5.3	75,016	5.9	53,463	4.8
Other North America	164,306	15.6	192,291	15.2	183,507	16.4
Oceania	6,101	0.6	7,384	0.6	6,546	0.6
South America	106,525	10.1	137,986	10.9	103,135	9.2
Unknown	1,394	0.1	2,734	0.2	5,303	0.5
Country:						
Mexico	148,640	14.1	173,749	13.7	161,445	14.4
China, People's Republic	76,655	7.3	87,307	6.9	69,933	6.2
Philippines	72,596	6.9	74,606	5.9	60,746	5.4
India	65,353	6.2	61,369	4.8	84,680	7.5
Colombia	33,187	3.2	43,144	3.4	25,566	2.3
Haiti	30,405	2.9	22,226	1.8	14,524	1.3
Cuba	29,104	2.8	45,614	3.6	36,261	3.2
Vietnam	28,691	2.7	30,691	2.4	32,784	2.9
Dominican Republic	28,024	2.7	38,068	3.0	27,503	2.5
Korea	22,405	2.1	24,386	1.9	26,562	2.4
El Salvador	21,127	2.0	31,782	2.5	21,359	1.9
Jamaica	19,375	1.8	24,976	2.0	18,345	1.6
Guatemala	17,908	1.7	24,133	1.9	16,818	1.5
Peru	17,699	1.7	21,718	1.7	15,676	1.4
Canada	15,495	1.5	18,207	1.4	21,878	1.9
United Kingdom	14,545	1.4	17,207	1.4	19,800	1.8
Brazil	14,295	1.4	17,903	1.4	16,662	1.5
Pakistan	13,492	1.3	17,418	1.4	14,926	1.3
Ethiopia	12,786	1.2	16,152	1.3	10,571	0.9
Nigeria	12,448	1.2	13,459	1.1	10,597	0.9
All other countries	358,185	34.0	462,014	36.5	415,621	37.0

SOURCE: Kelly Jefferys and Randall Monger, "Table 3. Legal Permanent Resident Flow by Region and Country of Birth: Fiscal Years 2005 to 2007," in *Annual Flow Report: U.S. Legal Permanent Residents: 2007*, U.S. Department of Homeland Security, Office of Immigration Statistics, March 2008, http://www.dhs.gov/xlibrary/assets/statistics/publications/LPR_FR_2007.pdf (accessed December 22, 2008)

FY 2007, 45% came from Asia. (See Figure 3.14.) North America (Canada, Mexico, Central America, and Island Nations) contributed 39% of these workers. Among Asian workers, 71% came from India. Mexico accounted for 83% of North American H-class workers.

H-1 VISA PROGRAM. According to the Department of Labor (DOL; http://www.foreignlaborcert.doleta.gov/h-1b.cfm), the H-1B program "allows an employer to temporarily employ a foreign worker in the U.S. on a nonimmigrant basis in a specialty occupation or as a fashion model of distinguished merit and ability. A specialty occupation requires the theoretical and practical application of a body of specialized knowledge and a bachelor's degree or the equivalent in the specific specialty (e.g., sciences, medicine and health care, education, biotechnology, and business specialties, etc.)." In 2007 the United States issued 461,730 H-1B visas. (See Table 3.16.) The H-1B1 program began in January 1, 2004, allowing employers to request specialty foreign workers from Chile and Singapore—called Free Trade Agreement Professionals. In 2007, 170 H-1B1

visas were issued. Additionally, 49 H-1C visas were issued to nurses under the Nursing Relief for Disadvantaged Areas program.

The DOL notes that a foreign worker is allowed to remain in H-1 status for up to six continuous years. After the H-1 visa expires, "the worker must remain outside the United States for one year before another [H-1] petition can be approved. Certain foreign workers with labor certification applications or immigrant visa petitions in process may stay in [H-1] status beyond the normal six-year limitation, in one-year increments." However, "adjustment of status to another nonimmigrant category or to legal permanent residency is not permitted."

IMMACT set a ceiling on H-1B admissions for initial employment at 65,000 beginning in FY 1992. Demand for H-1B workers grew, and the ceilings were increased through a series of legislative actions until the American Competitiveness in the 21st Century Act of 2000 returned the cap to 65,000 in FY 2004. When the H-1B1 visa was introduced in

TABLE 3.12

LPR by class and occupation, fiscal year 2007

Characteristic	Total	Family-sponsored preferences	Employment based preferences	Immediate relatives of U.S. citizens	Diversity	Refugees and asylees	Other
Gender							
Total	1,052,415	194,900	162,176	494,920	42,127	136,125	22,167
Male	471,377	90,869	83,237	192,230	23,802	69,563	11,676
Female	581,031	104,029	78,938	302,689	18,324	66,562	10,489
Unknown	7	2	1	1	1	—	2
Age							
Total	1,052,415	194,900	162,176	494,920	42,127	136,125	22,167
Under 1 year	10,209	642	298	8,044	600	—	625
1 to 4 years	29,110	6,435	3,215	13,927	2,591	2,683	259
5 to 9 years	50,705	14,489	9,519	16,184	2,442	7,831	240
10 to 14 years	68,184	21,278	11,932	23,282	2,009	9,136	547
15 to 19 years	91,166	27,160	12,775	33,105	2,150	13,899	2,077
20 to 24 years	101,099	17,988	6,321	53,765	6,501	14,770	1,754
25 to 29 years	121,014	11,892	13,113	73,600	8,309	12,829	1,271
30 to 34 years	136,508	18,495	34,340	59,084	6,676	15,389	2,524
35 to 39 years	113,790	18,601	30,806	39,438	4,277	16,377	4,291
40 to 44 years	85,853	17,665	19,203	27,145	2,598	15,642	3,600
45 to 49 years	63,673	15,520	11,073	22,498	1,727	10,533	2,322
50 to 54 years	50,044	12,093	5,594	22,811	1,180	7,051	1,315
55 to 59 years	40,266	7,136	2,443	25,506	648	3,830	703
60 to 64 years	32,284	3,295	1,054	25,161	262	2,182	330
65 to 74 years	43,367	1,992	449	37,779	140	2,766	241
75 years and over	15,137	217	41	13,590	17	1,206	66
Unknown	6	2	—	1	—	1	2
Broad age groups							
Total	1,052,415	194,900	162,176	494,920	42,127	136,125	22,167
Under 16 years	174,899	47,807	27,551	67,194	7,993	22,421	1,933
16 to 20 years	97,042	28,753	12,367	36,575	2,803	13,950	2,594
21 years and over	780,468	118,338	122,258	391,150	31,331	99,753	17,638
Unknown	6	2	—	1	—	1	2
Marital status							
Total	1,052,415	194,900	162,176	494,920	42,127	136,125	22,167
Single	387,252	117,222	60,621	113,780	21,721	63,629	10,279
Married	610,134	72,371	98,503	345,455	19,717	63,366	10,722
Widowed	28,011	1,297	291	23,589	133	2,500	201
Divorced/separated	22,307	3,588	2,244	10,048	535	5,213	679
Unknown	4,711	422	517	2,048	21	1,417	286
Occupation							
Total	1,052,415	194,900	162,176	494,920	42,127	136,125	22,167
Management, professional, and related occupations	106,763	12,323	52,803	26,219	10,346	4,822	250
Service occupations	53,218	11,441	6,411	17,565	4,889	12,258	654
Sales and office occupations	40,732	11,372	2,992	16,877	2,599	6,576	316
Farming, fishing, and forestry occupations	15,152	6,172	D	8,032	D	216	D
Construction, extraction, maintenance, and repair occupations	9,340	1,022	1,624	3,942	51	2,339	362
Production, transportation, and material moving occupations	45,529	13,119	2,537	19,157	1,050	8,656	1,010
Military	72	14	D	40	D	10	D
No occupation/not working outside home	507,200	112,973	62,887	260,273	17,235	49,507	4,325
Homemakers	146,284	26,828	17,869	93,762	1,837	5,442	546
Students or children	272,537	75,929	41,156	98,584	14,191	39,405	3,272
Retirees	9,300	178	141	8,067	6	854	54
Unemployed	79,079	10,038	3,721	59,860	1,201	3,806	453
Unknown	274,409	26,464	32,455	142,815	5,820	51,741	15,114

D Data withheld to limit disclosure.
—Represents zero.

SOURCE: Adapted from "Table 9. Persons Obtaining Legal Permanent Resident Status by Broad Classification of Admission and Selected Demographic Characteristics: Fiscal Year 2007," in *Yearbook of Immigration Statistics: 2007*, U.S. Department of Homeland Security, Office of Immigration Statistics, 2008, http://www.dhs.gov/xlibrary/assets/statistics/yearbook/2007/table09d.xls (accessed December 22, 2008)

2004, the 6,800 allowable H-1B1 visas were deducted from the total H-1B program. This left 58,200 H-1B visas available per year. On October 1, 2004, the first day of FY 2005, the USCIS announced that it had already received enough H-1B petitions to meet the FY 2005 annual cap. The H-1B Visa Reform Act of 2004 made an additional 20,000 visas avail-

FIGURE 3.12

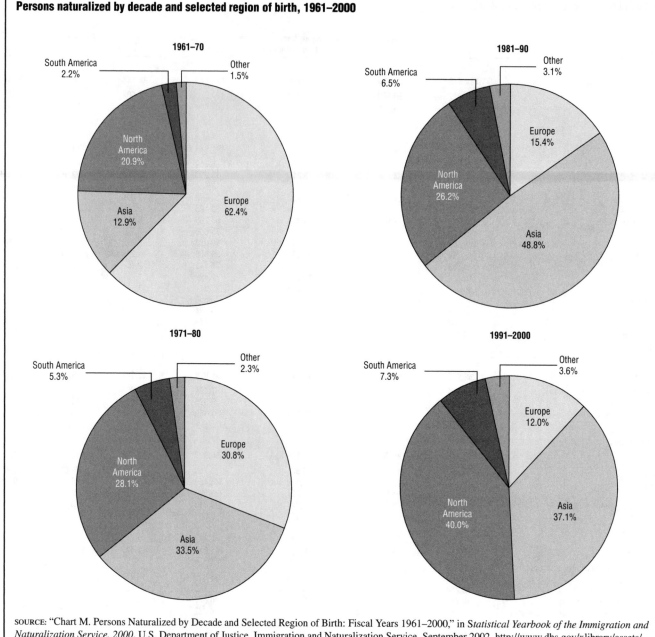

Persons naturalized by decade and selected region of birth, 1961–2000

SOURCE: "Chart M. Persons Naturalized by Decade and Selected Region of Birth: Fiscal Years 1961–2000," in *Statistical Yearbook of the Immigration and Naturalization Service, 2000*, U.S. Department of Justice, Immigration and Naturalization Service, September 2002, http://www.dhs.gov/xlibrary/assets/statistics/yearbook/2000/Yearbook2000.pdf (accessed December 27, 2008)

able for individuals with a master's degree or higher from a U.S. graduate institution. On March 12, 2008, the USCIS announced in "Fact Sheet: Changes to the FY 2009 H-1B Program" (http://www.uscis.gov/) changes to the H-1B program effective for FY 2009. Because demand exceeds the number of available H-1B visas, the USCIS will process applications by random selection from the pool of applications rather than by the order the applications were received.

ABUSE OF H-1B PROGRAM. Moira Herbst reports in "It's True: There's Fraud in the H-1B Visa Program" (*Business Week*, October 16, 2008) that a recent study by the USCIS found 13% of H-1B requests were fraudulent.

According to Herbst, critics charge that employers use the program to hire cheaper foreign labor rather than use American labor. Examples of fraud include H-1B workers who lacked the education or experience specified on the application and workers who were paid less than the prevailing wage for the position. In response to this study, the USCIS plans to examine more closely applications from small companies (25 employees or less), which were the group with the highest violation rate.

H-2 PROGRAM. The H-2 Temporary Agricultural Worker Program was authorized by the Immigration and Nationality Act of 1952 to provide a flexible response to seasonal agricul-

FIGURE 3.13

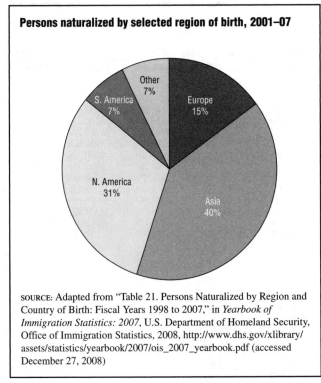

Persons naturalized by selected region of birth, 2001–07

SOURCE: Adapted from "Table 21. Persons Naturalized by Region and Country of Birth: Fiscal Years 1998 to 2007," in *Yearbook of Immigration Statistics: 2007*, U.S. Department of Homeland Security, Office of Immigration Statistics, 2008, http://www.dhs.gov/xlibrary/assets/statistics/yearbook/2007/ois_2007_yearbook.pdf (accessed December 27, 2008)

TABLE 3.13

Citizenship rates for immigrants from top 25 countries of birth, 2007

[In thousands]

	Total	Share who are citizens
Mexico*	11,671	19.8%
China	2,007	52.3%
India	1,704	38.5%
Philippines	1,665	60.3%
Vietnam	999	68.8%
El Salvador	998	25.8%
Cuba	980	47.6%
Former USSR	973	54.7%
Korea	906	43.4%
Dominican Republic	856	40.1%
Canada	699	43.2%
Guatemala	681	17.4%
Colombia	669	42.7%
United Kingdom	590	41.0%
Jamaica	550	60.4%
Germany	514	62.6%
Haiti	514	54.0%
Honduras	439	20.3%
Poland	427	51.1%
Italy	418	76.3%
Ecuador	411	37.2%
Iran	371	75.8%
Peru	354	39.0%
Brazil	338	24.9%
Japan	286	28.0%
World total	37,280	39.0%

*Includes 100,000 persons who indicated they are foreign-born, Hispanic, and Mexican, but who did not indicate a country of birth.

SOURCE: Adapted from Steven A. Camarota, "Table 5. Top-25 Countries of Birth in 2007," in *Immigrants in the United States, 2007: A Profile of America's Foreign-born Population*, Center for Immigration Studies, November 2007, http://www.cis.org/immigrants_profile_2007 (accessed December 15, 2008)

tural labor demands. Since 1964 it has been the only legal program in the United States for temporary foreign agricultural workers. In 1986 the H-2 program was amended to specify categories of workers. H-2A temporary workers perform agricultural services, H-2B workers perform other services, and H-2R workers are former H-2B workers authorized to return to the United States. Even though the H-2A temporary program is based on employer needs and has no set numerical limits, the H-2B program is capped at 66,000 new visas per year.

Agricultural employers who anticipate a shortage of domestic workers file an application for H-2A certification with the U.S. Department of Labor. Employers must certify that there are not enough U.S. workers able, qualified, and willing to do the work. The employer must also certify that the jobs are not vacant due to a labor dispute. The employer pays a $100 fee, plus $10 for each job certified, up to a maximum fee of $1,000 for each certification granted.

Hiring foreign workers under the H-2A program places a number of requirements on the employer, including advertising for and hiring qualified domestic workers, providing workers compensation insurance or equivalent insurance for all workers, and following specific pay and recordkeeping procedures. In some situations the employer may be required to pay for transportation and provide housing and meals for workers.

The employer of H-2A workers is required to pay all workers the higher of (1) both the state and/or the federal minimum wage, (2) the locally prevailing wage for the type of work, or (3) the Adverse Effect Wage Rate (AEWR), which is determined annually by the Labor Department for each state. The federal minimum wage was $6.55 per hour effective July 24, 2008, and $7.25 per hour effective July 24, 2009. In 2008 state minimum wage rates ranged from $2.65 in Kansas to $8.07 in Washington. (See Table 3.17; note that Alabama, Louisiana, Mississippi, South Carolina, and Tennessee had no minimum wage.) AEWR rates ranged from $8.41 in Arkansas, Louisiana, and Mississippi, to $10.44 in Iowa and Missouri, and to $10.86 in Hawaii.

The Labor Department reports a total of 7,491 employers and 76,818 workers were certified for the H-2A program in FY 2007. (See Table 3.18.) Ten states accounted for 60.3% of all H-2A workers requested for that year. In North Carolina, 1,256 employers were certified for the program, and they requested 9,286 workers (11.5% of all H-2A workers requested nationally). Just 80 employers were certified in Georgia, but they requested 6,886 workers. These two states together claimed one-fifth of all H-2A workers in 2007.

In "Identification of Foreign Countries Whose Nationals Are Eligible to Participate in the H-2A Visa Program"

TABLE 3.14

Nonimmigrant admissions by class of admission, fiscal years 2003–07

Class of admission	2003	2004	2005	2006	2007
TDS: Total all admissions[a]	180,500,000	180,200,000	175,300,000	175,100,000	171,400,000
Total I–94 admissions	27,849,443	30,781,330	32,003,435	33,667,328	37,149,651
Non-residents	24,735,380	27,568,652	28,747,652	30,198,154	33,301,754
Temporary visitors for pleasure[b]	19,981,833	22,653,699	23,701,858	24,788,438	27,486,177
Temporary visitors for pleasure (B2)	8,532,461	9,185,492	9,758,617	11,269,933	13,087,974
Visa waiver program—temporary visitors for pleasure (WT)	11,365,723	13,380,069	13,462,507	12,827,677	13,469,851
Guam visa waiver program—temporary visitors for pleasure to Guam (GT)	83,649	88,138	480,734	690,828	928,352
Temporary visitors for business[b]	4,198,988	4,576,783	4,684,164	5,030,779	5,418,884
Temporary visitors for business (B1)	2,245,350	2,352,404	2,432,587	2,673,309	2,928,875
Visa waiver program—temporary visitors for business (WB)	1,952,506	2,223,331	2,249,816	2,355,332	2,486,015
Guam visa waiver program—temporary visitors for business to Guam (GB)	1,132	1,048	1,761	2,138	3,994
Transit aliens	554,559	338,170	361,597	378,749	396,383
Aliens in continuous and immediate transit through the United States (C1)	239,681	322,187	343,609	357,682	376,451
Aliens in transit to the United Nations (C2)	2,181	2,283	2,379	2,854	2,914
Foreign government officials, their spouses, children, and attendants in transit (C3)	10,870	13,700	15,609	18,213	17,018
Transit without visa (C4)[c]	301,827	X	X	X	X
Commuter students	—	—	33	188	310
Canadian or Mexican national academic commuter students (F3)	—	—	33	188	307
Canadian or Mexican national vocational commuter students (M3)	—	—	—	—	3
Short-term residents	2,707,347	2,802,115	2,906,922	3,170,056	3,566,367
Temporary workers and families	1,431,472	1,507,769	1,572,863	1,709,268	1,932,075
Temporary workers and trainees	796,653	831,144	882,957	985,456	1,118,138
Temporary workers with "specialty occupation" (H1B)	360,498	386,821	407,418	431,853	461,730
Chile and Singapore Free Trade Agreement aliens (H1B1)	X	4	47	129	170
Registered nurses participating in the Nursing Relief forDisadvantaged Areas (H1C)	48	70	31	24	49
Seasonal agricultural workers (H2A)[d]	14,094	22,141	NA	46,432	87,316
Seasonal nonagricultural workers (H2B)[d]	102,833	86,958	NA	97,279	75,727
Returning H2B workers (H2R)[d]	X	X	NA	36,792	79,168
Trainees (H3)	2,370	2,226	2,938	4,134	5,540
Spouses and children of H 1, H2, or H3 (H4)	124,487	130,847	130,145	133,437	144,136
Workers with extraordinary ability or achievement (O1)	25,541	27,127	29,715	31,969	36,184
Workers accompanying and assisting in performance of O1 workers (O2)	5,321	6,332	7,635	9,567	10,349
Spouses and children of O1 and O2 (O3)	3,665	3,719	4,154	4,674	5,377
Internationally recognized athletes or entertainers (P1)	43,274	40,466	43,766	46,205	53,050
Artists or entertainers in reciprocal exchange programs (P2)	3,898	3,810	4,423	4,604	4,835
Artists or entertainers in culturally unique programs (P3)	8,869	10,038	10,836	12,630	11,900
Spouses and children of P1, P2, or P3 (P4)	1,667	1,853	1,938	2,067	2,223
Workers in international cultural exchange programs (Q1)	2,074	2,113	2,575	2,423	2,412
Workers in religious occupations (R1)	20,272	21,571	22,362	22,706	25,162
Spouses and children of R1 (R2)	6,105	6,443	6,712	7,330	6,881
North American Free Trade Agreement (NAFTA) professional workers (TN)	59,201	65,970	64,713	73,880	85,142
Spouses and children of TN (TD)	12,436	12,635	14,222	17,321	20,787
Intracompany transferees	434,281	456,583	455,350	466,009	531,073
Intracompany transferees (L1)	298,054	314,484	312,144	320,829	363,536
Spouses and children of L1 (L2)	136,227	142,099	143,206	145,180	167,537
Treaty traders and investors	168,508	182,934	192,824	216,842	238,936
Treaty traders and their spouses and children (E1)	44,090	47,083	D	50,230	51,722
Treaty investors and their spouses and children (E2)	124,418	135,851	143,786	164,795	177,920
Australian Free Trade Agreement principals, spouses and children (E3)	X	X	D	1,817	9,294
Representatives of foreign information media	32,030	37,108	41,732	40,961	43,928
Representatives of foreign information media and spouses and children (I1)	32,030	37,108	41,732	40,961	43,928
Students	662,966	656,373	663,919	740,724	841,673
Academic students (F1)	617,556	613,221	621,178	693,805	787,756
Spouses and children of F1 (F2)	37,112	35,771	33,756	35,987	40,178
Vocational students (M1)	7,361	6,989	8,378	10,384	13,073
Spouses and children of M1 (M2)	937	392	607	548	666
Exchange visitors	362,782	360,777	382,463	427,067	489,286
Exchange visitors (J1)	321,660	321,975	342,742	385,286	443,482
Spouses and children of J1 (J2)	41,122	38,802	39,721	41,781	45,804

(*Federal Register*, vol. 73, no. 244, December 18, 2008), the USCIS details the final rule changes to the H-2A program that are designed to streamline the hiring process for these workers. Key changes include easing the process for an H-2A worker to change employers and reducing from six months to three months the time a three-year H-2A worker must remain outside the United States before being eligible to return under H-2A rules. New requirements for employers include prohibition on charging workers certain fees as a condition of employment and requiring employers to notify the USCIS when an H-2A worker fails to show up for work, completes the job more than 30 days early, is terminated, or disappears from the work site.

Additionally, the USCIS identifies 28 approved countries from which H-2A workers may be recruited, effective January 17, 2009, such as Argentina, Belize, Chile, Costa Rica, Indonesia, Moldova, Romania, South Africa, Turkey,

TABLE 3.14

Nonimmigrant admissions by class of admission, fiscal years 2003–07 [CONTINUED]

Class of admission	2003	2004	2005	2006	2007
Diplomats and other representatives	249,454	276,817	287,484	292,846	303,290
Ambassadors, public ministers, career diplomatic or consular officers and their families (A1)	26,903	28,046	28,488	29,337	30,291
Other foreign government officials or employees and their families (A2)	109,699	122,809	126,827	127,296	131,583
Attendants, servants, or personal employees of A1 and A2 and their families (A3)	1,894	1,794	1,630	1,496	1,602
Principals of recognized foreign governments (G1)	12,231	13,189	13,606	14,523	15,099
Other representatives of recognized foreign governments (G2)	9,813	13,685	16,608	15,661	15,160
Representatives of nonrecognized or nonmember foreign governments (G3)	392	593	740	811	816
International organization officers or employees (G4)	74,343	80,515	82,826	85,119	88,374
Attendants, servants, or personal employees of representatives (G5)	1,610	1,373	1,336	1,411	1,477
North Atlantic Treaty Organization (NATO) officials, spouses, and children (N1 to N7)	12,569	14,813	15,423	17,192	18,888
Other classes	673	379	193	151	43
Expected long-term residents	109,157	103,893	84,802	76,783	76,158
Legal Immigration Family Equity (LIFE) Act	109,089	103,839	84,754	76,726	76,101
Fiancé(e)s of U.S. citizens (K1)	24,643	28,546	32,900	30,021	32,991
Children of K1 (K2)	3,652	4,515	5,127	4,926	5,516
Spouses of U.S. citizens, immigrant visa pending (K3)	12,774	17,864	16,249	14,739	15,065
Children of U.S. citizens, immigrant visa pending (K4)	2,960	4,253	4,098	3,692	3,430
Spouses of permanent residents, immigrant visa pending (V1)	22,509	17,866	10,157	9,321	6,960
Children of permanent residents, immigrant visa pending (V2)	20,496	15,239	7,159	6,070	5,435
Dependents of V1 or V2, immigrant visa pending (V3)	22,055	15,556	9,064	7,957	6,704
Other classes	68	54	48	57	57
Unknown	297,559	306,670	264,059	222,335	205,372

NA Not available.
X Not applicable.
D Data withheld to limit disclosure.
—Represents zero.
[a]Estimated admission totals rounded to the nearest hundred thousand.
[b]Due to the temporary expiration of the Visa Waiver Program from May through October 2000, data for temporary visitors by business and pleasure are not available for 2000 and 2001.
[c]C4 admissions were suspended as of 8/2/2003.
[d]Data are not available separately for 2005; during 2005 there were 129,327 admissions for all H2 classes (H2A, H2B, and H2R).
Note: Admissions represent counts of events, i.e., arrivals, not unique individuals. Admission totals exceed the number of nonimmigrants admitted. Excludes sea and air crew admissions (D1 and D2 visas) as well as the majority of short-term admissions from Canada and Mexico.

SOURCE: Adapted from "Table 25. Nonimmigrant Admissions by Class of Admission: Fiscal Years 1998 to 2007," in *Yearbook of Immigration Statistics: 2007*, U.S. Department of Homeland Security, Office of Immigration Statistics, 2008, http://www.dhs.gov/xlibrary/assets/statistics/yearbook/2007/ois_2007_yearbook.pdf (accessed December 27, 2008)

TABLE 3.15

Immigrant and nonimmigrant visa processing fees collected by the U.S. Department of State, fiscal year 2007

Affadavit of support fees	$23,000,000
Diversity lottery fees	$22,300,000
Machine readable visa fees	$981,233,000
Visa fingerprint fees	$1,600,000
H-1B and L fraud prevention fees	$31,800,000
Western hemisphere travel surcharge	$569,500,000
Enhance border security program fees	$526,825,000
Total fees	**$2,156,258,000**

SOURCE: Adapted from *Fiscal Year 2009 Budget in Brief*, U.S. Department of State, February 2008, http://www.state.gov/documents/organization/100033.pdf (accessed January 17, 2009)

and the United Kingdom. Future changes to the list will be published in the *Federal Register*. Workers from other countries will be considered by the DHS on a case-by-case basis.

Visas for Foreign-Born Athletes

The National Basketball Association (NBA) states in "NBA Players from around the World: 2007–08 Season" (August 7, 2008, http://www.nba.com/players/int_players _0708.html) that it ended the 2007–08 season with a 30-team official roster that included 76 international players from 31 countries and territories. Europe accounted for 59% of foreign-born NBA players. (See Figure 3.15.)

The increase of foreign-born players in U.S. Major League Baseball (MLB) can be tracked over more than 100 years. In 1900 just 2.7% of players came from other countries. (See Figure 3.16.) The share remained relatively low until after World War II (1939–1945), increased slowly into the 1990s, and peaked at 29.2% in 2005. Major League baseball opened its 2008 season with 28% foreign-born players.

MINOR LEAGUE TEAMS IN FOREIGN COUNTRIES. The article "Percentage of Foreign-Born MLB Players Drops from 29.0 to 28.0" (Associated Press, April 1, 2008) notes that in 2008, 37% of foreign-born MLB players came from the Dominican Republic. Jesse Sanchez reports in "Creating Complete, Healthy Players" (MLB.com, September 18, 2007) that 28 of the 30 major league teams owned baseball academies in the Dominican Republic in 2007. He also indicates that a recent study by Entrena Consulting group found baseball brought $84 million annually to the small island nation. The largest share, $52.5 million, was reinvested in the country by Dominican-born players who made it to the major leagues.

FIGURE 3.14

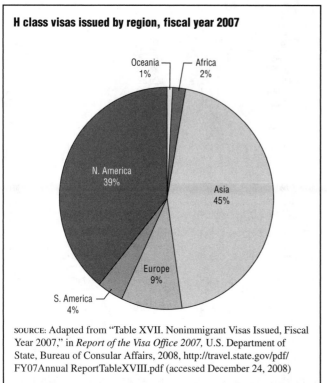

H class visas issued by region, fiscal year 2007

Oceania 1%
Africa 2%
N. America 39%
Asia 45%
Europe 9%
S. America 4%

SOURCE: Adapted from "Table XVII. Nonimmigrant Visas Issued, Fiscal Year 2007," in *Report of the Visa Office 2007,* U.S. Department of State, Bureau of Consular Affairs, 2008, http://travel.state.gov/pdf/FY07Annual ReportTableXVIII.pdf (accessed December 24, 2008)

In "Baseball Teams Worried Some Teams May Not Be Fielded Due to Visa Quotas" (Cox News Service, May 4, 2006), Meg Coker reports problems that major league teams encountered when they wanted to bring up players from their minor league teams based in foreign countries. These players did not qualify for the P-1 visa, which is reserved for artists, entertainers, and athletes who demonstrate an "internationally recognized" level of performance. Instead, the minor league players needed to apply for the H-2B visa. The problem was that the 66,000 annual cap on H-2B visas was quickly filled by employers hiring service industry and season agricultural workers. According to Coker, about 350 foreign-born minor league players were denied visas between 2004 and 2006.

CREATING OPPORTUNITIES FOR MINOR LEAGUE PROFESSIONALS, ENTERTAINERS, AND TEAMS THROUGH LEGAL ENTRY ACT OF 2006. On December 22, 2006, President Bush signed the Creating Opportunities for Minor League Professionals, Entertainers, and Teams through Legal Entry Act. The act amended the Immigration and Nationality Act (INA) by enlarging the scope of P-1 nonimmigrant visas and eliminating the "internationally recognized" performance standard. This change allows minor league athletes to apply for P-1 visas.

OLYMPIC ATHLETES. When the U.S. Olympic team marched into the opening ceremonies for the 2008 Beijing Olympic Games, Lopez Lomong (1985–), a refugee from Sudan, carried the U.S. flag. Domenick DiPasquale states in "U.S. Olympic Team Reflects America's Global Roots"

(July 30, 2008, http://www.america.gov/st/sports-english/2008/July/20080729175201fjreffahcs0.7992212.html) that the U.S. Olympic Committee (USOC) reported 33 foreign-born athletes were on the U.S. team. All were U.S. citizens.

Unlike professional sports organizations, the USOC requires that "a competitor must be a U.S. citizen in order to compete in trials or tryouts for the Olympic Games, the Paralympic Games or the Pan American Games," according to Anna Welch and Paul Green, in "An Overview of Immigration Issues" (June 11, 2008, http://assets.teamusa.org/). An athlete who gains U.S. citizenship after previously competing for another country may not be immediately eligible to compete for the United States. The Olympic Charter imposes a three-year waiting period for athletes who change citizenship. The waiting period can be reduced or canceled by the International Olympic Committee (IOC) Executive Board. The IOC considers how long the athlete has been a permanent resident of the new country and why the athlete requests to change nationality. Decisions about the waiting period require approval of the Olympic committee of the athlete's previous country and relevant International Federation.

ALIENS NOT ADMITTED TO THE UNITED STATES

State Department officials in foreign countries screen applicants and deny visas for a variety of reasons. Applicants denied visas are given the opportunity to "overcome" the issue(s) that caused the denial. The Bureau of Consular Affairs lists in *Report of the Visa Office 2007* the broad categories of reasons for such denials. The greatest share of initial denials fall under "Technical Status/INA regulations." (See Table 3.19.) Of the people applying for immigrant status, 67% were able to provide documentation to overcome eligibility issues that initially caused their visa denial. Only 22% of nonimmigrant applicants were able to overcome such technical status issues.

The "Other" category of visa denials includes practicing polygamists, international child abductors, former U.S. citizens who renounced citizenship to avoid taxation, draft evaders, and people denied by presidential proclamation. The Bureau of Consular Affairs notes that in 2007 seven immigrant visa applications and 450 nonimmigrant applications were denied based on presidential proclamations. Only eight nonimmigrants were able to overcome this type of denial. In "Presidential Proclamations" (2009, http://travel.state.gov/visa/frvi/reciprocity/reciprocity_3724.html), the State Department lists all the current proclamations, such as Proclamation 7750: To Suspend Entry as Immigrants or Nonimmigrants of Persons Engaged in or Benefiting from Corruption (January 12, 2004, http://edocket.access.gpo.gov/2004/pdf/04-957.pdf). This proclamation states that foreign public officials "who have committed, participated in, or are beneficiaries of corruption in the performance of public functions" that have "had serious adverse effects on

TABLE 3.16

Non-immigrant admissions by class of admission, fiscal year 2007

Class	Description	Total
	Total	37,149,651
A1	Foreign government officials and families: ambassadors, public ministers, career diplomats, or consular officers	30,291
A2	Foreign government officials and families: other foreign government officials or employees	131,583
A3	Foreign government officials and families: attendants, servants, or personal employees of A-1 and A-2 classes	1,602
B1	Temporary visitors: for business	2,928,875
B2	Temporary visitors: for pleasure	13,087,974
C1	Transit aliens: aliens in transit	376,451
C2	Transit aliens: aliens in transit to the United Nations	2,914
C3	Transit aliens: foreign government officials and families in transit	17,018
E1	Treaty traders and investors: treaty traders	51,722
E2	Treaty traders and investors: treaty investors	177,920
E3	Treaty traders and investors: Australian Free Trade Agreement	9,294
F1	Students and exchange visitors: academic students	787,756
F2	Students and exchange visitors: spouses and children of academic students	40,178
F3	Students and exchange visitors: Canadian or Mexican national academic commuter students	307
G1	Representatives to international organizations and families: principals of recognized foreign governments	15,099
G2	Representatives to international organizations and families: other representatives of recognized foreign governments	15,160
G3	Representatives to international organizations and families: representatives of nonrecognized or nonmember foreign governments	816
G4	Representatives to international organizations and families: international organization officers or employees	88,374
G5	Attendants, servants or personal employees of representatives	1,477
GB	Temporary visitors: for business, visa waiver, Guam	3,994
GT	Temporary visitors: for pleasure, visa waiver, Guam	928,352
H1B	Temporary workers and trainees: specialty occupations	461,730
H1B1	Temporary workers and trainees: Chile and Singapore Free Trade Agreement	170
H1C	Temporary workers and trainees: registered nurses participating in the Nursing Relief for Disadvantaged Areas	49
H2A	Temporary workers and trainees: seasonal agricultural workers	87,316
H2B	Temporary workers and trainees: seasonal nonagricultural workers	75,727
H2R	Temporary workers and trainees: returning H-2B workers	79,168
H3	Temporary workers and trainees: trainees	5,540
H4	Temporary workers and trainees: spouses and children of H-1, H-2, and H-3 workers	144,136
I1	Representatives of foreign information media and families	43,928
J1	Students and exchange visitors: exchange visitors	443,482
J2	Students and exchange visitors: spouses and children of exchange visitors	45,804
K1	LIFE Act: fiances(ees) of U.S. citizens	32,991
K2	LIFE Act: children of fiances(ees) of U.S. citizens	5,516
K3	LIFE Act: spouses U.S. citizens, visa pending	15,065
K4	LIFE Act: children of U.S. citizen, visa pending	3,430
L1	Intracompany transferees: principals	363,536
L2	Intracompany transferees: spouses and children of intracompany transferees	167,537
M1	Students and exchange visitors: vocational students	13,073
M2	Students and exchange visitors: spouses and children of vocational students	666
M3	Students and exchange visitors: Canadian or Mexican national vocational commuter student	*
N1 to N7	NATO officials and families	18,888
O1	Temporary workers and trainees: extraordinary ability or achievement	36,184
O2	Temporary workers and trainees: accompanying and assisting in performance of O-1 workers	10,349
O3	Temporary workers and trainees: spouses and children of O-1 and O-2 workers	5,377
P1	Temporary workers and trainees: internationally recognized athletes or entertainers	53,050
P2	Temporary workers and trainees: artists or entertainers in reciprocal exchange programs	4,835
P3	Temporary workers and trainees: artists or entertainers in culturally unique programs	11,900
P4	Temporary workers and trainees: spouses and children of P-1, P-2, and P-3 workers	2,223
Q1	Temporary workers and trainees: workers in international cultural exchange programs	2,412
R1	Temporary workers and trainees: workers in religious occupations	25,162
R2	Temporary workers and trainees: spouses and children of R-1 workers	6,881
TD	Temporary workers and trainees: spouses and children of NAFTA workers	20,787
TN	Temporary workers and trainees: NAFTA professional workers	85,142
V1	LIFE Act: spouses of permanent residents, visa pending	6,960
V2	LIFE Act: children of permanent residents, visa pending	5,435
V3	LIFE Act: dependents of V-1 and V-2, visa pending	6,704
WB	Temporary visitors: visa waiver, business	2,486,015
WT	Temporary visitors: visa waiver, pleasure	13,469,851
Other	All other classes	100
Unknown	Unknown	205,372

*Data withheld to limit disclosure.

Note: Admissions represent counts of events, i.e., arrivals, not unique individuals. Admission totals exceed the number of nonimmigrants admitted. Also, the majority of short-term admissions from Canada and Mexico are excluded.

SOURCE: Adapted from "Nonimmigrant Supplemental Table 1. Nonimmigrant Admissions (I–94 Only) by Class of Admission and Country of Citizenship: Fiscal Year 2007," in *Yearbook of Immigration Statistics: 2007* U.S. Department of Homeland Security, Office of Immigration Statistics, 2008, http://www.dhs.gov/xlibrary/assets/statistics/yearbook/2007/nimsuptable1d.xls (accessed December 16, 2008)

TABLE 3.17

Comparison of adverse effect wage rate with state and federal minimum wage rates, 2008

[As of March 2008, in dollars]

State	Adverse effect wage rate (AEWR)	State minimum wage rate	Amount by which the AEWR exceeds the state minimum	Federal minimum wage rate	Amount by which the AEWR exceeds the federal minimum
Alabama	8.53	—	8.53	5.85	2.68
Arizona	8.70	6.90	1.80	5.85	2.85
Arkansas	8.41	6.25	2.16	5.85	2.56
California	9.72	8.00	1.72	5.85	3.87
Colorado	9.42	7.02	2.40	5.85	3.57
Connecticut	9.70	7.65	2.05	5.85	3.85
Delaware	9.70	7.15	2.55	5.85	3.85
Florida	8.82	6.79	2.03	5.85	2.97
Georgia	8.53	5.15	3.38	5.85	2.68
Hawaii	10.86	7.25	3.61	5.85	5.01
Idaho	8.74	5.85	2.89	5.85	2.89
Illinois	9.90	7.50	2.40	5.85	4.05
Indiana	9.90	5.85	4.05	5.85	4.05
Iowa	10.44	7.25	3.19	5.85	4.59
Kansas	9.90	2.65	7.25	5.85	4.05
Kentucky	9.13	5.85	3.28	5.85	3.28
Louisiana	8.41	—	8.41	5.85	2.56
Maine	9.70	7.00	2.70	5.85	3.85
Maryland	9.70	6.15	3.55	5.85	3.85
Massachusetts	9.70	8.00	1.70	5.85	3.85
Michigan	10.01	7.15	2.86	5.85	4.16
Minnesota	10.01	6.15	3.86	5.85	4.16
Mississippi	8.41	—	8.41	5.85	2.56
Missouri	10.44	6.65	3.79	5.85	4.59
Montana	8.74	6.25	2.49	5.85	2.89
Nebraska	9.90	5.85	4.05	5.85	4.05
Nevada	9.42	6.33	3.09	5.85	3.57
New Hampshire	9.70	6.50	3.20	5.85	3.85
New Jersey	9.70	7.15	2.55	5.85	3.85
New Mexico	8.70	6.50	2.20	5.85	2.85
New York	9.70	7.15	2.55	5.85	3.85
North Carolina	8.85	6.15	2.70	5.85	3.00
North Dakota	9.90	5.85	4.05	5.85	4.05
Ohio	9.90	7.00	2.90	5.85	4.05
Oklahoma	9.02	5.85	3.17	5.85	3.17
Oregon	9.94	7.95	1.99	5.85	4.09
Pennsylvania	9.70	7.15	2.55	5.85	3.85
Rhode Island	9.70	7.40	2.30	5.85	3.85
South Carolina	8.53	—	8.53	5.85	2.68
South Dakota	9.90	5.85	4.05	5.85	4.05
Tennessee	9.13	—	9.13	5.85	3.28
Texas	9.02	5.85	3.17	5.85	3.17
Utah	9.42	5.85	3.57	5.85	3.57
Vermont	9.70	7.68	2.02	5.85	3.85
Virginia	8.85	5.85	3.00	5.85	3.00
Washington	9.94	8.07	1.87	5.85	4.09
West Virginia	9.13	6.55	2.58	5.85	3.28
Wisconsin	10.01	6.50	3.51	5.85	4.16
Wyoming	8.74	5.15	3.59	5.85	2.89

Note: Coverage may vary from one state to the next: reference will need to be made to each state's statute.

SOURCE: William G. Whitaker, "Table 2. Comparison of the Adverse Effect Wage Rate with State and Federal Minimum Wage Rates," in *Farm Labor: The Adverse Effect Wage Rate (AEWR)*, Congressional Research Service, March 26, 2008, http://www.nationalaglawcenter.org/assets/crs/RL32861.pdf (accessed January 15, 2009)

the national interests of the United States" are not permitted to enter the country. This proclamation also applies to the spouses, children, and dependent household members of these public officials.

Returns and Removals

Having a U.S. visa does not guarantee entry. A visa allows a traveler arriving at a U.S. port of entry to request permission to enter. Customs and Border Protection inspectors determine the admissibility of aliens who arrive at any of the approximately 300 U.S. ports of entry. Aliens who arrive without required documents, present improper or fraudulent documents, or who are on criminal wanted lists are deemed inadmissible. The Illegal Immigration Reform and Immigrant Responsibility Act (IIRIRA) of 1997 provides two options to the inadmissible alien: removal proceedings and returns (voluntary departure).

TABLE 3.18

Top ten states using H-2A workers, 2007

State	Employers		Workers		% all workers requested
	Requesting	Certified	Requested	Certified	
North Carolina	1,260	1,256	9,286	9,204	11.5%
Georgia	80	80	6,886	6,781	8.6%
Florida	110	101	6,291	5,588	7.8%
Kentucky	745	737	4,950	4,902	6.2%
Louisiana	367	364	4,265	4,248	5.3%
New York	277	276	3,952	3,950	4.9%
Arkansas	141	140	3,748	3,725	4.7%
California	295	282	3,530	3,098	4.4%
Virginia	536	533	2,809	2,787	3.5%
Tennessee	275	267	2,739	2,550	3.4%
Ten state total	4,086		48,456		60.3%
USA total	7,740	7,491	80,413	76,818	

SOURCE: Adapted from "H-2A National Summary, Fiscal Year 2007 Annual," U.S. Department of Labor, Employment and Training Administration, December 2008, http://www.foreignlaborcert.doleta.gov/h-2a_region2007.cfm (accessed December 24, 2008)

FIGURE 3.15

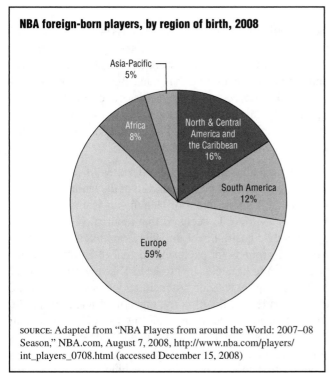

NBA foreign-born players, by region of birth, 2008

SOURCE: Adapted from "NBA Players from around the World: 2007–08 Season," NBA.com, August 7, 2008, http://www.nba.com/players/int_players_0708.html (accessed December 15, 2008)

FIGURE 3.16

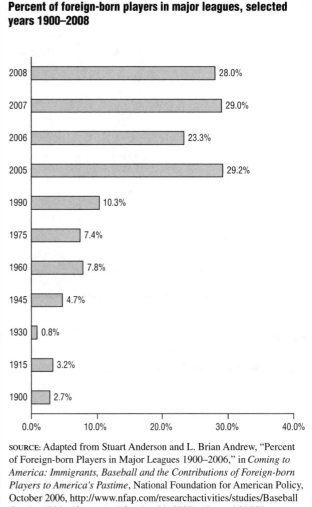

Percent of foreign-born players in major leagues, selected years 1900–2008

SOURCE: Adapted from Stuart Anderson and L. Brian Andrew, "Percent of Foreign-born Players in Major Leagues 1900–2006," in *Coming to America: Immigrants, Baseball and the Contributions of Foreign-born Players to America's Pastime*, National Foundation for American Policy, October 2006, http://www.nfap.com/researchactivities/studies/BaseballComing1006.pdf (accessed October 21, 2008); "Record 246 Players Born outside the U.S." MLB.com, April 3, 2007, http://mlb.mlb.com/news/press_releases/press_release.jsp?ymd=20070403&content_id=1877328&vkey=pr_mlb&fext=.jsp&c_id=mlb (accessed October 21, 2008); and "Percentage of Foreign-born MLB Players Drops from 29.0 to 28.0," Associated Press, April 1, 2008, http://sports.espn.go.com/mlb/news/storu?id=3324312 (accessed October 21, 2008). National Foundation for American Policy data also from Baseball Oracle and MLB.

Most removal proceedings involve a hearing before an immigration judge, which could result in removal or adjustment to a legal status, such as granting asylum. Removal proceedings can also involve fines or imprisonment. The IIRIRA empowered immigration officers to order an alien removed without a hearing or review through a process called expedited removal. This process applies to cases in which the officers determine that the alien is inadmissible because the alien engaged in fraud or misrepresentation or lacked proper documents. Returns are not based on an order of removal; the alien is offered the option to leave the country. Most such voluntary departures are undocumented people apprehended by the U.S. Border Patrol.

According to the Office of Immigration Statistics, in *Yearbook of Immigration Statistics: 2007*, 319,382 aliens were removed from the United States in FY 2007, an increase of 14% over the 280,974 removals in FY 2006. Of these removals, 99,900 (31%) were the result of criminal charges or criminal convictions. (See Figure 3.17.)

Aliens with Communicable Diseases

All immigrants, refugees, and certain nonimmigrants, including fiancés, coming to the United States must have a physical and mental examination before arriving in the country. In "Medical Examinations of Aliens (Refugees and

TABLE 3.19

Summary of immigrant and nonimmigrant visa ineligibilities and percent of applicants who overcame ineligibility, fiscal year 2007

	Immigrant			Nonimmigrant		
Grounds for visa refusal	Ineligibility finding	Ineligibility overcome	Percent overcome	Ineligibility finding	Ineligibility overcome	Percent overcome
Labor certification lacking	14,421	440	3%	0	0	
Smugglers	625	50	8%	1,445	225	16%
Drug use/trafficking	2,590	260	10%	8,563	4,865	57%
Misrepresentation	4,811	798	17%	7,437	1,359	18%
Terrorist activity	44	8	18%	296	140	47%
Removal order exists	1,770	361	20%	984	242	25%
Illegal activities	36	9	25%	193	21	11%
Medical	1,143	427	37%	350	170	49%
Past unlawful presence	17,536	7,091	40%	11,292	934	8%
Technical status/INA regulations	240,738	160,633	67%	2,085,489	461,984	22%
Public charge (indigent)	5,034	4,247	84%	560	43	8%
Other	130	114	88%	632	64	10%
Total	**288,878**	**174,438**		**2,117,241**	**470,047**	

Note: INA = Immigration and Nationality Act.

SOURCE: Adapted from "Table XX. Immigrant and Nonimmigrant Visa Ineligibilities (by Grounds for Refusal under the Immigration and Nationality Act, Unless Otherwise Indicated) Fiscal Year 2007," in *Report of the Visa Office 2007,* U.S. Department of State, Bureau of Consular Affairs, 2008, http://travel.state .gov/pdf/FY07AnnualReportTableXX.pdf (accessed December 24, 2008)

FIGURE 3.17

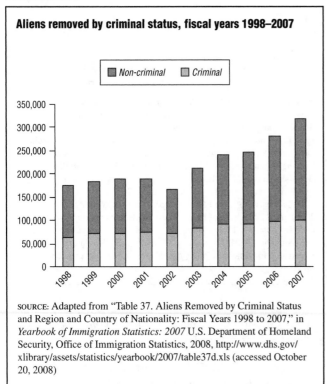

Aliens removed by criminal status, fiscal years 1998–2007

SOURCE: Adapted from "Table 37. Aliens Removed by Criminal Status and Region and Country of Nationality: Fiscal Years 1998 to 2007," in *Yearbook of Immigration Statistics: 2007* U.S. Department of Homeland Security, Office of Immigration Statistics, 2008, http://www.dhs.gov/ xlibrary/assets/statistics/yearbook/2007/table37d.xls (accessed October 20, 2008)

Immigrants)" (October 6, 2008, http://www.cdc.gov/ncidod/ dq/health.htm), the Centers for Disease Control and Prevention (CDC) provides information on the exam requirements. The exam must be conducted by a U.S.-approved panel physician. People already in the United States who apply for adjustment of status to permanent resident must have a physical and mental examination in the United States by a civil surgeon. The medical examination includes a skin test/ chest x-ray for tuberculosis and blood tests for syphilis and the human immunodeficiency virus (HIV) for people 15 years and older. Applicants under the age of 15 may be tested if there is reason to suspect any of these diseases. All immigrants are required to have an assessment for vaccine-preventable diseases: mumps, measles, rubella, polio, tetanus and diphtheria toxoids, pertussis, *Haemophilus influenzae* type B, meningitis and invasive disease, hepatitis B, varicella, and *pneumococcal pneumonia*.

Aliens with "communicable diseases of public health significance" are not permitted to enter the United States. In 1990 the U.S. Department of Health and Human Services, as part of IMMACT, declared that tuberculosis and AIDS were a public health threat. In 1993 Congress added HIV to the list of grounds for exclusion (denial of an alien's entry into the United States). In "Related Diseases" (December 7, 2007, http://www.cdc.gov/ncidod/dq/diseases.htm), the CDC provides the list of communicable diseases of public health concern. A communicable disease of public health concern is not a legal ground for deportation of immigrants already in the country. One particular concern about illegal aliens is that they bypass any screening or treatment for communicable diseases.

TUBERCULOSIS. The CDC monitors tuberculosis (TB) cases in the United States. In *Reported Tuberculosis in the United States, 2007* (September 2008, http://www.cdc.gov/ tb/surv/2007/pdf/fullreport.pdf), the CDC states that between 1993 and 2007 the number of TB cases among foreign-born people remained constant at 7,000 to 8,000 cases per year. (See Figure 3.18.) Among native-born people, TB cases decreased from more than 17,000 in 1993 to less than 5,500 in 2007. According to the CDC, this decrease in TB cases among native-born people caused the percentage of TB cases occurring in foreign-born people to rise from 29% in 1993 to 58% in 2007.

FIGURE 3.18

Number of TB cases in the United States, by foreign-born status, 1993–2007

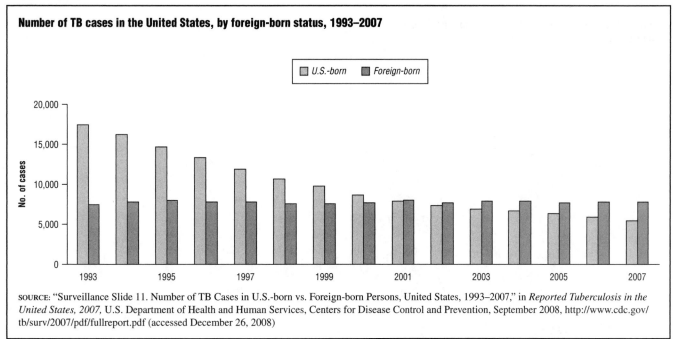

SOURCE: "Surveillance Slide 11. Number of TB Cases in U.S.-born vs. Foreign-born Persons, United States, 1993–2007," in *Reported Tuberculosis in the United States, 2007,* U.S. Department of Health and Human Services, Centers for Disease Control and Prevention, September 2008, http://www.cdc.gov/tb/surv/2007/pdf/fullreport.pdf (accessed December 26, 2008)

The number of states with 50% or greater of all TB cases occurring among foreign-born people doubled from 14 states in 1997 to 28 in 2007. (See Figure 3.19.) The CDC indicates that the number of states with at least 70% of cases among foreign-born people increased from two (Hawaii and Minnesota) in 1997 to thirteen (California, Colorado, Delaware, Massachusetts, Minnesota, Nebraska, New Hampshire, New Jersey, New York, Oregon, Rhode Island, Virginia, and Washington) in 2007.

Because TB is more prevalent and less treated in some countries, the rates of TB among immigrants from those countries is higher. The CDC states that the countries of birth producing the highest rates of TB have remained relatively constant since 1986, when the CDC began gathering this information. Seven out of 135 countries-of-birth account for 62% of TB cases among the foreign born in 2007. Mexico accounted for nearly one-fourth (24%) of cases. The other six countries with high TB rates were the Philippines (12%), India (8%), Vietnam (7%), China (5%), the Republic of Korea (3%), and Haiti (2%).

Of further concern to the CDC are cases of TB that prove resistant to standard drugs used to treat the disease. The proportion of TB patients with primary multidrug-resistant TB has decreased from 2.4% in 1993 to 1.1% in 2007. Since 1998 the percentage of native-born patients with multidrug-resistant TB has remained near 0.7%. However, the proportion occurring in foreign-born people increased from 25.5% in 1993 to 80% in 2007. The drug-resistant strains of TB require more patients to be placed on an initial treatment regimen of three or more drugs.

The CDC, in efforts to address the high rate of TB cases among the foreign born, is teaming up with other public health organizations, both nationally and internationally, to improve overseas screening of immigrants and refugees and to increase treatment follow-up.

FIGURE 3.19

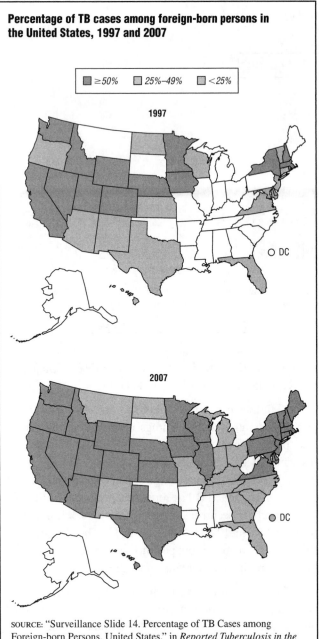

Percentage of TB cases among foreign-born persons in the United States, 1997 and 2007

≥50%   25%–49%   <25%

1997

2007

SOURCE: "Surveillance Slide 14. Percentage of TB Cases among Foreign-born Persons, United States," in *Reported Tuberculosis in the United States, 2007,* U.S. Department of Health and Human Services, Centers for Disease Control and Prevention, September 2008, http:// www.cdc.gov/tb/surv/2007/pdf/fullreport.pdf (accessed December 26, 2008)

CHAPTER 4
THE WORLDWIDE REFUGEE CHALLENGE

In the October 2006 issue of *Refugees* (http://www.unh cr.org/publ/PUBL/4523caa32.pdf), the magazine of the Office of the United Nations High Commissioner for Refugees (UNHCR), Rupert Colville reflects on the 50th anniversary of the Hungarian revolution—"the first major refugee relief operation of its kind" since the UNHCR was established by the UN General Assembly on December 14, 1950. The UNHCR grew out of the post–World War II efforts to deal with some 40 million people displaced by the war.

On October 23, 1956, Hungarian citizens overthrew their communist government. Twelve days later the Soviet army crushed the revolution. Thousands of people were killed, arrested, or missing. Frightened Hungarians poured across the border into Austria. Within just nine weeks, 200,000 Hungarians became refugees. The UNHCR and the French Red Cross took action to house refugees in Austria using camps with barracks recently vacated by post–World War II peacekeeping forces. The UNHCR set to work resettling the refugees. By the end of 1959, 180,000 refugees had been resettled in 37 countries. The UNHCR reported that the United States accepted the largest share (40,650, or 23%) of the refugees. As of spring 2009, according to the U.S. Department of State ("U.S. Gives $9.3 Million to Help Displaced Pakistanis," April 2, 2009, http://www.state.gov/r/pa/prs/ps/2009/04/121232.htm), one of the most recent initiatives by the UNHCR was to manage, along with the International Committee of the Red Cross, a $9.3 million contribution from the U.S. government to help Pakistanis displaced by their country's conflict.

WHO IS A REFUGEE?

Every year millions of people around the world are displaced by war, famine, civil unrest, and political turmoil. Others are forced to flee their country to escape the risk of death and torture at the hands of persecutors on account of race, religion, nationality, membership in a particular social group, or political opinion.

The United States works with other governmental, international, and private organizations to provide food, health care, and shelter to millions of refugees throughout the world. Resettlement in another country, including the United States, is considered for refugees in urgent need of protection, refugees for whom other long-term solutions are not feasible, and refugees able to join close family members. The United States gives priority to the safe, voluntary return of refugees to their homelands. This policy, recognized in the Refugee Act of 1980, is also the preference of the UNHCR.

The UNHCR reports in *2007 Global Trends: Refugees, Asylum-Seekers, Returnees, Internally Displaced and Stateless Persons* (June 2008, http://www.unhcr.org/statistics/STATISTICS/4852366f2.pdf) that 731,000 refugees voluntarily repatriated (returned to their homeland) in 2007. The main countries of return included Afghanistan (374,000), Sudan (130,700), the Democratic Republic of the Congo (60,000), Iraq (45,400), and Liberia (44,400). If repatriation is not feasible, refugees can be resettled in countries within their geographic region or in more distant countries, such as the United States.

According to the UNHCR, in 2007 a total of 75,300 refugees were admitted for permanent resettlement by 14 countries. The United States continued to take the lead in receiving refugees referred by the UNHCR by accepting 48,300 cases in 2007. Other major refugee-receiving countries were Canada (11,200), Australia (9,600), Sweden (1,800), and Norway (1,100).

Legally Admitting Refugees

Before World War II (1939–1945) the U.S. government had no arrangements for admitting people seeking refuge. The only way oppressed people were able to enter the United States was through regular immigration procedures.

After World War II refugees were admitted through special legislation passed by Congress. The Displaced Persons

Act of 1948, which admitted 400,000 East Europeans displaced by the war, was the first U.S. refugee legislation. The Immigration and Nationality Act (INA) of 1952 did not specifically mention refugees, but it did allow the U.S. attorney general parole authority (temporary admission) for oppressed people, such as Hungarians after their unsuccessful uprising in 1956. Other legislation—the Refugee Relief Act of 1953, the Fair Share Refugee Act of 1960, and the Indochinese Refugee Act of 1977—responded to particular world events and admitted specific groups.

Refugees were legally recognized for the first time in the Immigration and Nationality Act Amendments of 1965 with a preference category reserved for refugees from the Middle East or from countries ruled by a communist government.

Refugee Act of 1980

The Refugee Act of 1980 established a geographically and politically neutral adjudication standard for refugee status. The act redefined the term *refugee* as:

> (A) any person who is outside any country of such person's nationality or, in the case of a person having no nationality, is outside any country in which such person last habitually resided, and who is unable or unwilling to return to, and is unable or unwilling to avail himself or herself of the protection of, that country because of persecution or a well-founded fear of persecution on account of race, religion, nationality, membership in a particular social group, or political opinion, or (B) in such circumstances as the President after appropriate consultation... may specify, any person who is within the country of such person's nationality or, in the case of a person having no nationality, within the country in which such person is habitually residing, and who is persecuted or who has a well-founded fear of persecution on account of race, religion, nationality, membership in a particular social group, or political opinion.

The Refugee Act of 1980 required the president, at the beginning of each fiscal year, to determine the number of refugees to be admitted without consideration of any overall immigrant quota. The 1980 law also regulated U.S. asylum policy.

REFUGEES AND ASYLEES. The Refugee Act of 1980 made a distinction between refugees and asylees. A refugee is someone who applies for protection while outside the United States; an asylee is someone who is already in the United States when he or she applies for protection.

HOW MANY ARE ADMITTED?

The United States has resettled refugees for more than 50 years. The range is wide, from a peak of roughly 135,000 refugee arrivals in 1992 to a low of about 25,000 in 2002. (See Figure 4.1.) Kelly J. Jefferys and Daniel C. Martin of the U.S. Department of Homeland Security's (DHS) Office of Immigration Statistics note in *Annual Flow Report: Refugees and Asylees, 2007* (July 2008, http://www.dhs.gov/

FIGURE 4.1

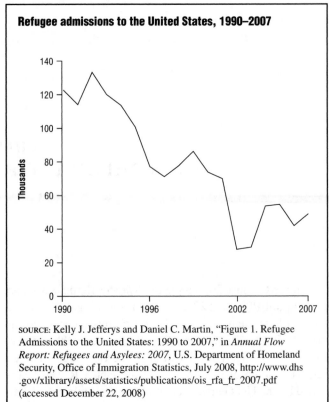

Refugee admissions to the United States, 1990–2007

SOURCE: Kelly J. Jefferys and Daniel C. Martin, "Figure 1. Refugee Admissions to the United States: 1990 to 2007," in *Annual Flow Report: Refugees and Asylees: 2007*, U.S. Department of Homeland Security, Office of Immigration Statistics, July 2008, http://www.dhs.gov/xlibrary/assets/statistics/publications/ois_rfa_fr_2007.pdf (accessed December 22, 2008)

xlibrary/assets/statistics/publications/ois_rfa_fr_2007.pdf) that this decline is partly due to changes in security procedures after the September 11, 2001, terrorist attacks and tighter admission requirements resulting from the Uniting and Strengthening America by Providing Appropriate Tools Required to Intercept and Obstruct Terrorism Act of 2001 (also known as the Patriot Act) and the READ ID Act of 2005.

A total of 48,217 people were admitted to the United States during fiscal year (FY) 2007. (See Table 4.1.) The leading countries of origin for refugees were Burma (Myanmar; 28.8%), Somalia (14.5%), and Iran (11.4%).

California has consistently been the state receiving the largest share of refugees, with 14% in 2005 and 13.9% in 2007. (See Table 4.2.) In 2005 and 2006 Minnesota was a close second, with 11.8% and 11.1%, respectively. In 2007 Minnesota's share of refugee resettlements dropped to 6.6%, whereas resettlements in Texas rose from 6% in 2005 to 9.1% in 2007.

Annual Refugee Admissions Limits

The admission of refugees to the United States and their resettlement are authorized by the INA. From FYs 2005 to 2007 the total U.S. refugee ceiling was 70,000 people distributed by world regions. (See Table 4.3.) The allocation for people from Africa increased from 20,000 in FY 2006 to 22,000 in FY 2007, whereas the allocation for Asia dropped from 15,000 in FY 2006 to 11,000 in FY

TABLE 4.1

Refugee arrivals by country of nationality, fiscal years 2005–07

[Ranked by 2007 country of nationality]

Country	2007 Number	2007 Percent	2006 Number	2006 Percent	2005 Number	2005 Percent
Total	**48,217**	**100.0**	**41,150**	**100.0**	**53,738**	**100.0**
Burma	13,896	28.8	1,612	3.9	1,447	2.7
Somalia	6,969	14.5	10,357	25.2	10,405	19.4
Iran	5,481	11.4	2,792	6.8	1,856	3.5
Burundi	4,545	9.4	466	1.1	214	0.4
Cuba	2,922	6.1	3,143	7.6	6,360	11.8
Russia	1,773	3.7	6,003	14.6	5,982	11.1
Iraq	1,608	3.3	202	0.5	198	0.4
Liberia	1,606	3.3	2,402	5.8	4,289	8.0
Ukraine	1,605	3.3	2,483	6.0	2,889	5.4
Vietnam	1,500	3.1	3,039	7.4	2,009	3.7
Other	6,312	13.1	8,651	21.0	18,089	33.7

SOURCE: Kelly J. Jefferys and Daniel C. Martin, "Table 3. Refugee Arrivals by Country of Nationality: Fiscal Years 2005 to 2007," in *Annual Flow Report: Refugees and Asylees: 2007*, U.S. Department of Homeland Security, Office of Immigration Statistics, July 2008, http://www.dhs.gov/xlibrary/assets/statistics/publications/ois_rfa_fr_2007.pdf (accessed December 22, 2008)

TABLE 4.2

Refugee arrivals by state of residence, fiscal years 2005–07

[Ranked by 2007 state of residence]

State	2007 Number	2007 Percent	2006 Number	2006 Percent	2005 Number	2005 Percent
Total	**48,217**	**100.0**	**41,150**	**100.0**	**53,738**	**100.0**
California	6,699	13.9	5,163	12.5	7,505	14.0
Texas	4,394	9.1	2,764	6.7	3,243	6.0
Minnesota	3,198	6.6	4,578	11.1	6,357	11.8
New York	2,978	6.2	2,303	5.6	2,561	4.8
Florida	2,691	5.6	2,582	6.3	4,799	8.9
Washington	2,215	4.6	2,458	6.0	2,841	5.3
Arizona	1,992	4.1	1,649	4.0	1,868	3.5
Illinois	1,872	3.9	1,227	3.0	1,463	2.7
North Carolina	1,805	3.7	1,228	3.0	1,259	2.3
Georgia	1,609	3.3	1,442	3.5	1,870	3.5
Other	18,764	38.9	15,756	38.3	19,972	37.2

SOURCE: Kelly J. Jefferys and Daniel C. Martin, "Table 5. Refugee Arrivals by State of Residence: Fiscal Years 2005 to 2007," in *Annual Flow Report: Refugees and Asylees: 2007*, U.S. Department of Homeland Security, Office of Immigration Statistics, July 2008, http://www.dhs.gov/xlibrary/assets/statistics/publications/ois_rfa_fr_2007.pdf (accessed December 22, 2008)

TABLE 4.3

Refugee admissions ceilings, fiscal years 2005–07

Region	Ceiling 2007	Ceiling 2006	Ceiling 2005
Total	**70,000**	**70,000**	**70,000**
Africa	22,000	20,000	20,000
East Asia	11,000	15,000	13,000
Europe/Central Asia	6,500	15,000	9,500
Latin America/Caribbean	5,000	5,000	5,000
Near East/South Asia	5,500	5,000	2,500
Unallocated reserve	20,000	10,000	20,000

SOURCE: Kelly J. Jefferys and Daniel C. Martin, "Table 1. Refugee Admissions Ceilings: Fiscal Years 2005 to 2007," in *Annual Flow Report: Refugees and Asylees: 2007*, U.S. Department of Homeland Security, Office of Immigration Statistics, July 2008, http://www.dhs.gov/xlibrary/assets/statistics/publications/ois_rfa_fr_2007.pdf (accessed December 22, 2008)

2007. For FY 2008 the ceiling increased to 80,000, with 70,000 of these numbers allocated among the regions of the world and the remaining 10,000 accounting for the "unallocated reserve." Refugee numbers that are unused in a fiscal year do not carry over to the following year.

In the Proposed Refugees Admissions, the president specifies that certain otherwise qualified people may be considered refugees of special humanitarian concern to the United States, even though they are still within their countries of nationality. For example, Rhoda Margesson, Jeremy M. Sharp, and Andorra Bruno of the Congressional

Research Service explain in *Iraqi Refugees and Internally Displaced Persons: A Deepening Humanitarian Crisis?* (August 15, 2008, http://fpc.state.gov/documents/organization/110399.pdf) that in FY 2008 the allocation for the Near East/South Asia region (which includes Iraq) was 28,000. This allocation included vulnerable Iraqis plus Bhutanese and Iranian religious and ethnic minorities. The UNHCR reports in the press release "Trauma Survey in Syria Highlights Suffering of Iraqi Refugee" (January 22, 2008, http://www.unhcr.org/news/NEWS/479616762.html) that by January 2008 more than 2 million Iraqis left their homes for neighboring states, mainly Syria and Jordan, and an additional 2.2 million were displaced within Iraq.

Material Support Denials

The 2001 Patriot Act and the 2005 REAL ID Act prohibit granting entrance to the United States to anyone who has given material support (money or other support) to terrorists or terrorist organizations. In "The 'Material Support' Problem: An Uncertain Future for Thousands of Refugees and Asylum Seekers" (*Bender's Immigration Bulletin*, vol. 10, December 15, 2005), Melanie Nezer of the Hebrew Immigrant Aid Society in Washington, D.C., argues that people who had been "coerced under extreme duress to make payments to armed groups on the State Department's list of foreign terrorist organizations" are being denied admission to the United States as refugees. Nezer cites as an example Colombian refugees who gave money to the United Self-Defense Forces of Colombia, the Revolutionary Armed Forces of Colombia, or the National Liberation Army. Payments to these groups were made under threat of torture or death to self or a loved one. Making such payments became a necessity of survival for many Colombians. Nezer contends that such nonvoluntary material support should not deny these refugees admission to the United States.

Processing Priority System

The United States has established three priority categories for admitting refugees.

PRIORITY 1: INDIVIDUAL REFERRALS. This category is available to individuals with compelling protection needs or those for whom no other durable solution exists and who are identified and referred to the program by the UNHCR, a U.S. embassy, or a designated nongovernmental organization (NGO). This processing priority is available to people of any nationality.

PRIORITY 2: GROUP REFERRALS. This category is used for groups of special humanitarian concern to the United States that are designated for resettlement processing. It includes specific groups (which can be defined by their particular nationalities, clans, ethnicities, religions, location, or a combination of such characteristics) identified by the State Department in consultation with the U.S. Citizenship and Immigration Services (USCIS), NGOs, the UNHCR, and other experts.

PRIORITY 3: FAMILY REUNIFICATION CASES. This category is used for spouses, unmarried children under the age of 21, parents of people admitted to the United States as refugees or granted asylum, or people who were lawful permanent residents or U.S. citizens and were initially admitted to the United States as refugees or granted asylum. In FY 2007 Priority 3 eligibility was extended to nationals of particular countries based on the UNHCR's annual assessment of refugees in need of resettlement, prospective or ongoing repatriation efforts, and U.S. foreign policy interests. These Priority 3 countries are Afghanistan, Burma, Burundi, Colombia, Congo (Brazzaville), Cuba, the Democratic People's Republic of Korea, the Democratic Republic of Congo, Eritrea, Ethiopia, Haiti, Iran, Iraq, Rwanda, Somalia, Sudan, and Uzbekistan.

Profile of Refugees Admitted

Table 4.4 profiles FYs 2005 to 2007 refugee admissions by age, gender, and marital status. Even though the share of refugees aged 17 and under decreased from 40.6% in FY 2005 to 37.8% in FY 2007, refugees aged 18 to 24 increased from 17% to 18.8% and aged 25 to 34 rose from 15.1% to 16.7%. The share of spouses and children in the refugee population declined from 62.3% in FY 2005 to 58.7% in FY 2007. (See Table 4.5.)

WHO IS AN ASYLUM SEEKER?

Like a refugee, an asylee is someone who wants safe haven in another country. The only difference is the location of the alien when he or she applies for refugee or asylee status: A refugee is outside the United States when applying for refuge, whereas an asylee is already in the United States, perhaps on an expired tourist visa or at a port of entry. Just like a refugee applying for entrance into the country, an asylee seeks the protection of the United States because of persecution or a well-founded fear of persecution.

After being the second most important destination for new asylum seekers in 2005 and 2006 (48,900 and 50,800

TABLE 4.4

Refugee arrivals by age, gender, and marital status, fiscal years 2005–07

	2007		2006		2005	
Age	Number	Percent	Number	Percent	Number	Percent
Total	**48,217**	**100.0**	**41,150**	**100.0**	**53,738**	**100.0**
0 to 17 years	18,202	37.8	15,430	37.5	21,838	40.6
18 to 24 years	9,088	18.8	8,057	19.6	9,141	17.0
25 to 34 years	8,058	16.7	6,365	15.5	8,138	15.1
35 to 44 years	5,585	11.6	4,942	12.0	6,460	12.0
45 to 54 years	3,552	7.4	3,059	7.4	3,821	7.1
55 to 64 years	2,192	4.5	1,782	4.3	2,237	4.2
65 years and over	1,540	3.2	1,515	3.7	2,103	3.9
Gender						
Male	25,201	52.3	21,188	51.5	27,484	51.1
Female	23,016	47.7	19,962	48.5	26,254	48.9
Marital status						
Married	17,101	35.5	14,457	35.1	19,557	36.4
Single	28,739	59.6	24,555	59.7	31,590	58.8
Other	2,377	4.9	2,138	5.2	2,591	4.8

SOURCE: Kelly J. Jefferys and Daniel C. Martin, "Table 4. Refugee Arrivals by Age, Gender, and Marital Status: Fiscal Years 2005 to 2007," in *Annual Flow Report: Refugees and Asylees: 2007*, U.S. Department of Homeland Security, Office of Immigration Statistics, July 2008, http://www.dhs.gov/xlibrary/assets/statistics/publications/ois_rfa_fr_2007.pdf (accessed December 22, 2008)

TABLE 4.5

Refugee arrivals by category of admission, fiscal years 2005–07

	2007		2006		2005	
Category of admission	Number	Percent	Number	Percent	Number	Percent
Total	**48,217**	**100.0**	**41,150**	**100.0**	**53,738**	**100.0**
Principal applicant	19,911	41.3	16,384	39.8	20,260	37.7
Dependents	28,306	58.7	24,766	60.2	33,478	62.3
Spouse	7,414	15.4	6,055	14.7	8,511	15.8
Child	20,892	43.3	18,711	45.5	24,967	46.5

SOURCE: Kelly J. Jefferys and Daniel C. Martin, "Table 2. Refugee Arrivals by Category of Admission: Fiscal years 2005 to 2007," in *Annual Flow Report: Refugees and Asylees: 2007*, U.S. Department of Homeland Security, Office of Immigration Statistics, July 2008, http://www.dhs.gov/xlibrary/assets/statistics/publications/ois_rfa_fr_2007.pdf (accessed December 22, 2008)

claims, respectively), the United States became the main receiving country in 2007. The UNHCR reports in *2007 Global Trends* that out of the 548,000 new asylum claims lodged worldwide in 2007, an estimated 50,700 (about 10%) were submitted in the United States. Rather than reflecting an increase in new asylum seekers, the United States' top position comes as a result of fewer asylum seekers going to South Africa in 2007. South Africa, the top destination in 2006 with 53,400 asylum requests, was in second position in 2007 with 45,600 new claims. Sweden was the third-largest recipient during 2007 (36,400 claims), mostly due to the arrival of Iraqi asylum seekers. Other important destination countries for asylum seekers were France (29,400), the United Kingdom (27,900), Canada (27,900), and Greece (25,100).

Asylees in the United States include sailors who jumped ship while their boat was docked in a U.S. port, athletes who asked for asylum while participating in a sports event, and women who based their claim on a fear of being compelled to undergo a coercive population-control procedure such as abortion or sterilization. Any alien physically present in the United States or at a port of entry can request asylum in the United States. It is irrelevant whether the person is a legal or illegal alien. Like refugees, asylum applicants do not count against the worldwide annual U.S. limitation of immigrants.

In the press release "Asylum Protection in the United States" (April 28, 2005, http://www.usdoj.gov/eoir/press/05/AsylumProtectionFactsheetQAApr05.htm), the U.S. Department of Justice notes that certain individuals are barred from obtaining asylum, including those who:

- Have firmly resettled in another country prior to arriving in the United States;

- Have ordered, incited, assisted, or otherwise participated in the persecution of any person on account of race, religion, nationality, membership in a particular social group, or political opinion;

- Were convicted of a particularly serious crime (includes aggravated felonies);

- Committed a serious nonpolitical crime outside the United States;

- Pose a danger to the security of the United States;

- Are members or representatives of a foreign terrorist organization; or

- Have engaged in or incited terrorist activity.

How Many Asylees?

Critics charge that many people seek asylum in the United States to avoid dismal economic conditions at home rather than the legitimate reasons to seek asylum under U.S. law: to escape political or religious persecution or because of a well-founded fear of physical harm or death. In addition, some illegal aliens try to obtain the legal right to work by filing for asylum. People granted asylum are authorized to work in the United States and are also eligible for a Social Security card and for social services benefits.

Under the INA, as amended, a person can be granted asylum only if he or she establishes a well-founded fear of persecution on account of one of five protected grounds: race, religion, nationality, membership in a particular social group, or political opinion. Some people charge that the United States constantly changes its definition of what constitutes "membership in a particular social group" to accommodate the growing number of asylum seekers.

According to the USCIS, in "Membership in a Particular Social Group" (1999, http://www.uscis.gov/propub/ProPubVAP.jsp?dockey=0d78ecc050f6c88adac192048403eb71), regulation changes proposed in 2000 included this def-

inition: "A particular social group is composed of members who share a common, immutable characteristic, such as sex, color, kinship ties, or past experience, that a member either cannot change or that is so fundamental to the identity or conscience of the member that he or she should not be required to change it."

Those who believe the term should be interpreted broadly argue that the intent of the law is to provide a catch-all to include all the types of persecution that can occur. Those with a narrow view see the law as a means of identifying and protecting individuals from known forms of harm, not in anticipation of future types of abuse.

Filing Claims

Asylum seekers must apply for asylum within one year from the date of last arrival in the United States. If the application is filed past the one-year mark, asylum seekers must show changed circumstances that materially affect their eligibility or extraordinary circumstances that delayed filing. They must also show that they filed within a reasonable amount of time given these circumstances. The Justice Department identifies two types of asylum claims: affirmative and defensive. Aliens in the United States can apply for asylum by filing an Application for Asylum (Form I-589) with the USCIS. Initiating this process is called an affirmative asylum claim. Aliens who have been placed in removal proceedings and who are in immigration court can request asylum through the Executive Office of Immigration Review. This last-resort effort is called a defensive asylum claim.

Affirmative and Defensive Asylum Claims

Figure 4.2 shows the pattern of affirmative and defensive asylum claims from 1990 to 2007. The total volume of both types of asylum claims in the early 1990s was less than 10,000, perhaps because so many people were being admitted as refugees in that period. Defensive asylum claims increased steadily from less than 3,000 in 1994 to a high of more than 13,000 in 2003. Affirmative claims rose dramatically from about 4,000 in 1991 to a peak of more than 28,000 in 2001.

The number of affirmative and defensive asylum claims granted differ by countries of origin. China is the leading country of origin for both types of claims—in FY 2007 it represented 14.6% of affirmative claims granted (see Table 4.6) and 35.4% of defensive claims granted (see Table 4.7). By contrast, Haitian asylees were granted more affirmative claims (8.6%) than defensive claims (4.6%) in FY 2007.

Challenges of Immigration Courts

Nina Bernstein reports in "In New York Immigration Court, Asylum Roulette" (*New York Times*, October 8, 2006) that there are several allegations of vast disparity between judges' decisions on asylum cases. Bernstein notes examples

FIGURE 4.2

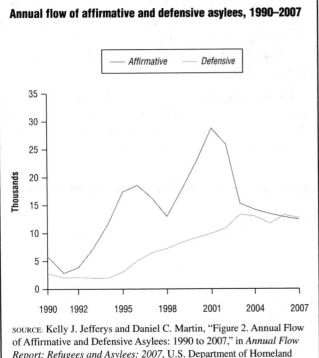

Annual flow of affirmative and defensive asylees, 1990–2007

SOURCE: Kelly J. Jefferys and Daniel C. Martin, "Figure 2. Annual Flow of Affirmative and Defensive Asylees: 1990 to 2007," in *Annual Flow Report: Refugees and Asylees: 2007*, U.S. Department of Homeland Security, Office of Immigration Statistics, July 2008, http://www.dhs.gov/xlibrary/assets/statistics/publications/ois_rfa_fr_2007.pdf (accessed December 22, 2008)

TABLE 4.6

Affirmative asylees by country of nationality, fiscal years 2005–07

[Ranked by 2007 country of nationality]

Country	2007 Number	2007 Percent	2006 Number	2006 Percent	2005 Number	2005 Percent
Total	**12,463**	**100.0**	**12,855**	**100.0**	**13,414**	**100.0**
China	1,821	14.6	1,514	11.8	2,214	16.5
Colombia	1,497	12.0	2,189	17.0	2,212	16.5
Haiti	1,073	8.6	2,428	18.9	2,285	17.0
Venezuela	855	6.9	1,084	8.4	951	7.1
Indonesia	567	4.5	428	3.3	95	0.7
Guatemala	547	4.4	477	3.7	246	1.8
Ethiopia	497	4.0	431	3.4	462	3.4
El Salvador	431	3.5	501	3.9	179	1.3
Iraq	409	3.3	175	1.4	192	1.4
Cameroon	302	2.4	228	1.8	382	2.8
All other countries, including unknown	4,464	35.8	3,400	26.4	4,196	31.3

SOURCE: Kelly J. Jefferys and Daniel C.Martin, "Table 7. Affirmative Asylees by Country of Nationality: Fiscal Years 2005 to 2007," in *Annual Flow Report: Refugees and Asylees: 2007*, U.S. Department of Homeland Security, Office of Immigration Statistics, July 2008, http://www.dhs.gov/xlibrary/assets/statistics/publications/ois_rfa_fr_2007.pdf (accessed December 22, 2008)

such as "90 percent of asylum cases granted by one judge and 9 percent [by another judge] down the hall." Concerning asylum cases, "the wrong decision can be a death sentence. In others, banishment hangs in the balance, with the prospect of families split up or swept into harm's way." Bernstein also

TABLE 4.7

Defensive asylees by country of nationality, fiscal years 2005–07

[Ranked by 2007 country of nationality]

Country	2007 Number	2007 Percent	2006 Number	2006 Percent	2005 Number	2005 Percent
Total	**12,807**	**100.0**	**13,352**	**100.0**	**11,757**	**100.0**
China	4,540	35.4	4,061	30.4	3,014	25.6
Colombia	683	5.3	779	5.8	1,151	9.8
Haiti	587	4.6	570	4.3	653	5.6
Albania	420	3.3	506	3.8	610	5.2
India	357	2.8	450	3.4	311	2.6
Ethiopia	349	2.7	344	2.6	266	2.3
Guinea	324	2.5	358	2.7	257	2.2
Venezuela	315	2.5	279	2.1	153	1.3
Iraq	276	2.2	191	1.4	94	0.8
Egypt	231	1.8	240	1.8	194	1.7
All other countries, including unknown	4,725	36.9	5,574	41.7	5,054	43.0

SOURCE: Kelly J. Jefferys and Daniel C.Martin, "Table 8. Defensive Asylees by Country of Nationality: Fiscal Years 2005 to 2007," in *Annual Flow Report: Refugees and Asylees: 2007*, U.S. Department of Homeland Security, Office of Immigration Statistics, July 2008, http://www.dhs.gov/xlibrary/assets/statistics/publications/ois_rfa_fr_2007.pdf (accessed December 22, 2008)

acknowledges the challenges faced by immigration judges, in that they have to "cope with an intricate web of laws, changing conditions in distant lands, and a mix of false and truthful testimony in 227 tongues vulnerable to an interpreter's mistake as small as pronouncing 'rebels' like 'robbers.'"

In 2008 the U.S. Government Accountability Office conducted a study of immigration courts and judges. The resulting report *U.S. Asylum System: Significant Variation Existed in Asylum Outcomes across Immigration Courts and Judges* (September 2008, http://www.gao.gov/new.items/d08940.pdf) states:

> The likelihood of being granted asylum differed for affirmative and defensive cases and varied depending on the immigration court in which the case was heard. Overall, the grant rate for affirmative cases (37 percent) was significantly higher than the grant rate for defensive cases (26 percent). The affirmative asylum grant rate ranged from 6 percent in Atlanta to 54 percent in New York City. The grant rate for defensive cases ranged from 7 percent in Atlanta to 35 percent in San Francisco and New York City.... As an example of differences in asylum outcomes across immigration courts, affirmative applicants in the San Francisco immigration court were 12 times more likely to be granted asylum than affirmative applicants in the Atlanta immigration court, even after we controlled for the statistically significant effects of applicants' nationality, time period of the decision, [use of legal] representation, filing within 1 year of entry, and claiming dependents.

Expedited Removal

Under the expedited removal provisions of the Illegal Immigration Reform and Immigrant Responsibility Act of

1996, any alien subject to expedited removal because of fraud, misrepresentation, or a lack of valid documents must be questioned by an immigration officer regarding the fear of being persecuted at home. Aliens who express such a fear are detained until an asylum officer can determine the credibility of the fear. Aliens found to have a credible fear are referred to an immigration judge for a final determination and are generally released until their case is heard. In some instances an alien is detained while his or her case is pending before an immigration judge. If the fear is deemed not credible, the alien is refused admission and removed.

Critics charge that the expedited removal process denies aliens a fair chance to fully present their asylum claims, places unprecedented authority in the hands of asylum officers, is conducted so quickly that mistakes are inevitable, limits an alien's right to review a deportation order, and results in the wrongful expulsion of individuals with legitimate fears of persecution. An alien who is deported under the expedited removal process is barred from returning to the United States for five years.

VICTIMS OF TRAFFICKING AND VIOLENCE

The Trafficking Victims Protection Act (TVPA) of 2000 makes victims of severe forms of trafficking eligible for benefits and services to the same extent as refugees. In addition, the law attempts to identify and prosecute traffickers. The Trafficking Victims Protection Reauthorization Act of 2003 mandated informational awareness campaigns and created a new civil action provision that allows victims to sue their traffickers in federal district court. It also required the U.S. attorney general to give an annual report to Congress on the results of U.S. government activities to combat trafficking. The Trafficking Victims Protection Reauthorization Act of 2006 appropriated over $361 million in funding through FY 2007. The William Wilberforce Trafficking Victims Protection Reauthorization Act of 2008 was signed into law in December of that year, authorizing appropriations for FY 2008–2011.

The TVPA designated the U.S. Department of Health and Human Services (HHS) as the agency responsible for helping victims of human trafficking become eligible to receive benefits and services so they may rebuild their lives safely in the United States. The TVPA authorizes "certification" of adult victims to receive certain federally funded or federally administered benefits and services, such as cash assistance, medical care, food stamps, and housing. Though not required to be certified by the HHS, minors who are determined to be victims of severe forms of trafficking receive "letters of eligibility" for the same types of services.

The U.S. attorney general states in *Attorney General's Report to Congress on U.S. Government Activities to Combat Trafficking in Persons Fiscal Year 2007* (June 2008, http://www.usdoj.gov/ag/annualreports/tr2007/agreporthumantrafficking2007.pdf) that in FY 2007 the Office of Ref-

TABLE 4.8

Certifications and letters of eligibility issued, 2001–07

Fiscal year	Minors	Adults	Total
2001	4	194	198
2002	18	81	99
2003	6	145	151
2004	16	147	163
2005	34	197	231
2006	20	214	234
2007	33	270	303
Total	**131**	**1,248**	**1,379**

SOURCE: "Certifications and Letters of Eligibility," in *Attorney General's Annual Report to Congress and Assessment of the U.S. Government Activities to Combat Trafficking in Persons, Fiscal Year 2007,* U.S. Department of Justice, May 2008, http://www.usdoj.gov/ag/annualreports/tr2007/agreporthumantrafficking2007.pdf (accessed January 4, 2008)

ugee Resettlement issued a total of 303 letters: 270 certification letters to adults and 33 eligibility letters to minors. This was the greatest total number of letters issued since the TVPA was implemented. (See Table 4.8.) In FY 2007, 30% of victims certified were male, whereas only 6% were certified in FY 2006. The attorney general also states that "FY 2007 letters were provided to victims or their representatives in 29 states plus the District of Columbia and Saipan, a 35 percent increase from FY 06. Certified victims came from over 50 countries, spanning the Americas, Asia, Africa, and Europe. Forty-one percent of victims originated in Latin America and the Caribbean, and an additional 41 percent of victims originated in Asia."

Trafficking victims in the United States are eligible for Continued Presence (CP) or T (nonimmigrant visa) status. CP authorizes the victim to remain in the United States as a potential witness in the investigation and prosecution of traffickers. Victims who are over the age of 18 and have complied with reasonable requests for assistance in the investigation and prosecution of acts of trafficking may apply for a T visa. The T visa allows the victim to remain in the United States for three years and then apply for lawful permanent residence. The U.S. attorney general reports that there were 125 requests for CP status in FY 2007. The requesting victims came from 24 countries, with the highest number of victims coming from Mexico, El Salvador, and China. (See Table 4.9.) Since 2001, 1,974 T visas have been awarded by the United States. A total of 230 people applied for T visas in FY 2007. (See Table 4.10.) A total of 279 requests for T visas were approved, including carryover from previous years.

Monitoring Foreign Governments

The TVPA requires the State Department to monitor the efforts of foreign governments to eliminate trafficking. The State Department identifies governments in full compliance with TVPA (Tier I), governments in compliance with minimum standards (Tier II), governments who have

TABLE 4.9

Requests for Continued Presence (CP) visas, fiscal year 2007

CP requests in FY 07	Number awarded	Number withdrawn	Requests for extensions	Extensions authorized	Countries represented	Countries with highest number of victims	Cities with most CP requests
125	122	3	5	5	24	Mexico, El Salvador, and China	Los Angeles, Newark, Houston and New York

SOURCE: "CP Requests in FY2007," in *Attorney General's Annual Report to Congress and Assessment of the U.S. Government Activities to Combat Trafficking in Persons, Fiscal Year 2007,* U.S. Department of Justice, May 2008, http://www.usdoj.gov/ag/annualreports/tr2007/agreporthumantrafficking2007.pdf (accessed January 4, 2008)

TABLE 4.10

Applications for T visas, fiscal year 2007

Applications for T visas	FY 2007
Victims	
Applied	230
Approved*	279
Denied	70
Family of victims	
Applied	149
Approved*	261
Denied	52

*Some approvals are from prior fiscal year(s) filings.

SOURCE: "Applications for T Visas, FY2007," in *Attorney General's Annual Report to Congress and Assessment of the U.S. Government Activities to Combat Trafficking in Persons, Fiscal Year 2007,* U.S. Department of Justice, May 2008, http://www.usdoj.gov/ag/annualreports/tr2007/agreporthumantrafficking2007.pdf (accessed January 4, 2008)

shown minimum standards of compliance (Tier II Watch List), and those who have not taken serious action to stop human trafficking (Tier III). Fourteen countries were listed as Tier III in 2008. (See Table 4.11.) According to the State Department, in *Trafficking in Persons Report 2008* (June 2008, http://www.state.gov/documents/organization/105501.pdf), there were 5,682 prosecutions and 3,427 convictions of alleged traffickers worldwide in 2007. There were also 28 new or amended pieces of antitrafficking legislation implemented by other countries during that year.

Further efforts to combat human trafficking include the U.S. Department of State post of Ambassador-at-Large to Monitor and Combat Trafficking in Persons. President Barack Obama (1961–) nominated Luis C. de Baca for the post in March 2009, stating, as quoted by a White House press release (March 24, 2009, http://www.whitehouse.gov/the_press _office/President-Obama-Announces-Another-Key-State-Department-Post/), that "he will be an indispensable part of our team as we work tirelessly to stand up for human rights and the rule of law."

VICTIMS OF TORTURE

In a report to the U.S. Senate on the Torture Victims Relief Reauthorization Act of 2007 (October 9, 2007, http://

TABLE 4.11

Tier placement of countries, 2008

Tier 1

Australia	Finland	Lithuania	Slovenia
Austria	France	Luxembourg	Spain
Belgium	Georgia	Macedonia	Sweden
Canada	Germany	Madagascar	Switzerland
Colombia	Hong Kong	Netherlands	United Kingdom
Croatia	Hungary	New Zealand	
Czech Republic	Italy	Norway	
Denmark	Korea, Republic of	Poland	

Tier 2

Afghanistan	Ghana	Malta	Sierra Leone
Angola	Greece	Mauritania	Singapore
Bangladesh	Honduras	Mauritius	Slovak Republic
Belarus	Indonesia	Mexico	Suriname
Belize	Israel	Mongolia	Tanzania
Benin	Ireland	Morocco	Taiwan
Bolivia	Jamaica	Nepal	Thailand
Bosnia & Herzegovina	Japan	Nicaragua	Timor-Leste
Brazil	Kazakhstan	Nigeria	Togo
Bulgaria	Kenya	Pakistan	Turkey
Burkina Faso	Kyrgyz Republic	Paraguay	Uganda
Cambodia	Laos	Peru	Ukraine
Chile	Latvia	Philippines	United Arab Emirates
Djibouti	Lebanon	Portugal	Uruguay
Ecuador	Liberia	Romania	Vietnam
El Salvador	Macau	Rwanda	Yemen
Estonia	Malawi	Senegal	
Ethiopia	Mali	Serbia	

Tier 2 watch list

Argentina	Congo, Rep. Of	Guinea-Bissau	South Africa
Armenia	Costa Rica	Guyana	Sri Lanka
Azerbaijan	Cyprus	India	Tajikistan
Albania	Cote d'Ivoire	Jordan	Tanzania
Bahrain	Dominican Republic	Libya	Venezuela
Burundi	Egypt	Malaysia	Uzbekistan
Cameroon	Equatorial Guinea	Montenegro	Zambia
Central African Republic	Gabon	Mozambique	Zimbabwe
Chad	The Gambia	Niger	
China (PRC)	Guatemala	Panama	
Congo (DRC)	Guinea	Russia	

Tier 3

Algeria	Iran	Oman	Sudan
Burma	Kuwait	Papua New Guinea	Syria
Cuba	Moldova	Qatar	
Fiji	North Korea	Saudi Arabia	

SOURCE: "Tier Placements," in *Trafficking in Persons Report*, U.S. Department of State, Office to Monitor Trafficking in Persons, June 4, 2008, http://www.state.gov/g/tip/rls/tiprpt/2008/ (accessed January 5, 2009)

frwebgate.access.gpo.gov/cgi-bin/getdoc.cgi?dbname=110 _cong_reports&docid=f:sr194.110.pdf), the Congressional Budget Office states:

According to Amnesty International, over 150 countries worldwide engage in torture. Estimates indicate that there may be up to 100 million torture victims worldwide, with approximately 400,000–500,000 foreign victims residing in the United States. In 1998, Congress passed the Torture Victims Relief Act (P.L. 105-320) to authorize appropriations for domestic and foreign programs and centers to provide treatment and assistance to victims of torture.... In 2006, the Victims' Torture Fund of the U.S. Agency for International Development supported programs in 28 countries.... Within the United States, programs administered by the Office of Refugee Resettlement provided direct services to 3,220 victims of torture.

In March 2009 a bill was introduced to amend the Torture Victims Relief Reauthorization Act to allow for appropriations for FY 2010–FY 2011 that would include help for programs and centers that treat torture victims.

REFUGEE ADJUSTMENT TO LIFE IN THE UNITED STATES

The State Department's Bureau of Population, Refugee, and Migration explains in *FY 2008 Summary of Major Activities* (October 24, 2008, http://www.state.gov/documents/organization/111547.pdf) that the U.S. government expected to spend over $1.4 billion to help process and resettle refugees in FY 2008. (See Figure 4.3.) The bulk of this budget ($1.1 billion) supported overseas assistance. The costs of processing, transporting, and assisting refugees approved for reset-

FIGURE 4.3

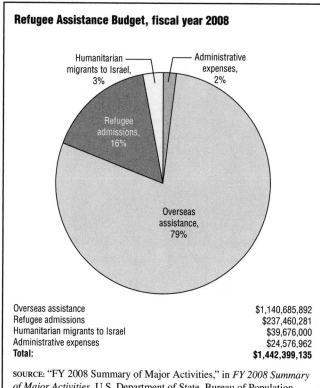

Refugee Assistance Budget, fiscal year 2008

Humanitarian migrants to Israel, 3%
Administrative expenses, 2%
Refugee admissions, 16%
Overseas assistance, 79%

Overseas assistance	$1,140,685,892
Refugee admissions	$237,460,281
Humanitarian migrants to Israel	$39,676,000
Administrative expenses	$24,576,962
Total:	**$1,442,399,135**

SOURCE: "FY 2008 Summary of Major Activities," in *FY 2008 Summary of Major Activities*, U.S. Department of State, Bureau of Population, Refugees, and Migration, October 24, 2008, http://www.state.gov/documents/organization/111547.pdf (accessed January 5, 2009)

tlement in the United States totaled $237.5 million. The State Department makes funds available for the transportation of refugees resettled in the United States. The cost of transportation is provided to refugees in the form of a loan. Beginning six months after their arrival, refugees become responsible for repaying these loans over time.

NGOs recruit church groups and volunteers from local communities to provide a variety of services and to contribute clothing and household furnishings to meet the needs of arriving refugees. They also become mentors and friends of the refugees, providing orientation to community services, offering supportive services such as tutoring children after school, and teaching families how to shop and handle other essential functions of living in the community.

Mutual assistance associations, many of which have national networks, provide opportunities for refugees to meet their countrymen who are already settled in the United States. These associations also help refugees connect with their ethnic culture through holiday and religious celebrations.

Benefits to Assist Transition

Ongoing benefits for the newly arrived refugees include transitional cash assistance, health benefits, and a wide variety of social services, which are provided through grants from the Office of Refugee Resettlement. English-language training is a basic service offered to all refugees. The primary focus is preparation for employment through skills training, job development, orientation to the workplace, and job counseling. Early employment leads not only to early economic self-sufficiency for the family but also helps establish the family in its new country and community. Special attention is paid to ensure that women have equal access to training and services leading to job placement. Other services include family strengthening, youth and elderly services, adjustment counseling, and mental health services.

Support for Elderly and Disabled Refugees

Refugees who are elderly or disabled receive benefits from the Social Security Administration, the same as U.S. citizens. However, changes by Congress in the late 1990s limit the eligibility of noncitizens to their first seven years in the United States. Time limits for noncitizens do not apply once they become U.S. citizens. The refugee program offers citizenship classes to assist refugees who want to study for the citizenship test.

Unaccompanied Children

According to the National Center for Immigrant and Refugee Children (2008, http://www.refugees.org/article.aspx?id=1260), more than 7,000 unaccompanied immigrant youth come to the United States every year. Many are fleeing gang violence, domestic abuse, poverty, or human trafficking. They want to be united with friends or family. The majority of these children fight for the right to stay in this country, but most go through immigration proceedings without speaking with an attorney.

Children who do not have parents in the United States and who are granted asylum are eligible for the Specialized Refugee Foster Care Program. This program is coordinated by the Lutheran Immigration and Refugee Service and the U.S. Conference of Catholic Bishops. Benefits include financial support for housing, food, clothing, and other necessities; case management by a social worker; medical care; independent living skills training; education and English as a second language; tutoring and mentoring; job skills training and career counseling; mental health services; ongoing family tracing; cultural activities and recreation; special education where needed; and legal assistance.

CHAPTER 5
ILLEGAL ALIENS

BARRIERS TO LEGAL IMMIGRATION: TIME AND MONEY

Even in times of economic chaos, the United States is the best place to work. However, Stuart Anderson and David Miller of the National Foundation for American Policy explain in *Legal Immigrants: Waiting Forever* (May 2006, http://www.competeamerica.org/resource/h1b_glance/NFAP _Study.pdf) that "those who 'play by the rules' are likely to wait many years" to enter the United States. The word is out around the world that there are jobs in the United States. Anderson and Miller note that even the lowest-paying jobs in the United States far exceed what workers can earn in most parts of the world, even if employment were available in impoverished countries. Many aliens who enter the United States accept high risk and sometimes great expense for a chance to work. Their families often follow.

Waiting Time for Legal Entry Documents

The annual limit on the number of U.S. employment-based legal admissions is well below the number requested by potential immigrants seeking employment. This has created backlogs in some categories. Anderson and Miller indicate that waiting times for new employer-sponsored skilled workers and professionals to receive green cards exceeds five years. The demand for green cards for "other workers" (that is, for workers who are not sponsored by an employer, are not highly educated, and who do not possess specialized skills) exceeded the established annual limits to such an extent that the U.S. Department of State set cutoff dates and only processed applications received before that date. This resulted in visas for "other worker" applicants being "unavailable" for part of the year. The wait time for priority workers from China and India is one year, whereas it is immediate for workers from Mexico, the Philippines, and all other countries. (See Table 5.1.) Highly educated workers with specialty skills from China and India had been so heavily recruited that wait times ranged from one to three years. All other workers can wait from three to five

years. Anderson and Miller note that a worker being sponsored by a U.S. employer goes into a state of limbo while waiting for a green card. With no knowledge of when the card will arrive, the worker cannot make firm plans, secure housing, or travel freely; in most cases the worker cannot even change jobs in his or her home country.

According to the Asian Pacific American Legal Center of Southern California (APALC), the wait time for families to immigrate together is excessive and forces them apart for years. In *A Devastating Wait: Family Unity and the Immigration Backlogs* (2008, http://www.apalc.org/pdffiles/ Immigration%20v14.pdf), the APALC estimates that 4 million to 5 million spouses, children, and siblings of U.S. citizens and green card residents wait in enormous backlogs for visas that will reunite them with their loved ones. A backlog of visas—experienced in many immigration categories, but especially for family members—currently separates immigrants from spouses and their young children for over five years and separates elderly parents, adult children, and siblings for as many as 23 years. (See Table 5.2.)

Because of the long waits, all kinds of difficult scenarios arise. Senior citizens may learn to their despair that a spouse's recent death invalidated immigration applications for their children, forcing them to reapply and wait an additional 8 to 15 years. Family members receive their visas after many years in the backlog, only to learn that their children can no longer immigrate with them because they recently turned 21 years old and must now apply separately as adults.

The United States also issues nonimmigrant visas for foreign nationals to transact business or travel as tourists in the United States. The wait times for nonimmigrant visas differ depending on where in the world someone applies at an American consular post. For example, in Beijing, China, visas to visit the United States are processed in 39 days and student visas take 22 days. (See Table 5.3.) In Hanoi, Vietnam, these same visas take only one day.

TABLE 5.1

Wait time for employment-based immigrants to have visa application processed, February 2009

	China	India	Mexico	Phillipines	All other countries
1st preference: Priority workers	Available immediately to qualified applicants	Available immediately to qualified applicants	Available immediately to qualified applicants	Available immediately to qualified applicants	Available immediately to qualified applicants
2nd preference: Advanced degree holders and persons of exceptional ability	Processing applications received before January 2005	Processing applications received before January 2004	Available immediately to qualified applicants	Available immediately to qualified applicants	Available immediately to qualified applicants
3rd preference: Skilled workers and professionals	Processing applications received before October 2002	Processing applications received before October 2001	Processing applications received before April 2003	Processing applications received before May 2005	Processing applications received before May 2005
Other workers	Processing applications received before October 2002	Processing applications received before October 2001	Processing applications received before October 2001	Processing applications received before March 2003	Processing applications received before March 2003

SOURCE: Adapted from "A. Employment-Based Preferences," in *Visa Bulletin for February 2009*, vol. 5, no. IX, U.S. Department of State, Bureau of Consular Affairs, January 9, 2009, http://travel.state.gov/visa/frvi/bulletin/bulletin_4417.html# (accessed January 15, 2009)

TABLE 5.2

Wait time for family-sponsored immigrants to have visa application processed, February 2009

	China	India	Mexico	Philippines	All other countries
1st preference: Unmarried adult children of U.S. citizens	6 year wait	6 year wait	17 year wait	16 year wait	6 year wait
2nd preference A: Spouses and minor children of permanent residents	5 year wait	5 year wait	8 year wait	5 year wait	5 year wait
2nd preference B: Unmarried adult children of permanent residents	9 year wait	9 year wait	17 year wait	12 year wait	9 year wait
3rd preference: Married adult children of U.S.citizens	9 year wait	9 year wait	17 year wait	18 year wait	9 year wait
4th preference: Siblings of U.S.citizens	12 year wait	11 year wait	14 year wait	23 year wait	11 year wait

SOURCE: Adapted from "A. Family-Sponsored Preferences," in *Visa Bulletin for February 2009*, vol. 5, no. IX, U.S. Department of State, Bureau of Consular Affairs, January 9, 2009, http://travel.state.gov/visa/frvi/bulletin/bulletin_4417.html# (accessed January 15, 2009)

TABLE 5.3

Wait times for visa interviews at key consular posts, January 2009

[In work days]

Consular post	Visitor Visa	Student and exchange visitors (excluding A,G,K, and V class)	All other non-immigrant visas
Beijing	39	22	39
Bogota	16	1	16
Frankfurt	15	15	11
Hanoi	1	1	1
Manila	15	3	15
Mexico City	1	1	1
Mumbai (Bombay)	14	14	14
Tel Aviv	2	Same day	Same day
Tokyo	3	3	3

SOURCE: Adapted from "Visa Wait Times," U.S. Department of State, Bureau of Consular Affairs, January 2009, http://www.travel.state.gov/visa/temp/wait/tempvisitors_wait.php (accessed January 15, 2009)

Cost of a U.S. Visa

Foreign visitors or immigrants who want to travel to the United States pay a variety of fees to obtain their visas. Fees for visa services are collected by the State Department's Bureau of Consular Affairs. Fees for services related to immigration status are collected by the U.S. Citizenship and Immigration Services (USCIS).

TEMPORARY NONIMMIGRANT VISA SERVICES. Visas are classified by the type of nonimmigrant visitor. A foreign government official has an A visa, and a student has an F visa. (See Table 5.4.) The State Department charges visa issuance fees based on reciprocity (what another country charges a U.S. citizen for a similar type of visa). For example, most countries welcome tourists and the money they spend, so they charge them no visa fees. Most U.S. B visas (temporary visitors for business or pleasure) have no fee. Yemen is one of the few countries that charges a visa fee to U.S. business or pleasure visitors, including travelers and airline crewmembers passing through on the way to another country. Thus, the State Department charges reciprocal visa fees of $30 for these classifications of people from Yemen to enter the United States. The State Department's Visa Reciprocity Tables (January 16, 2009, http://travel.state.gov/visa/reciprocity/index.htm) identify reciprocal visa fees and special requirements by country.

TABLE 5.4

U.S. nonimmigrant visa classifications

Category	Description
A	Foreign government officials
B	Temporary visitors for business or pleasure
C	Aliens in transit (airplane passenger passing through to another country)
D	Crew members (airplanes, ships)
E	Treaty traders and treaty investors
F	Academic students
G	Foreign government officials to international organizations
H	Temporary workers
I	Foreign media representatives
J	Exchange visitors
K	Fiance of a U.S. citizen
L	Intracompany transferee
M	Vocational and language students
N	Parent or child of certain "special immigrants"
NAFTA	North American Free Trade Agreement representatives
NATO	North Atlantic Treaty Organization representatives
O	Workers with extraordinary ability
P	Athletes and entertainers
Q	International cultural exchange visitors
R	Religious workers
S	Witness or informant of criminal organization or terrorism
T	Victims of severe forms of trafficking in persons
U	Victims of certain crimes
V	Nonimmigrant spouse of child of a U.S. permanent resident
TPS	Temporary protected status

SOURCE: Adapted from "Immigration Classification and Visa Categories," U.S. Citizenship and Immigration Services, http://www.uscis.gov/portal/site/uscis/menuitem.5af9bb95919f35e66f614176543f6d1a/?vgnextoid=e6c08875d714d010VgnVCM10000048f3d6a1RCRD (accessed January 15, 2009)

In "Fees for Visa Services" (January 16, 2009, http://travel.state.gov/visa/temp/types/types_1263.html), the State Department discusses the charges and other fees for processing visas and related documents. Examples of common fees are:

- Nonimmigrant visa application processing fee, Form DS-156 (nonrefundable): $131.00

- Border crossing card—10-year (aged 15 and over) nonrefundable: $131.00

- Border crossing card—for Mexican citizen (under age 15) if parent or guardian has or is applying for a border crossing card (nonrefundable): $13

WHO IS AN ILLEGAL ALIEN?

An illegal alien is a person who is not a U.S. citizen and who is in the United States in violation of U.S. immigration laws. Illegal aliens are also known as immigrants, migrants, or workers who are unauthorized, undocumented, or paperless. Some people mistakenly assume that the term *illegal alien* refers specifically to Mexicans who have crossed the U.S.-Mexican border without authorization. Even though Mexicans account for a large share of the unauthorized entrants to the United States, illegal aliens can come from anywhere in the world.

An illegal alien could be one of the following:

- An undocumented alien who entered the United States without a visa, often between land ports of entry

- A person who entered the United States using fraudulent documentation

- A person who entered the United States legally with a temporary visa and then stayed beyond the time allowed (often called a nonimmigrant overstay or a visa overstay)

- A legal permanent resident who committed a crime after entry, became subject to an order of deportation, but failed to depart

Survey of Hispanics on Immigration Situation

In the United States Hispanics are often presumed to be immigrants and subject to a certain degree of harassment. The Pew Hispanic Center conducted a nationwide survey of 2,015 Hispanic adults in 2008, and the results were published by Mark Hugo Lopez and Susan Minushkin in *Hispanics See Their Situation in U.S. Deteriorating; Oppose Key Immigration Enforcement Measures* (September 18, 2008, http://pewhispanic.org/files/reports/93.pdf). Lopez and Minushkin state that in 2008, 50% of all Latinos said the situation of Latinos in the United States was worse than it had been the previous year. One out of 10 Hispanic adults (8% of the native-born U.S. citizens and 10% of the immigrants) reported having been stopped by the police or other authorities and asked about their immigration status in the previous 12 months.

According to Lopez and Minushkin, the situation is causing Hispanics to feel pessimistic at a time when the economy is slowing and there is greater enforcement of immigration laws by the United States. In 2007 and 2008 Pew asked the same question: "Compared to one year ago, do you think that the situation of Hispanics in this country is better, worse or about the same?" Foreign-born Hispanics thought the environment became much worse. Their assessment went from 42% worse in 2007 to 63% worse in 2008. (See Figure 5.1.) All Hispanics thought the situation in the United States became much worse in 2008 (50%) than in 2007 (33%).

ESTIMATES OF THE ILLEGAL ALIEN POPULATION

Because illegal aliens do not readily identify themselves out of fear of deportation, it is almost impossible to determine how many illegal aliens are in the United States. Various sources estimate between 10 million and 20 million, but these estimates are little more than educated guesses. They are politically influenced and have wide variance among the estimates. This is an indication of their unreliability. The number of illegal aliens varies somewhat between the winter and summer months based on the number of people in agricultural work.

FIGURE 5.1

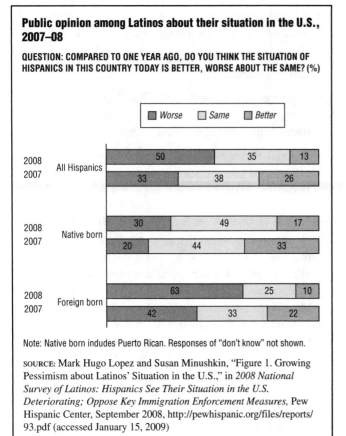

Public opinion among Latinos about their situation in the U.S., 2007–08

QUESTION: COMPARED TO ONE YEAR AGO, DO YOU THINK THE SITUATION OF HISPANICS IN THIS COUNTRY TODAY IS BETTER, WORSE ABOUT THE SAME? (%)

■ Worse   □ Same   ■ Better

	Worse	Same	Better
2008 All Hispanics	50	35	13
2007 All Hispanics	33	38	26
2008 Native born	30	49	17
2007 Native born	20	44	33
2008 Foreign born	63	25	10
2007 Foreign born	42	33	22

Note: Native born includes Puerto Rican. Responses of "don't know" not shown.

SOURCE: Mark Hugo Lopez and Susan Minushkin, "Figure 1. Growing Pessimism about Latinos' Situation in the U.S.," in *2008 National Survey of Latinos: Hispanics See Their Situation in the U.S. Deteriorating; Oppose Key Immigration Enforcement Measures,* Pew Hispanic Center, September 2008, http://pewhispanic.org/files/reports/93.pdf (accessed January 15, 2009)

Immigrants Returning to Native Countries

With the economic downturn in the United States in 2008, many immigrants were returning to their native lands. Miriam Jordan reports in "Latest Immigration Wave: Retreat" (*Wall Street Journal,* October 2, 2008) that after years of growth, illegal immigration to the United States from Mexico and Central America had slowed sharply. At the same time, say demographers and immigrant advocates, more Latin American immigrants were apparently returning home.

In *Trends in Unauthorized Immigration: Undocumented Inflow Now Trails Legal Inflow* (October 2, 2008, http://pewhispanic.org/files/reports/94.pdf), Jeffrey S. Passel and D'Vera Cohn of the Pew Hispanic Center estimate that there were 11.9 million unauthorized immigrants living in the United States in March 2008. (See Figure 5.2.) The size of the unauthorized population appeared to have declined since 2007. Passel and Cohn estimate that from 2000 to 2004 inflows of unauthorized immigrants averaged 800,000 per year; from 2005 to 2008 the inflows dropped to 500,000 per year, with a decreasing year-to-year trend. As the global economic crisis continued to deepen in the United States, the number of illegal immigrants declined for the first time in 2008, a trend that is expected to continue. Of the illegal immigrants in the United States, 59% were born in Mexico, with another 22% born in other Latin American nations. (See Figure 5.3.)

In the fact sheet "Modes of Entry for the Unauthorized Migrant Population" (May 22, 2006, http://pewhispanic.org/files/factsheets/19.pdf), the Pew Hispanic Center estimates that half of all illegal aliens living in the United States originally entered the country legally through a port of entry such as an airport or border crossing point. They came on visas or border crossing cards (good for frequent short visits and commuting back and forth to work) and simply did not leave. According to Passel and Cohn, from 2005 to 2008 about 1.6 million new undocumented immigrants arrived (see Table 5.5), compared with 2.1 million legal permanent residents.

Steven A. Camarota and Karen Jensenius of the Center for Immigration Studies (CIS) indicate in *Homeward Bound: Recent Immigration Enforcement and the Decline in the Illegal Alien Population* (July 2008, http://www.cis.org/trends_and_enforcement) that as the flow of all other adult immigrants started to taper off in May 2008, the number of less educated Hispanic immigrants (aged 18 to 40) dropped 11%, a dramatic decrease from August 2007. (See Figure 5.4.) This group includes Spanish-speaking farm workers, construction laborers, and restaurant helpers who are usually the first to get laid off when the economy slows down. Camarota and Jensenius's report of the drop in Hispanic immigrants in the United States came before the federal government reported a significant jump in unemployment rates late in 2008 and early 2009.

In "Is Illegal Tide of Immigrants Finally Easing?" (*Investor's Business Daily,* January 16, 2009), Michael Barone cites U.S. Census Bureau estimates that in the 2007–08 period net immigration was 14% lower than the average for the 2000–07 period. He notes that these figures do not cover the period after June 30, 2008, when the effects of the recession became more pronounced. Barone explains that "people move . . . in pursuit of dreams—or to escape nightmares. One of those dreams—home ownership in America—now seems much less attainable than it did just six months ago, with thousands of foreclosures and with subprime loans to low-income buyers presumably a thing of the past." He predicts the economy will continue to drive the decline in immigration.

Immigrant Children in the United States Alone

Amy Thompson of the Center for Public Policy Priorities notes in *A Child Alone and without Papers* (September 2008, http://www.cppp.org/repatriation/A%20Child%20Alone%20and%20Without%20Papers.pdf) that every year the United States apprehends some 43,000 unaccompanied and undocumented children under the age of 18. Many of the children (most from Mexico and Honduras) arrive without a parent or legal guardian. Many of these children enter the United States to overcome poverty. Others come to flee violence or the sex trade. Most of these children who come into custody are removed from the United States by federal authorities and repatriated to their country of origin. In

FIGURE 5.2

Estimates of the U.S. unauthorized immigrant population, 2000–08

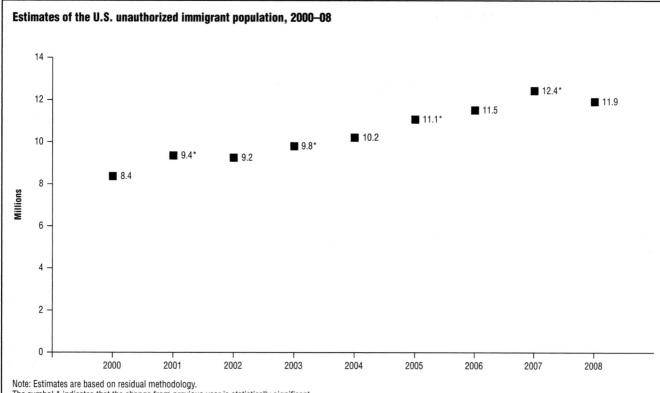

Note: Estimates are based on residual methodology.
The symbol * indicates that the change from previous year is statistically significant

SOURCE: Jeffrey S. Passel and D'Vera Cohn, "Figure 1. Estimates of the U.S. Unauthorized Immigrant Population, 2000–2008," in *Trends in Unauthorized Immigration: Undocumented Inflow Now Trail Legal Inflow,* Pew Hispanic Center, October 2, 2008, http://pewhispanic.org/files/reports/94.pdf (accessed January 15, 2009)

FIGURE 5.3

Estimated U.S. unauthorized immigrant population, by region and country of birth, 2008

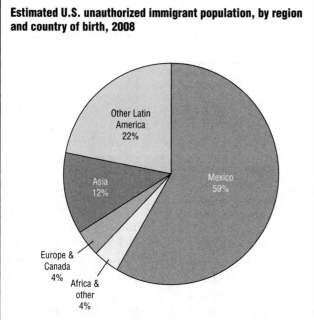

Note: Estimates are based on residual methodology.

SOURCE: Jeffrey S. Passel and D'Vera Cohn, "Figure 2. Estimated U.S. Unauthorized Immigrant Population by Region and Country of Birth, 2008," in *Trends in Unauthorized Immigration: Undocumented Inflow Now Trails Legal Inflow,* Pew Hispanic Center, October 2, 2008, http:// pewhispanic.org/files/reports/94.pdf (accessed January 15, 2009)

TABLE 5.5

Estimates of the U.S. unauthorized immigrant population, by period of arrival, 1980–March 2008

[Millions]

Period	Number	Percent
Total	**11.9**	**100%**
2005–2008	1.6	13%
2000–2004	3.7	31%
1995–1999	3.1	26%
1990–1994	2.0	16%
1980–1989	1.6	13%

Note: Estimates are based on residual methodology.
Numbers rounded independently and may not add to total shown. Estimates represent persons in the U.S. in unauthorized status as of March 2008. They do not represent the status at entry or the magnitude of unauthorized immigration during the period.

SOURCE: Jeffrey S. Passel and D'Vera Cohn, "Table 2. Estimates of the U.S. Unauthorized Immigrant Population by Period of Arrival, March 2008," in *Trends in Unauthorized Immigration: Undocumented Inflow Now Trails Legal Inflow,* Pew Hispanic Center, October 2, 2008, http://pewhispanic.org/ files/reports/94.pdf (accessed January 15, 2009)

2007, 35,546 Mexican children were returned to Mexico. (See Table 5.6.)

FEDERAL RESPONSE TO ILLEGAL ALIENS

Spencer S. Hsu reports in "Immigration Raid Jars a Small Town" (*Washington Post*, May 18, 2008) that on

FIGURE 5.4

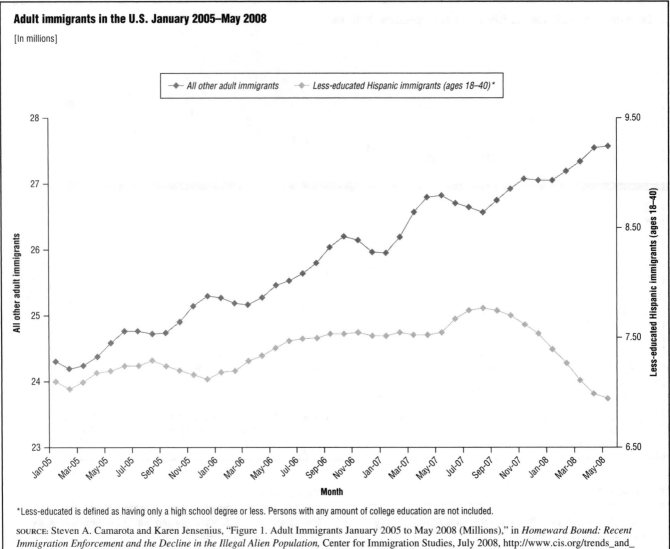

Adult immigrants in the U.S. January 2005–May 2008

[In millions]

◆ *All other adult immigrants*   ◆ *Less-educated Hispanic immigrants (ages 18–40)* *

*Less-educated is defined as having only a high school degree or less. Persons with any amount of college education are not included.

SOURCE: Steven A. Camarota and Karen Jensenius, "Figure 1. Adult Immigrants January 2005 to May 2008 (Millions)," in *Homeward Bound: Recent Immigration Enforcement and the Decline in the Illegal Alien Population,* Center for Immigration Studies, July 2008, http://www.cis.org/trends_and_enforcement (accessed January 15, 2009)

TABLE 5.6

Repatriated Mexican migrants under age 18, 2007

Delegation	Location of origin			Total
	Local	State	Interior Mexico	
Coahuila	270	137	891	1,298
Tamaulipas	748	329	2,915	3,992
Sonora	717	739	10,283	11,739
Chihuahua	1,139	742	4,224	6,105
Baja California	804	161	11,447	12,105
Total	**3,678**	**2,108**	**29,760**	**35,546**
Percent	**10.1**	**5.9**	**84.0**	**100**

Note: Above numbers refer to events where minors maybe repatriated more than one time a year.

SOURCE: Amy Thompson, "Repatriation of Minor Mexican Migrants Based on Residential Status January–December 2007," in *A Child Alone and without Papers: Appendix A—2007 INM Data on Unaccompanied Children,* Center for Public Policy Priorities, November 13, 2008, http://www.cppp.org/repatriation/Appendix%20A.pdf (accessed January 15, 2009). Data from the National Institute of Migration, Mexico.

May 12, 2008, U.S. Immigration and Customs Enforcement (ICE) agents descended on Agriprocessors Inc., a kosher meat processing facility in Postville, Iowa. ICE agents carried out federal search warrants on the Agriprocessors site and arrested 389 workers. Hsu states that "according to an affidavit filed by an ICE agent in conjunction with this week's arrests, 76 of the 968 employees on the company's payroll over the last three months of 2007 used false or suspect Social Security numbers. The affidavit cited unnamed sources who alleged that some company supervisors employed 15-year-olds, helped cash checks for workers with fake documents, and pressured workers without documents to purchase vehicles and register them in other names." Eventually, nearly 300 pleaded guilty.

In September 2008 the Iowa attorney general's office charged the owners of Agriprocessors and their human resources division with over 9,000 misdemeanor violations of Iowa's child labor laws. Simultaneously, the federal gov-

TABLE 5.7

Poverty and near poverty among illegal aliens, 2007

	Poverty				In or near poverty[a]			
	Illegal aliens only		Illegal aliens plus U.S.-born children under 18[b]		Illegal aliens only		Illegal aliens plus U.S.-born children under 18[b]	
	Percent	Number	Percent	Number	Percent	Number	Percent	Number
Colorado	35%	59	35%	82	69%	117	75%	178
Texas	30%	507	32%	755	65%	1,105	68%	1,580
Florida	23%	235	25%	311	54%	546	57%	723
California	21%	586	23%	867	58%	1,644	62%	2,323
Arizona	21%	119	24%	196	69%	401	73%	604
North Carolina	20%	74	23%	105	50%	179	54%	246
New York	18%	102	19%	130	50%	278	54%	359
New Jersey	18%	75	19%	97	41%	175	43%	220
Maryland	15%	39	17%	52	38%	102	40%	124
Washington	14%	38	17%	59	40%	111	45%	157
Georgia	13%	63	14%	91	43%	213	48%	299
Virginia	12%	32	14%	44	43%	111	44%	141
Nevada	12%	19	14%	31	47%	75	50%	109
Massachusetts	11%	23	13%	33	37%	82	42%	109
Illinois	10%	46	11%	70	43%	209	51%	321
Nation	**21%**	**2,380**	**23%**	**3,434**	**55%**	**6,213**	**59%**	**8,677**

Note: Estimates are only for those who responded to the survey.
[a]In or near-poverty defined as income under 200% of the poverty threshold.
[b]Includes U.S.-born children of illegal aliens.

SOURCE: Steven A. Camarota, "Table 24. Poverty and Near Poverty among Illegal Aliens," in *Immigrants in the United States, 2007: A Profile of America's Foreign-born Population,* Center for Immigration Studies, November 2007, http://www.cis.org/articles/2007/back1007.pdf (accessed January 15, 2009)

ernment filed charges against two human resources managers for harboring illegal aliens.

Postville was not the only big immigration raid in 2008. A high-profile workplace seizure of illegal immigrants took place in May 2008 at Pilgrim's Pride chicken plants in five states where ICE agents detained more than 300 individuals. In August 2008 ICE conducted its biggest raid, when it detained 600 illegals at Howard Industries in Laurel, Mississippi.

STATE RESPONSES TO ILLEGAL IMMIGRANTS

Steven A. Camarota of the CIS states in *Immigrants in the United States, 2007: A Profile of America's Foreign-Born Population* (November 2007, http://www.cis.org/articles/2007/back1007.pdf) that:

> [I]mmigrants and their young children (under 18) now account for one-fifth of the school-age population, one-fourth of those in poverty, and nearly one-third of those without health insurance, creating enormous challenges for the nation's schools, healthcare system, and physical infrastructure. The low educational attainment of many immigrants, 31 percent of whom have not completed high school, is the primary reason so many live in poverty, use welfare programs, or lack health insurance, not their legal status or an unwillingness to work.

Illegals use social welfare programs even though they do not collect many cash benefits. They use food assistance programs (e.g., food stamps and free lunch) and Medicaid but seldom apply for cash programs. Camarota explains that a large percentage of illegals hold jobs but their employment is in positions that pay low wages because of their educational level. Only 24% of them have completed high school, and 19% have an education beyond high school. Camarota estimates that in 2007 there were 8.7 million illegals living at or near the poverty level in the United States, including children under the age of 18. (See Table 5.7.)

Regional Response to Southwest Border Issues

The US/Mexico Border Counties Coalition commissioned the Institute for Policy and Economic Development to examine the economic condition of the 24 U.S. counties that are contiguous with Mexico. (See Figure 5.5.) The resulting report was published by Dennis L. Soden et al. in *At the Cross Roads: US/Mexico Border Counties in Transition* (March 2006, http://www.bordercounties.org/index.asp?Type=B_BASIC&SEC={62E35327-57C7-4978-A39A-36A8E00387B6}). Soden et al. address the question: "If the 24 southwest border counties were a 51st state, how would they compare to the other 50 states?"

Between 1990 and 2004 the 24 U.S. border counties collectively experienced a 29.3% growth rate. By 2006 there were 6.7 million residents. The border counties were home to 5% of the foreign-born residents of the United States; nearly 72% of the foreign-born living in the border counties were from Mexico.

Soden et al. point out that the immigrants living in this region have an enormous impact on the United States: If the 24 border counties comprised the 51st state, then that state would rank 2nd in percentage of population under age 18, 2nd in unemployment, 4th in military employment, 12th in

FIGURE 5.5

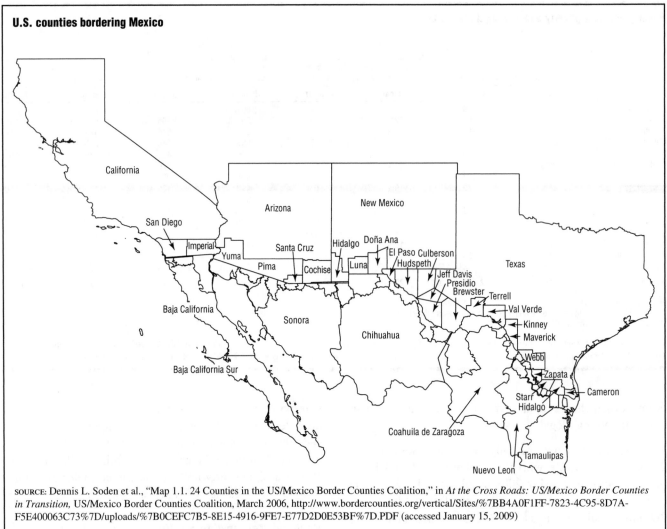

U.S. counties bordering Mexico

SOURCE: Dennis L. Soden et al., "Map 1.1. 24 Counties in the US/Mexico Border Counties Coalition," in *At the Cross Roads: US/Mexico Border Counties in Transition,* US/Mexico Border Counties Coalition, March 2006, http://www.bordercounties.org/vertical/Sites/%7BB4A0F1FF-7823-4C95-8D7A-F5E400063C73%7D/uploads/%7B0CEFC7B5-8E15-4916-9FE7-E77D2D0E53BF%7D.PDF (accessed January 15, 2009)

incidence of the acquired immunodeficiency syndrome (AIDS), 13th in population, 16th in violent crime, and 29th in total federal government expenditures. (See Table 5.8.) Given these statistics, Soden et al. suggest that the 24 U.S. border counties be treated collectively as the 51st state.

Many of the immigrants living in this region as well as in other parts of the country are here illegally. According to Camarota, in 2007 there were an estimated 11.3 million illegal immigrants in the United States. (See Table 5.9.) These illegals made up 30% of the share of the foreign born. Some states had a high proportion of illegals among the foreign born (Arizona at 65%), whereas other states had a lower proportion (New York at 13%).

Even with the large number of illegals, the Congressional Budget Office (CBO) estimates in *The Impact of Unauthorized Immigrants on the Budgets of State and Local Governments* (December 2007, http://www.cbo.gov/ftpdocs/87xx/doc8711/12-6-immigration.pdf) that the amount that state and local governments spend on services for unauthorized immigrants represents a small percentage of the total amount spent by these governments to provide such services

to residents in their jurisdictions. The CBO indicates that spending for unauthorized immigrants accounts for less than 5% of the total state and local spending for these services.

States Less Hospitable toward Illegals

Not every American sees illegals as a small burden on American society. In 2007 Arizona passed one of the toughest immigration laws in the country. As noted earlier, Camarota estimates that 65% of all foreign-born residents of the state were illegal. (See Table 5.9.) Arizona also has the highest percentage (12%) of undocumented workers as a share of the workforce of all states, more than double the national average. Then-Governor Janet Napolitano (1957–) signed into law the Legal Arizona Workers Act (LAWA) of 2007, which became effective on January 1, 2008. LAWA provides for the suspension and revocation of the business licenses of Arizona employers who knowingly employ illegal immigrants. It also requires employers to verify the work status of newly hired workers through E-Verify (http://www.dhs.gov/xprevprot/programs/gc_1185221678150.shtm), the federal employment verification program.

TABLE 5.8

If the 24 U.S. counties bordering Mexico were the 51st state, how would they compare to the rest of the nation?

1st in federal crimes, primarily due to drug and immigration arrests by federal agencies
2nd in incidence of tuberculosis
2nd in percentage of population under age 18
2nd in unemployment (5th with San Diego County included)
3rd in deaths due to hepatitis
3rd in concentration of Hispanics
4th in military employment
5th in diabetes-related deaths
7th in incidence of adult diabetes
10th in employment of federal civilians
12th in government and government enterprise employment
12th in incidence of AIDS
13th in population
16th in violent crime
22nd in allocation of federal highway planning and construction expenditures
22nd in home ownership
29th in receipt of total federal government expenditures
37th in low birth weight babies
39th in infant mortality
42nd in percent of teen pregnancy
45th in home affordability (37th with San Diego County included)
46th in percentage of adults with four-year college degree (27th with San Diego County included)
50th in insurance coverage for adults and children
51st in percent of population that has completed high school (50th with San Diego)
51st in per capita income (40th with San Diego County included)
51st in number of health care professionals

Note: San Diego County is a major metropolitan area and an anomaly to the other 23 border counties in many respects.

SOURCE: Adapted from Dennis L. Soden, "One Page Report Highlights," in *At the Cross Roads: US/Mexico Border Counties in Transition*, US/Mexico Border Counties Coalition, March 2006, http://www.bordercounties.org/vertical/Sites/%7BB4A0F1FF-7823-4C95-8D7A-F5E400063C73%7D/uploads/%7B01CF6553-9553-4457-BA23-50B41E06536B%7D.PDF (accessed January 15, 2009)

In 2007 various business and civic associations and non-profit corporations filed two lawsuits challenging LAWA on the ground that it infringes on federal immigration powers. They also claimed that LAWA lacks adequate due process protection for Arizona employers.

One of the businesses that joined the lawsuits was MCL Industries, which owns 24 Burger King restaurants in Arizona that employ 600 employees. Each year MCL hires 900 new employees to maintain this workforce. Arizona law requires MCL to use E-Verify to validate the legal status of employees. If MCL knowingly employs two unauthorized aliens in a three-year period, it may lose its business license in Arizona.

Mitchell C. Laird, the president of MCL Industries, testified on behalf of the U.S. Chamber of Commerce before the House Subcommittee on Social Security of the Committee on Ways and Means on May 6, 2008 (http://waysand means.house.gov/media/pdf/110/larid.pdf). He said that Arizona's law was unfavorable legislation because it gave Arizona employers regulations that were unclear. Employers felt uneasy about their responsibilities and liabilities under the new Arizona law. He also testified that compliance was costly.

In *Immigration Enforcement: Weaknesses Hinder Employment Verification and Worksite Enforcement Efforts* (August 2005, http://www.gao.gov/new.items/d05813.pdf), the U.S. Government Accountability Office (GAO) indicated "that a mandatory dial-up version of the pilot program for all employers would cost the federal government, employers, and employees about $11.7 billion total per year, with employers bearing most of the costs." Laird estimated that up to 10% of all I-9 forms (documents that indicate each new employee, both citizen and noncitizen, is authorized to work in the United States) had errors in their initial submission to their administrative offices. In most cases, the store managers do not detect these errors that are made by employees while filling out their personal information. MCL received a higher than normal rejection response rate from E-Verify, which caused further administrative delay. If the employer made a mistake by rejecting a potential employee, this mistake could lead to discriminatory hiring practices and lawsuits.

Laird said that because E-Verify became mandatory in Arizona, applications at MCL Industries Burger King stores dropped. He said restaurant owners throughout Arizona experienced a shortage of employees. Laird told Congress that employers needed a single, federal workforce enforcement policy that was fast, accurate, and reliable under real-world working conditions and that did not create incentives for employers to treat applicants unequally based on their citizenship.

STATE LAWS DIRECTED AT ILLEGALS. According to the National Council of State Legislatures, in "2007 Enacted State Legislation Related to Immigrants and Immigration" (August 5, 2007, http://www.ncsl.org/programs/immig/2007 Immigration831.htm), the Oklahoma Taxpayer and Citizen Protection Act of 2007:

Restricts access to driver's licenses, ID cards and other licenses. It terminates several forms of public assistance and places tighter restrictions on higher education benefits and provides for exceptions with respect to emergency care, disaster assistance and certain immunizations. Requires state and local government's law enforcement to enforce federal immigration law (Memorandum of Understanding). The law makes it a felony to harbor, transport, conceal or shelter unauthorized immigrants and provides for fines. It creates a rebuttable presumption that unauthorized immigrants are a flight risk with respect to bond determinations. It requires the verification of employment eligibility using the electronic employment verifications system (EEVS) and provides for a discrimination cause of action for the discharge of a U.S. citizen while retaining an unauthorized immigrant on the payroll.

The Oklahoma statute (2007, http://webserver1.lsb.state.ok.us/2007-08SB/SB417_int.rtf) states:

Illegal immigration is causing economic hardship and lawlessness in this state, and that illegal immigration is encouraged when public agencies within this state

TABLE 5.9

Estimated number of illegal aliens in the U.S., 2007

[In thousands]

	Illegal-alien population	Illegals as a share of the foreign-born	Illegals as a share of total state population	Illegals as a share of workers	Number of illegals holding a job	Number of less-educated adult natives not holding a job (18 to 64) [a, b]	Number of native teens (15 to 17) not holding a job [b]
Arizona	579	65%	9%	12%	339	511	196
California	2,840	28%	8%	10%	1,733	1,846	1,323
L.A. County	997	27%	10%	14%	628	461	397
Colorado	170	39%	4%	4%	96	229	182
Florida	1,012	29%	6%	7%	634	1,162	539
Georgia	504	53%	5%	7%	320	787	320
Illinois	480	28%	4%	5%	288	804	403
Maryland	268	37%	5%	6%	177	362	210
Massachusetts	220	25%	3%	4%	134	338	221
Nevada	160	35%	6%	9%	110	161	90
New Jersey	429	23%	5%	6%	251	476	289
New York	552	13%	3%	4%	331	1,343	654
North Carolina	363	58%	4%	6%	245	793	314
Texas	1,702	50%	7%	9%	974	1,654	811
Virginia	259	30%	3%	4%	152	526	231
Washington	277	38%	4%	5%	172	410	217
Nation	**11,328**	**30%**	**4%**	**5%**	**6,850**	**22,344**	**10,104**

Note: Estimates are only for those who responded

[a]Less-educated is defined as either being a high school dropout or having a high school diploma with no additional schooling.

[b]Figures are for persons who are unemployed or not in the labor force. Those who are unemployed are not working, but are looking for work. Those not in the labor force are not working, nor are they looking for work.

SOURCE: Steven A. Camarota, "Table 21. Estimated Number of Illegal Aliens in the Current Population Survey (Thousands)," in *Immigrants in the United States, 2007: A Profile of America's Foreign-born Population,* Center for Immigration Studies, November 2007, http://www.cis.org/articles/2007/back1007.pdf (accessed January 15, 2009)

provide public benefits without verifying immigration status. This state further finds that illegal immigrants have been harbored and sheltered in this state, and encouraged and induced to reside in this state through the issuance of identification cards without verification of immigration status, and that these practices impede and obstruct federal immigration law, undermine the security of our borders, and impermissibly restrict the privileges and immunities of the citizens of Oklahoma. Therefore, the State of Oklahoma declares that it is a compelling public interest of this state to discourage illegal immigration by requiring all public agencies within this state to cooperate with federal immigration authorities.

In "Strict Immigration Law Rattles Okla. Businesses" (*USA Today,* January 10, 2008), Emily Bazar reports that the act forced many Hispanics to leave Oklahoma. As a result, restaurants and grocery stores reported fewer customers, and hotels and cotton gins lost workers. José Alfonso, the senior pastor at Iglesia Piedra Angular (Cornerstone Hispanic Church) in Tulsa, estimated his church had lost 15% of its 425-member congregation. The Greater Tulsa Hispanic Chamber of Commerce reported that based on reports of school enrollments, church attendance, and bus companies with service to Mexico, an estimated 15,000 to 25,000 illegal immigrants had left Tulsa County. Many of the immigrants moved to the adjacent states of Arkansas or Missouri.

IMMIGRANT RESPONSES TO GOVERNMENT RAIDS

In *Hispanics See Their Situation in U.S. Deteriorating,* Lopez and Minushkin note that in 2007, 81% of all Hispanics believed the federal government should be responsible for identifying undocumented or illegal immigrants rather than the local police. Concerning workplace raids, 20% supported them, whereas 76% did not support them. (See Figure 5.6.) Both foreign-born (84%) and native-born (64%) Hispanics disapproved of workplace raids.

Some immigrants who have been detained and interrogated because of these ICE raids have sued the federal government. For example, Bazar reports in "Citizens Sue after Detentions, Immigration Raids" (*USA Today,* June 25, 2008) that Nitin Dhopade, a naturalized U.S. citizen from India, was swept up in an ICE raid that resulted in the arrest of 138 suspected illegal immigrants at Micro Solutions Enterprises (MSE), where Dhopade worked as an accountant. Also swept up in the raid were other U.S. citizens and legal residents.

Bazar notes that Dhopade believed he was a victim of racial profiling by ICE. He claimed an ICE agent questioned him about his immigration status and his ability to speak English "because of my skin color. None of the white folks in the office...that I know of were asked for proof of citizenship. To be asked for proof of citizenship, in this

FIGURE 5.6

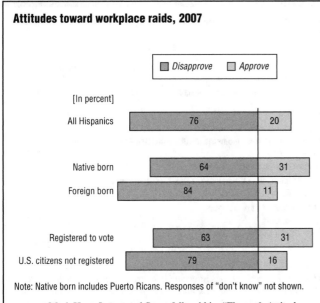

Attitudes toward workplace raids, 2007

Note: Native born includes Puerto Ricans. Responses of "don't know" not shown.

SOURCE: Mark Hugo Lopez and Susan Minushkin, "Figure 6. Attitudes toward Workplace Raids," in *2008 National Survey of Latinos: Hispanics See Their Situation in the U.S. Deteriorating; Oppose Key Immigration Enforcement Measures*, Pew Hispanic Center, September 2008, http://pewhispanic.org/files/reports/93.pdf (accessed January 15, 2009)

country, it's an insult. This is the United States of America. This country does not require that."

According to Bazar, in April 2008 the Center for Human Rights and Constitutional Law filed a lawsuit for damages on behalf of 114 MSE employees, all citizens or legal permanent residents. Alleging that they were subjected to "false imprisonment" and "detention without justification," they each sought $5,000 in damages from the federal government.

Bazar also reports the arrest of Jesus Garcia, who worked for a Pilgrim's Pride processing plant in Texas. ICE agents went to Garcia's home and said that Garcia, a green card holder, was using the wrong Social Security number. He was handcuffed and spent more than 30 hours in ICE custody along with two coworkers, both citizens. When he was released, ICE agents told him that he was not the person they wanted. Garcia said the mishap cost him three days of work. "I worked hard to get my residency. And to take me to jail just over a mistake?" Believing that he, too, was a victim of racial profiling, Garcia decided to sue the federal government.

Fear of Deportation

In "Illegal Immigrants Opted to Stay during Gustav" (Associated Press, September 2, 2008), Peter Prengaman explains that when the city was ordered to be evacuated shortly before Hurricane Gustav made landfall, most of its illegal immigrants chose to stay. Carlos Mendoza, a 21-year-old illegal immigrant from Honduras who stayed behind, said, "We know that people died during Katrina, but we had

no choice but to stay here. . . . Many stayed because of fear." Emergency officials offered to transport residents to safety and promised not to identify illegal immigrants. Regardless, the fear of being arrested or deported kept undocumented people from accepting the free ride. Immigrants' rights groups estimate the city has up to 30,000 illegal immigrants.

Damien Cave reports in "States Take New Tack on Illegal Immigration" (*New York Times*, June 9, 2008) that many Hispanic immigrants who helped rebuild towns in Florida after Hurricane Ivan in 2004 either left the state or went into hiding after enforcement officials started making immigration raids. Even low unemployment (3.6%) in 2007 in Gulf Coast counties from Pensacola to Tallahassee did not encourage illegals to come into the area because of the immigration raids.

Those who stayed in rural Florida saw a change in attitude. As the economy slowed in 2008, local officials increased arrests. Because only the federal government can prosecute someone for immigration violations, in rural Santa Rosa County, Sheriff Wendell Hall arrested illegal workers for identity theft offenses such as using stolen Social Security numbers. He detained 13 workers at Panhandle Growers and another group at Emerald Coast Interiors, a boat-cushion factory. Officers located many of the illegals cooking in local restaurants. In the months following the raids, Cave indicates that hundreds of Hispanic families (both legal and illegal) left the county.

MONITORING WHO COMES AND GOES

Then-Secretary of Homeland Security Michael Chertoff (1953–; http://www.dhs.gov/xnews/speeches/sp_122963252 9576.shtm), announced in a speech at Georgetown University on December 18, 2008, that 500 miles (805 km) of fence secure the southern perimeter along the U.S.-Mexican border. With improved technological security, the barrier includes both physical and electronic fencing, where monitoring is done by cameras. He said that through a program called US-VISIT the U.S. Border Patrol records the fingerprints of all non-American and non-Canadian visitors entering the United States and checks those prints in real time against terrorist and criminal watch lists while maintaining rigorous privacy protections. To prevent the use of fraudulent or stolen licenses, the U.S. Department of Homeland Security (DHS) does not accept driver's licenses as documentation for entrance into the United States.

Chertoff estimated that each day at airports, seaports, and border crossings the DHS screens more than 2 million air travelers, 300,000 cars, and 70,000 shipping containers. In addition, the department "work[s] with the private sector to secure thousands of pieces of critical infrastructure, whether they be bridges and dams or chemical plants and cyber systems." Chertoff was replaced as Homeland Security secretary by Janet Napolitano on January 21, 2009, after President Barack Obama (1961–) was sworn into office. In

April 2009 she named Alan Bersin, a former U.S. attorney, as "border czar." Bersin's duties include decreasing illegal border crossings as well as reducing border violence spurred by drug cartels in Mexico.

Nonimmigrant Overstays

Despite congressional initiatives to track foreign visitors after the 1993 World Trade Center bombing, and again after the September 11, 2001, terrorist attacks, by 2006 the United States was not able to determine whether temporary foreign visitors had actually left the country. Section 110 of the Illegal Immigration Reform and Immigrant Responsibility Act (IIRIRA) of 1996 mandated that the U.S. Immigration and Naturalization Service (INS) develop an automated system to track the entry and exit of all noncitizens entering or leaving all ports of entry, including land borders and seaports. The INS, the Canadian government, and the airline industry, among others, opposed Section 110. According to the INS, it lacked the resources to put in place such an integrated system. The Canadian government claimed that filling out the entry form (Form I-94) and having it checked by INS inspectors would cause large backups at the border. The airlines considered Section 110 an additional reporting burden.

US-VISIT—AN ELECTRONIC TRACKING SYSTEM. On June 15, 2000, Congress passed the Immigration and Naturalization Service Data Management Improvement Act to amend Section 110 of the IIRIRA. It required the implementation of an electronic system—U.S. Visitor and Immigrant Status Indicator Technology (US-VISIT)—using available data to identify lawfully admitted unauthorized immigrants who might have overstayed their visits. The proposed system would scan visitors' fingerprints and check them against databases of known terrorists and criminals. It would also scan passports and record entries and departures. Beginning on January 31, 2008, the United States ended the practice of accepting oral declarations of citizenship at the border.

The DHS notes in "Fact Sheet: DHS End-of-Year Accomplishments" (December 18, 2008, http://www.dhs .gov/xnews/releases/pr_1229609413187.shtm) that U.S. Customs and Border Protection (CBP) officers collect biometrics from foreign visitors applying for admission into the United States at 183 air- and seaports and at 168 land border ports of entry. They have the ability to collect 10 fingerprints from arriving foreign visitors, enabling the DHS to check visitors' full set of fingerprints against the Federal Bureau of Investigation's Criminal Master File and latent fingerprints collected from terrorist training camps, safe houses, and battlefields around the world.

US-VISIT EXIT SYSTEM. In *Homeland Security: U.S. Visitor and Immigrant Status Indicator Technology Program Planning and Execution Improvements Needed* (December 2008, http://www.gao.gov/new.items/d0996.pdf), the GAO reports that even though the DHS spent $475 million on US-

TABLE 5.10

Department of Homeland Security budget for identity management, fiscal year 2008

Core mission areas/projects	Fiscal year 2008 total (dollars in millions)
Provide identity management and screening services	
Biometric support	$7.9
Data integrity	6.4
Law enforcement and intelligence	1.5
Develop and enhance biometric identity collection and data sharing	
Unique Identity	228.0
Comprehensive biometric exit—air/sea	13.0
Provide information technology support to mission service	
Operations and maintenance	103.0
Enhance program management	
Mission support	109.2
Management reserve	6.0
Total	**$475.0**

SOURCE: "Summary of Fiscal Year 2008 Expenditure Plan Budget," in *Homeland Security: U.S. Visitor and Immigrant Status Indicator Technology Program Planning and Execution Improvements Needed*, U.S. Government Accountability Office, December 2008, http://www.gao.gov/new.items/d0996.pdf (accessed January 15, 2009)

VISIT in 2008, the system still did not work the way it was envisioned. (See Table 5.10.) The air and sea exit expenditures exceeded original cost estimates for various reasons. Commercial airlines and cruise ships bore most of the costs because they were forced to allow passengers to confirm arrival and check-in online before entering the airport or sea terminal, or to check in and print a boarding pass at a kiosk. The greatest challenge was in the time and efficiency of collecting fingerprints. The air carriers commented that the passenger-agent contact required under the US-VISIT regulations slowed down the travel process, created flight delays, and made air- and seaports crowded when travelers were rushed. The GAO notes that according to one carrier's estimates, the proposed US-VISIT regulations added one to two minutes of processing time per passenger, and collectively added an estimated three to five hours per international flight. The proposed air and sea exit solution, according to data provided by the DHS, afforded less security and privacy than other alternatives, because it relied on private carriers to collect, store, and transmit passenger data.

Visa Waiver Program

According to the press release "Vast Majority of Visa Waiver Countries Meet Security Upgrade to e-Passports" (October 26, 2006, http://www.dhs.gov/xnews/releases/pr _1161876358429.shtm), the DHS reports that each year approximately 15 million people travel to the United States without a visa to stay 90 days or less for business or pleasure. The State Department explains in "Visa Waiver Program (VWP)" (January 16, 2009, http://www.travel.state .gov/visa/temp/without/without_1990.html) that citizens of any of the 35 countries participating in the Visa Waiver Program (VWP) can enter the United States on a passport

TABLE 5.11

U.S. Coast Guard alien interdictions, by country of origin, fiscal years 1997–2008

FY	Haiti	Dominican Republic	Cuba	Peoples Republic of China	Mexico	Ecuador	Other	Total
Oct-09	84	240	76	0	0	0	19	419
2008	1,582	688	2,199	1	47	220	65	4,802
2007	1,610	1,469	2,868	73	26	125	167	6,338
2006	1,198	3,011	2,810	31	52	693	91	7,886
2005	1,850	3,612	2,712	32	55	1,149	45	9,455
2004	3,229	5,014	1,225	68	86	1,189	88	10,899
2003	2,013	1,748	1,555	15	0	703	34	6,068
2002	1,486	177	666	80	32	1,608	55	4,104
2001	1,391	659	777	53	17	1,020	31	3,948
2000	1,113	499	1,000	261	49	1,244	44	4,210
1999	1,039	583	1,619	1,092	171	298	24	4,826
1998	1,369	1,097	903	212	30	0	37	3,648
1997	288	1,200	421	240	0	0	45	2,194

SOURCE: Adapted from "USCG Migrant Interdictions," in *Alien Migrant Interdiction*, U.S. Coast Guard, October 15, 2008, http://www.uscg.mil/hq/cg5/cg531/AMIO/FlowStats/currentstats.asp (accessed January 15, 2009)

issued by their country of citizenship. Representatives of the foreign press, radio, film, or other information media cannot use the visa waiver when traveling for professional pursuits.

PASSPORT REQUIREMENTS. In the Enhanced Border Security and Visa Entry Reform Act of 2002, as amended, Congress mandated that machine-readable, biometric passports would be required for all VWP travelers by October 26, 2006. Children would no longer be able to travel on their parents' passports. This change required VWP countries to certify that they had programs in place to issue their citizens machine-readable passports that incorporated biometric identifiers and complied with standards established by the International Civil Aviation Organization.

The new passports are identified by an international e-Passport logo on the cover and contain a secure contactless chip with the passport holder's biographic information and a biometric identifier. Biometric data are measurable physical characteristics or personal behavioral traits used to recognize the identity or verify the claimed identity of an enrollee. Among the features that can be measured are face, fingerprints, hand geometry, handwriting, iris, retina, vein, and voice. The size of the passport and photograph, and the arrangement of data fields, especially the two lines of data, have to be exact to be read by an Optical Character Reader.

TRACKING SECURITY RISKS. The National Security Entry-Exit Registration System was launched in 2003 to track nonimmigrant visitors coming from designated countries and others who meet a combination of intelligence-based criteria that identify them as potential security risks. State Department offices in foreign countries identify such people when issuing visas. These individuals are required to register on arrival at a port of entry, participate in an interview with the Bureau of Citizenship and Immigration before being allowed into the country, and report any change of address, employment, or educational institution

while in the country. They are also required to register on departure and are restricted to using certain designated ports of entry/departure. This system focuses only on the preidentified security risk visitors.

BORDERS ON THE WATER

The U.S. Coast Guard (USCG) is responsible for preventing unauthorized people from entering the United States by water. The USCG reports in "USCG Migrant Interdictions" (October 15, 2008, http://www.uscg.mil/hq/cg5/cg531/AMIO/FlowStats/currentstats.asp) that it intercepted 4,802 illegal entry attempts in fiscal year (FY) 2008. (See Table 5.11.) Most aliens attempting to enter the country by water came from Central America and the Caribbean. The largest number of interdictions, 2,199, came from Cuba. The next highest number of interdictions were all from South and Central America, such as from Haiti (1,582), the Dominican Republic (688), and Ecuador (220).

In 1994 the United States made an informal agreement with Cuba. This U.S.-Cuba Immigration Accord (http://www.state.gov/www/regions/wha/cuba/fs_000828_migration_accord.html) focused on Cuban migrants seeking to enter the United States. In a related agreement (informally called "wet-foot, dry-foot"), Cuban migrants intercepted at sea by the USCG would be returned to Cuba. Migrants who presented a "well-founded fear of persecution" would be sent to another country for asylum. Cuba agreed not to persecute returning migrants. Cuban migrants who made it to U.S. soil would be allowed to stay. After one year they would be eligible to apply for legal residence.

Cuban migrants continue to attempt entry into the United States. The USCG (October 15, 2008, http://www.uscg.mil/hq/cg5/cg531/AMIO/FlowStats/currentstats.asp) notes that even though the total number of interdictions have declined since FY 2004, the number of Cuban interdictions jumped from 1,225 in FY 2004 to 2,712 in FY 2005 and peaked at 2,868 in FY 2007. Cubans represented 11% of total interdictions in 2004 and 45% in FY 2007 and FY 2008.

PATROLLING U.S. LAND BORDERS

The U.S. Border Patrol, the mobile, uniformed law enforcement arm of the CBP, is responsible for the detection and apprehension of illegal aliens and smugglers of aliens at or near U.S. land borders.

The Southwestern Border

The biggest illegal entry problems occur along the nearly 2,000-mile (3,219-km) U.S.-Mexican border. The CBP reports in "Border Wait Times" (2009, http://apps.cbp.gov/bwt/index.asp) that the four states bordering Mexico (Texas, New Mexico, Arizona, and California) have 39 land ports of entry. In *Health in the Americas 2007* (October 2007, http://www.paho.org/hia/homeing.html), the Pan American Health Organization estimates the population of the U.S.-Mexico border area to be 13 million, with more than 6.1 million residing on the Mexican side of the border.

The importance of protecting the U.S.-Mexican border was elevated in 2008 and 2009 when drug violence in Mexico surged. CNN reported ("Obama to Beef Up Mexico Border Policy, March 25, 2009, http://www.cnn.com/2009/POLITICS/03/24/obama.mexico.policy) that, in 2008, 6,500 Mexicans were killed by drug cartels, and the violence threatened to spill into U.S. soil. The Obama administration pledged to address the crisis: "The new federal plan, developed by the departments of Justice and Homeland Security, calls for doubling the number of border security task force teams and moving a significant number of other federal agents, equipment and resources to the border." Following this statement, U.S. Secretary of State Hillary Rodham Clinton (1947–) traveled to Mexico endorsing the stepped-up border protection policy.

In addition to the violence associated with the shared U.S.-Mexico border, hundreds of Americans have been kidnapped in conjunction with Mexican drug cartels or human trafficking of drugs. Furthermore, some illegal immigrants enter the country to grow drugs, such as marijuana, on federal lands, including some national parks. All of these factors have prompted many to call for increased border security.

Secure Fence Act of 2006

The United States began using barrier fencing during the 1990s to deter illegal entry and drug smuggling, particularly to prevent vehicle entry. In *Border Security: Barriers along the U.S. International Border* (May 13, 2008, http://www.fas.org/sgp/crs/homesec/RL33659.pdf), Blas Nuñez-Nito and Yule Kim of the Congressional Research Service note that the 14-mile (22.5-km) fence at San Diego, California, the nation's busiest border port of entry, was the first

to be constructed. It was strengthened by increased Border Patrol staffing. However, Nuñez-Nito and Kim indicate that increased enforcement in San Diego had "little impact on overall apprehensions" of illegal entrants, because the border barrier simply shifted illegal traffic to more remote areas. An unintended consequence of this shift in migration paths was an increase in migrant deaths in the desert.

According to Nuñez-Nito and Kim, the Border Patrol's San Diego sector extends about 66 miles (106.2 km) from the Pacific Ocean of the international border with Mexico and encompasses 7,000 square miles (18,130 square km) of territory. This sector is located north of Tecate and Tijuana, Mexico, and does not contain any natural barriers that deter unauthorized migrants and smugglers from passing through. The primary San Diego fence covers the first 14 miles (22.5 km), starting from the Pacific Ocean, and was constructed of 10-foot-high (3-m-high) welded steel. The operations here are labeled "Operation Gatekeeper" and employ a three-tiered fence system first conceived at Sandia Laboratory, in Albuquerque, New Mexico, to detect intruders early and delay them as long as possible. It channels border crossers to geographic locations such as Tucson and Yuma in Arizona, San Diego, and other sector stations. (See Figure 5.7.) The fence improved the apprehensions at these stations with 620,000 apprehensions in FY 2004, up from about 425,000 apprehensions in FY 2002.

In a further effort to close the porous southwestern border, President George W. Bush signed the Secure Fence Act of 2006, which authorized the construction of hundreds of miles of additional fencing along the U.S.-Mexican border and added more vehicle barriers, checkpoints, and lighting to help prevent people from entering the country illegally. Nuñez-Nito and Kim explain that the Secure Fence Act required the DHS to fence five additional stretches: the 20 miles (32.2 km) around Tecate; from Calexico, California, to Douglas, Arizona; from Columbus, New Mexico, to El Paso, Texas; from Del Rio, Texas, to Eagle Pass, Texas; and from Laredo, Texas, to Brownsville, Texas. The 370-mile (595.5-km) portion of the U.S.-Mexican border between Calexico and Douglas is a "priority area," and the act required the DHS to install an "interlocking surveillance camera system" by May 30, 2007.

To get the fence built, the U.S. attorney general and the secretary of homeland security waived the National Environmental Policy Act of 1969 and the Endangered Species Act of 1973, to the extent the attorney general determined necessary to ensure expeditious construction of the barriers authorized to be constructed. This resulted in many lawsuits from environmental protection groups that slowed down the actual construction of the fence.

The act also authorized the DHS to increase the use of advanced technology such as cameras, satellites, and unmanned aerial vehicles to reinforce infrastructure at the border. The DHS secretary was directed to conduct a study

FIGURE 5.7

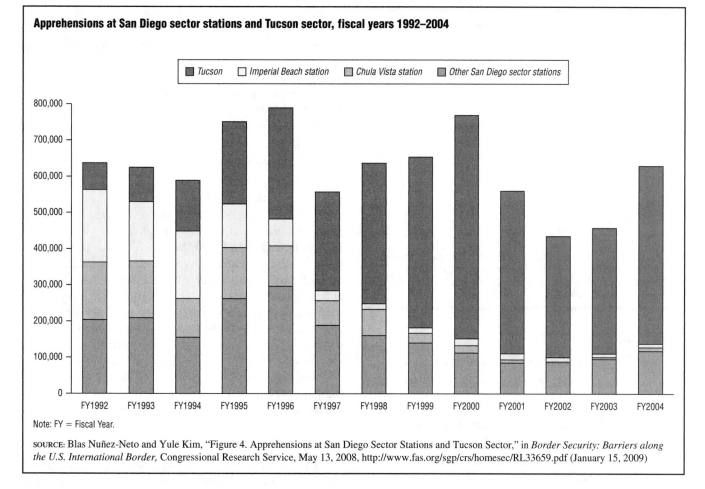

Apprehensions at San Diego sector stations and Tucson sector, fiscal years 1992–2004

Legend: ■ Tucson □ Imperial Beach station ▨ Chula Vista station ▨ Other San Diego sector stations

Note: FY = Fiscal Year.

SOURCE: Blas Nuñez-Neto and Yule Kim, "Figure 4. Apprehensions at San Diego Sector Stations and Tucson Sector," in *Border Security: Barriers along the U.S. International Border,* Congressional Research Service, May 13, 2008, http://www.fas.org/sgp/crs/homesec/RL33659.pdf (January 15, 2009)

on the construction of a state-of-the-art barrier system along the U.S.-Canadian border.

In December 2008 the CBP announced that border fence construction had surpassed the 500-mile (804.6-km) mark (December 2008, http://www.cbp.gov/xp/cgov/newsroom/news_releases/archives/2008_news_releases/december_2008/12192008.xml). The DHS indicates in "Southwest Border Fence" (December 30, 2008, http://www.dhs.gov/xprevprot/programs/border-fence-southwest.shtm) that as of December 19, 2008, 286 miles (460 km) of pedestrian border fence and 267 miles (430 km) of vehicle border fence, for a total of 553 miles (890 km) of fence, were completed. However, the American Border Patrol, an independent, nonprofit corporation based in Arizona, conducted its own border survey, and criticized the CBP's announcement as exaggerated. According to the American Border Patrol, the CBP's statistics included more than 240 miles (386 km) of vehicle barrier systems and 278 miles (447 km) of pedestrian fences that did not meet the legal mandate for 15-foot-high (4.5-meter), double-layered fencing outlined in the Secure Fence Act (http://www.americanborderpatrol.com/).

The ineffectiveness of the vehicle barriers was indicated by reports that traffickers penetrated U.S. border security by simply bringing a portable ramp to the vehicle barrier and driving over the top of the fence. In addition, Nuñez-Nito and Kim note that an "unintended consequence of the border fencing has been the proliferation of tunnels dug underneath the border." For example, the Border Patrol found one tunnel near San Diego that "was almost a kilometer long and was built from reinforced concrete—evidence of a rather sophisticated smuggling operation." The Border Patrol reports that fencing is most effective in urban areas, where populated neighborhoods are only a short distance away for border crossers.

The Northern Border

According to the International Boundary Commission, the U.S.-Canadian border is the longest undefended border in the world. Unlike the U.S.-Mexican border that is actively patrolled by CBP personnel to prevent illegal migration and drug trafficking, most of the U.S.-Canadian border is open. It crosses through mountainous terrain and heavily forested areas. (See Table 5.12.) Significant portions cross remote prairie farmland through Alaska, the Great Lakes, and the St. Lawrence River besides the maritime components of the boundary at the Atlantic, Pacific, and Arctic oceans.

TABLE 5.12

Length of U.S.-Canada land and water boundaries by state

[In descending order in miles]

State	Boundary length
Alaska	1,538
Michigan	721
Maine	611
Minnesota	547
Montana	545
New York	445
Washington	427
North Dakota	310
Ohio	146
Vermont	90
New Hampshire	58
Idaho	45
Pennsylvania	42
Total	**5,525**

SOURCE: Janice Cheryl Beaver, "Table 1. Length of U.S.-Canada Land and Water Boundary by State," in *U.S. International Borders: Brief Facts*, Congressional Research Service, November 9, 2006, http://www.fas.org/sgp/crs/misc/RS21729.pdf (accessed January 15, 2009)

The border also runs through the middle of the Akwesasne Nation and even divides some communities in Vermont and Quebec.

Despite its seemingly low-level threat to U.S. security—especially when compared with the U.S.-Mexico border—the U.S.-Canada border attracted attention at the turn of the 21st century and beyond with some incidents of concern. In late 1999 Ahmed Ressam, an al-Qaeda terrorist who became known as the Millennium Bomber, was captured upon his entry into the United States on a Canadian ferry near Seattle, Washington, with explosives he planned to use to bomb the Los Angeles airport on New Year's Eve of that year. In a later incident in 2006, according to Brian Todd for CNN.com ("Bust Shows Gaps in U.S.-Canada Border," April 13, 2006, http://edition.cnn.com/2006/WORLD/americas/04/12/human.smugglers/index.html), "fourteen U.S. and Canadian residents have been indicted by a U.S. grand jury on charges related to human smuggling." Todd explained: "As debate rages over securing the U.S. border with Mexico, authorities . . . had dismantled a human-smuggling ring that was running illegal immigrants into the United States through Canada. . . . The ring was responsible for importing dozens of Indian and Pakistani immigrants . . . . At least 50 illegal immigrants have been arrested."

IDENTIFICATION OF THOSE WHO ENTER

The Intelligence Reform and Terrorism Prevention Act of 2004 required the DHS and the State Department to implement a plan requiring all travelers, U.S. citizens, and foreign nationals to present a passport or other identity and citizenship documents when entering the United States. The proposed plan was called the Western Hemisphere Travel Initiative (WHTI; February 3, 2009, http://travel.state.gov/travel/cbpmc/cbpmc_2223.html). Beginning on January 23, 2007, all people, including U.S. citizens, traveling by air between the United States and Canada, Mexico, Central and South America, the Caribbean, and Bermuda were required to present a valid passport, Air NEXUS card, USCG Merchant Mariner Document, or an Alien Registration Card. On January 1, 2008, the requirements expanded to include arrivals by land or sea (including ferries).

The U.S. Passport Card

According to the State Department, in "U.S. Passport Card" (December 19, 2008, http://travel.state.gov/passport/ppt_card/ppt_card_3926.html), the production of the U.S. Passport Card began on July 14, 2008, and by December 2008 over 700,000 of them had been issued. It is a photo identification document that can be used to enter the United States from Canada, Mexico, the Caribbean, and Bermuda at land border crossings or sea ports of entry. It may not be used for air travel. It is valid for 10 years for adults and 5 years for minors (under the age of 16). The cost is $45 for adults and $35 for minors. Adults who already have a fully valid passport book may apply for the U.S. passport card by mail and pay only $20. The State Department explains that the passport card uses state-of-the-art security features to prevent against counterfeiting and forgery.

The NEXUS Card

The NEXUS card was established in 2002 as part of the U.S.-Canada Shared Border Accord. In "NEXUS Program Description" (January 12, 2009, http://www.cbp.gov/xp/cgov/travel/trusted_traveler/nexus_prog/nexus.xml), the CBP states that the NEXUS card allows pre-screened and approved travelers faster processing time with special NEXUS lanes at the border. There is a $50 fee for a NEXUS application, which must be approved by both the United States and Canada. The NEXUS card became acceptable for land and sea travel under WHTI effective June 1, 2009.

The Border Policy Research Institute and Western Washington University conducted a study that focused on the characteristics of cross-border travel in the Cascade Gateway (Washington state in the United States and Lower Mainland in British Columbia, Canada), and the results were published by Melissa Miller, Hugh Conroy, and David Davidson in *International Mobility and Trade Corridor (IMTC) Project Passenger Intercept Survey Final Report* (September 2008, http://resources.wcog.org/border/pis_2008finalreport.pdf). Miller, Conroy, and Davidson state that 87% of all cross-border trips by U.S. residents and 93% by Canadian residents were for non-work-related purposes. Recreation and vacation were the most frequent reasons for cross-border travel in both summer and winter. Shopping accounted for 17% of summer crossings and 27% of winter crossings (tied with recreation). (See Figure 5.8.)

FIGURE 5.8

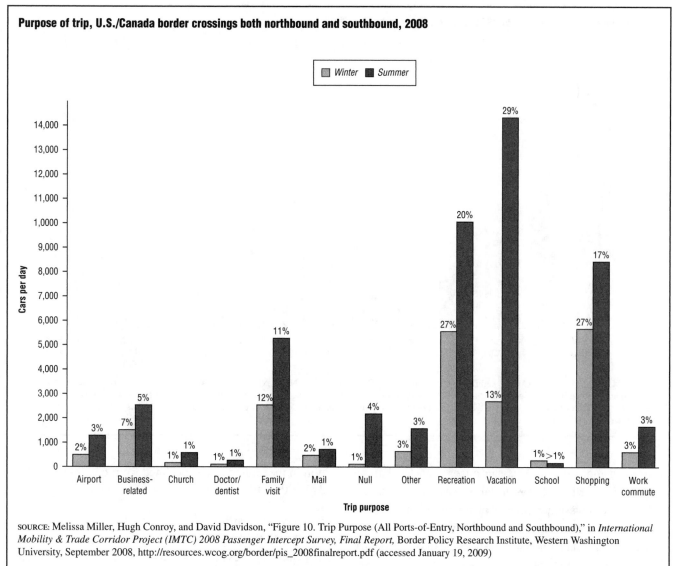

Purpose of trip, U.S./Canada border crossings both northbound and southbound, 2008

SOURCE: Melissa Miller, Hugh Conroy, and David Davidson, "Figure 10. Trip Purpose (All Ports-of-Entry, Northbound and Southbound)," in *International Mobility & Trade Corridor Project (IMTC) 2008 Passenger Intercept Survey, Final Report,* Border Policy Research Institute, Western Washington University, September 2008, http://resources.wcog.org/border/pis_2008finalreport.pdf (accessed January 19, 2009)

According to Miller, Conroy, and Davidson, 45% of all border-crossers crossed once per month, whereas 60% of NEXUS card holders crossed once per week or more. Surveyors asked drivers in the general lane why they were not enrolled in the NEXUS program so they could use the quicker NEXUS lane. One-third of respondents (33%) said they did not cross the border often enough to make the card worthwhile, and 24% were not familiar with the program. (See Figure 5.9.) Other reasons included the hassle of filing the application and the cost of the card.

American Attitudes toward New Regulations

According to a Zogby International poll (http://www.zogby.com/news/readnews.cfm?ID=1239) that was released on January 19, 2007, most Americans welcomed the passport rules. A 76% majority believed a valid passport should be required for all travelers entering the United States from Canada and Mexico. The new passport requirements made no difference in travel plans for 85% of Americans traveling to Canada and 86% traveling to Mexico.

MEXICO'S UNIQUE RELATIONSHIP WITH THE UNITED STATES

In no other place in the world does a nation as wealthy as the United States share a border with a nation as poor as Mexico. Huge disparities exist between the rich and poor people of Mexico, so it is understandable that Mexico's poor are attracted to the United States.

An Open Border

Before the 20th century, Mexicans moved easily back and forth across completely open borders to work in the mines, on the ranches, and on the railroad. Just 734 Mexicans immigrated between 1890 and 1899, but a decade later 31,188 came between 1900 and 1909. (See Table 1.1 in Chapter 1.) The flow of immigrants to the United States from Mexico rose to 185,334 between 1910 and 1919 and then increased to 498,945 between 1920 and 1929.

A large amount of illegal immigration also occurred. Some historians estimate that during the 1920s there might

FIGURE 5.9

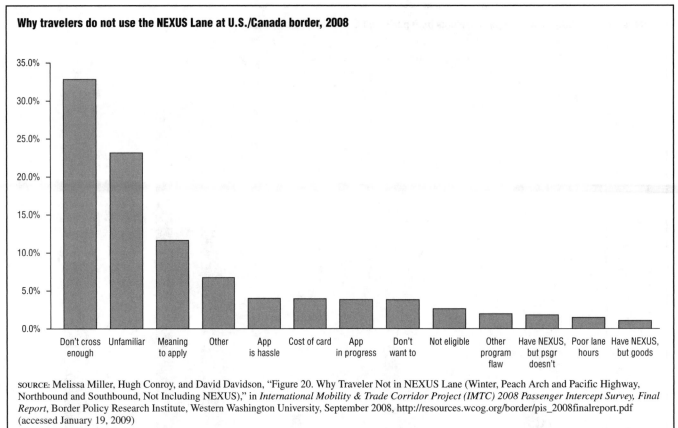

Why travelers do not use the NEXUS Lane at U.S./Canada border, 2008

SOURCE: Melissa Miller, Hugh Conroy, and David Davidson, "Figure 20. Why Traveler Not in NEXUS Lane (Winter, Peach Arch and Pacific Highway, Northbound and Southbound, Not Including NEXUS)," in *International Mobility & Trade Corridor Project (IMTC) 2008 Passenger Intercept Survey, Final Report*, Border Policy Research Institute, Western Washington University, September 2008, http://resources.wcog.org/border/pis_2008finalreport.pdf (accessed January 19, 2009)

have been more illegal Mexican aliens than legal immigrants. The need for Mexican labor was so great that in 1918 the commissioner-general of immigration exempted Mexicans from meeting most immigration conditions, such as head taxes (small amounts paid to come into the country) and literacy requirements.

Illegal Aliens and the Great Depression

From the latter 1800s up until the 1920s the United States maintained a small force of mounted guards to deter alien smuggling, but this force was inadequate to stop the increasing numbers of illegal aliens. To stem this flow of aliens, the federal government established in 1924 the U.S. Border Patrol as part of the Immigration Bureau. The efforts of the Border Patrol contributed to a sharp increase in the number of aliens deported during the mid-1920s and 1930s.

In 1929 administrative control along the U.S.-Mexican border was significantly tightened as the Great Depression (1929–1939) led many Americans to blame the nation's unemployment on the illegal aliens. Consequently, thousands of Mexicans—both legal immigrants and illegal aliens—were repatriated (sent back to Mexico). According to David Spener of Trinity University, in *Mexican Migration to the United States, 1882–1992: A Long Twentieth Century of Coyotaje* (October 2005, http://www.ccis-ucsd.org/publications/wrkg124.pdf), the Mexican-born population in the United States declined from 639,000 in 1930 to 377,000 in 1940.

Bracero Program

World War II (1939–1945) brought the country out of the Great Depression. Industry expanded and drew rural laborers into the cities. Other workers were drafted and sent overseas to fight in the war. Once more, the United States needed laborers, especially farm workers, so the nation again turned to Mexico. Fred L. Koestler notes in the *Handbook of Texas Online* (August 18, 2008, http://www.tshaonline.org/handbook/online/articles/BB/omb1.html) that the Bracero Program was a negotiated treaty between the United States and Mexico that permitted the entry of Mexican farm workers on a temporary basis under contract to U.S. employers. The entire program lasted from 1942 to 1964 and involved approximately 4.5 million Mexican workers.

Sophia Tareen reports in "Mexican Ministry Satisfied with Braceros Agreement" (Associated Press, October 17, 2008) that 2.5 million *braceros* (manual laborers) who worked in U.S. agricultural and railroad-building jobs as part of the Bracero Program won a $14.5 million settlement in October 2008 for money withheld from their paychecks and sent to the Mexican government. The money was part of a class-action suit filed against the Mexican government and three Mexican banks.

North American Free Trade Agreement

In December 1993 the North American Free Trade Agreement (NAFTA) was passed to eliminate trade and investment barriers among the United States, Canada, and Mexico over a 15-year period. NAFTA was intended to promote economic growth in each country so that, in the long run, the number of illegal immigrants seeking to enter the United States for work would diminish. NAFTA broke new ground by linking Mexico (a developing economy) with the United States and Canada (two major industrialized nations) in a pact to increase trade and investment. It established procedures for Canadian and Mexican citizens who were professional businesspeople to temporarily enter the United States to render services for pay.

NAFTA was established by the federal government to increase sales and profits for U.S. businesses, thus strengthening the economy. It was also designed to enhance the access of transnational capital from the United States to inexpensive Mexican labor and Canadian natural resources. Since then, the United States signed the Security and Prosperity Partnership in March 2005, which deepens these relations and expands the U.S.-Mexican-Canadian trade agenda to control of energy reserves.

ILLEGAL ALIENS AND CRIME

In "Information on Certain Illegal Aliens Arrested in the United States" (Government Accountability Office, 2005, http://www.gao.gov/new.items/d05646r.pdf), researchers studied "55,322 aliens [who] had entered the country illegally and were still illegally in the country at the time of their incarceration in federal and state prison or local jail during fiscal year 2003." Among the findings presented were number of arrests, types of crimes committed, and location of the crimes. The researchers learned that "[the imprisoned illegal aliens] were arrested at least a total of 459,614 times, averaging about 8 offenses per illegal alien. Ninety-seven percent had more than 1 arrest. About 38 percent had between 2 and 5 arrests, 32 percent had between 6 and 10 arrests, and 26 percent had over 11 arrests. Eighty-one percent of all arrests occurred after 1990." The GAO also noted that not all arrests were pros-

ecuted; of those that were prosecuted, not all led to a conviction.

The GAO further reports that the total number of alleged criminal offenses covered in the arrests numbered 691,890. Drugs (24%) topped the list of offenses, followed by immigration violations (21%), traffic violations (8%), assault (7%), obstruction of justice (7%), burglary (6%), larceny/theft (5%), and fraud/forgery/counterfeiting (4%). Weapons violations and motor vehicle theft registered 3% apiece, while sex offenses, robbery, and stolen property numbered 2% each. Murder was cited in only 1% of the offenses. The state with the most arrests of illegal aliens was California (58%), followed by Texas (14%) and Arizona (8%).

In spite of having the most arrests of illegal aliens, California—a state with a large immigrant population—has shown that immigrants do not pose a larger crime threat than native-born citizens. Kristen F. Butcher et al., in the Public Policy Institute of California's report *California Counts: Population Trends and Profiles* ("Crime, Corrections, and California: What Does Immigration Have to Do with It?," vol. 9, no. 3, February 2008, http://www.ppic.org/content/pubs/cacounts/CC_208KBCC.pdf), found that "the foreign-born, who make up about 35 percent of the adult population in California, constitute only about 17 percent of the adult prison population. Thus, immigrants are underrepresented in California prisons compared to their representation in the overall population. In fact, U.S.-born adult men are incarcerated at a rate over two-and-a-half times greater than that of foreign-born men." Butcher et al. acknowledge, however, that their "data do not reveal the precise [legal or illegal] immigration status of the foreign-born." Nonetheless, because data exist for naturalized citizens and noncitizens—and illegal immigrants are noncitizens—the researchers were able "to provide some insight into whether institutionalization rates for illegal immigrants are likely to be higher than they are for the foreign-born overall." Butcher et al. concluded that "institutionalization rates for noncitizens are dramatically lower than for the U.S.-born, as were the rates for the foreign-born overall. Indeed, U.S.-born institutionalization rates are almost 10 times higher."

CHAPTER 6
THE COST OF IMMIGRATION

WEIGHING THE COSTS AND BENEFITS OF IMMIGRATION

Immigration is a hotly contested issue. Immigration supporters contend that immigrants contribute considerable sums of money to the public coffers and that, in an aging society, immigration is the only hope for a secure economic future. By contrast, immigration opponents argue that immigrants cost taxpayers far more than they contribute.

Edwin S. Rubenstein of the Manhattan Institute calculates in "The Economic and Fiscal Impact of Immigration: A New Analysis" (*Social Contract*, vol. 18, no. 2, winter 2007–2008) that in fiscal year (FY) 2007 each immigrant cost U.S. taxpayers $9,139 in tax-funded expenses and each immigrant household of four cost $36,000. He estimates that immigrant children in kindergarten to 12th-grade classes for English language learners cost about $3.9 billion annually. Concerning criminal aliens held in U.S. prisons, Rubenstein states that it cost $1.5 billion in FY 2008.

The Congressional Budget Office Studies the Cost of Unauthorized Immigrants

The Congressional Budget Office (CBO) states in *The Impact of Unauthorized Immigrants on the Budgets of State and Local Governments* (December 2007, http://www.cbo.gov/ftpdocs/87xx/doc8711/12-6-Immigration.pdf) that "most efforts to estimate the fiscal impact of immigration in the United States have concluded that, in aggregate and over the long term, tax revenues of all types generated by immigrants—both legal and unauthorized—exceed the cost of the services they use."

The CBO notes that unauthorized immigrants are prohibited from receiving most federal benefits but that state and local governments are required to provide certain services regardless of immigration status. Primarily, these services include education, health care, and law enforcement. According to the CBO, these services offered to unauthorized immigrants make up a fraction of state and local spending.

After reviewing 29 reports that attempted to determine how the budgets of state and local governments are affected by unauthorized immigrants, the CBO concludes:

- State and local governments have limited options for "avoiding or minimizing" the cost of providing services to unauthorized immigrants.

- The amount spent on unauthorized immigrants is minimal when compared with the total cost of providing such services to all residents.

- Tax revenues generated by unauthorized immigrants are not sufficient to offset the cost of services provided.

- Federal aid to state and local governments does not fully offset the cost of these services to unauthorized immigrants.

Legal and illegal immigrants are more likely than U.S. natives to not have health insurance. Therefore, they are forced to rely on emergency room care. However, the CBO cites testimony by the Oklahoma Health Care Authority that Medicaid services provided to unauthorized immigrants between FYs 2003 and 2006 accounted for less than 1% of the total dollars spent.

The CBO also considers a number of state studies. In Colorado the annual costs of education, Medicaid, and corrections for unauthorized immigrants were between $217 million and $225 million, compared with between $159 million and $194 million in state and local taxes collected from unauthorized immigrants. The Missouri Budget Project estimated in 2006 the state paid between $17.5 million and $32.6 million to educate unauthorized immigrant children, whereas the immigrants paid between $29 million and $57 million in state income, property, and excise taxes. However, local school districts spent between $26.5 million and $49.3 million in educational costs for these children.

The Medicare Prescription Drug, Improvement, and Modernization Act of 2003 appropriated $250 million

FIGURE 6.1

Rates of welfare use, poverty, and lack of health insurance for all immigrants, immigrants in the U.S. 12 years or more, and natives, 2007

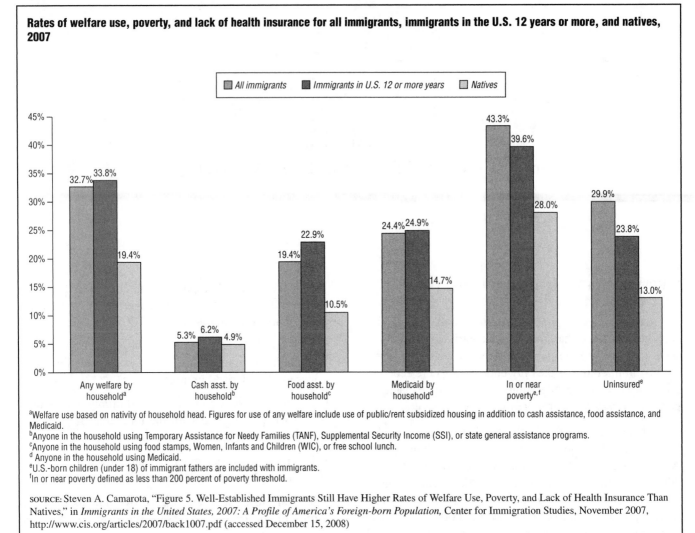

[a]Welfare use based on nativity of household head. Figures for use of any welfare include use of public/rent subsidized housing in addition to cash assistance, food assistance, and Medicaid.
[b]Anyone in the household using Temporary Assistance for Needy Families (TANF), Supplemental Security Income (SSI), or state general assistance programs.
[c]Anyone in the household using food stamps, Women, Infants and Children (WIC), or free school lunch.
[d] Anyone in the household using Medicaid.
[e]U.S.-born children (under 18) of immigrant fathers are included with immigrants.
[f]In or near poverty defined as less than 200 percent of poverty threshold.

SOURCE: Steven A. Camarota, "Figure 5. Well-Established Immigrants Still Have Higher Rates of Welfare Use, Poverty, and Lack of Health Insurance Than Natives," in *Immigrants in the United States, 2007: A Profile of America's Foreign-born Population,* Center for Immigration Studies, November 2007, http://www.cis.org/articles/2007/back1007.pdf (accessed December 15, 2008)

annually from FYs 2005 to 2008 to assist hospitals and health care providers with the cost of care for unauthorized immigrants. The CBO explains that two-thirds of the funds were divided among the states based on the number of unauthorized immigrants living in the state, and the remainder would be split among the states with the highest share of aliens arrested by federal officials.

Economic Gap between Immigrants and Natives

According to Steven A. Camarota of the Center for Immigration Studies, in *Immigrants in the United States, 2007: A Profile of America's Foreign-Born Population* (November 2007, http://www.cis.org/articles/2007/back1007 .pdf), analysts once believed immigrants spent 12 to 14 years working before they closed the economic gap with U.S. natives. That is no longer the case. Figure 6.1 shows that immigrants who have lived in the United States 12 years or more still have greater use of welfare, housing assistance, Temporary Assistance to Needy Families (TANF), Supplemental Security Income (SSI), state assistance programs, food stamps, the Women Infants and Children (WIC)

nutrition program, free school lunches, and Medicaid than native-born residents. These same immigrants are also more likely than natives to live in or near poverty and lack health insurance.

Camarota notes that "there is no way to know whether today's immigrants will take the same number of years to close the gap with natives, or even if they ever will. But given the [limited] education of recently arrived immigrants, it is not reasonable to expect that their income or rates of poverty, un-insurance, and welfare use will converge with natives any time soon. We do know that unskilled immigrants never come close to closing the gap with natives even when they have lived in the United States for many years."

IMMIGRANTS LIVING IN POVERTY. Table 6.1 considers the share of immigrants living in or near poverty. In 2007, 15.2% of immigrants lived in poverty, compared with 11.4% of natives. Immigrant children under the age of 18 were more likely to live in poverty (22.6%) than native children (16%). Table 6.1 also shows the great variation in

TABLE 6.1

Rates of poverty and near poverty by immigrants and their U.S. born children, by country of birth, 2007

	Poverty		In or near poverty	
Country	Immigrants	Immigrants and their U.S.- born children[a]	Immigrants	Immigrants and their U.S.-born children[a]
Dominican Republic	27.9%	31.2%	58.1%	61.7%
Mexico	22.2%	24.5%	60.4%	63.9%
Guatemala	21.3%	24.3%	59.4%	61.8%
Honduras	19.6%	19.5%	50.7%	52.0%
Jamaica	18.7%	20.1%	40.0%	43.6%
Haiti	17.8%	22.4%	43.4%	49.2%
Korea	16.7%	14.0%	30.4%	27.6%
Cuba	15.7%	14.9%	36.8%	37.2%
El Salvador	14.5%	17.1%	44.7%	46.5%
Vietnam	12.9%	13.1%	31.2%	32.1%
Ecuador	11.2%	10.2%	38.0%	42.5%
Columbia	11.0%	12.0%	31.1%	31.8%
China	10.4%	10.4%	28.4%	28.7%
Germany	10.3%	8.2%	22.6%	21.8%
Brazil	10.1%	9.1%	33.8%	33.5%
Japan	9.1%	7.2%	18.9%	17.8%
Peru	9.0%	9.3%	29.9%	29.7%
Italy	8.9%	6.8%	27.5%	28.3%
Iran	7.8%	7.2%	27.9%	26.2%
India	7.2%	7.2%	17.5%	16.9%
United Kingdom	7.1%	7.7%	18.0%	18.6%
Former USSR	7.0%	6.9%	27.9%	27.3%
Canada	6.7%	8.2%	17.0%	19.7%
Poland	5.9%	5.4%	23.2%	25.3%
Philippines	4.2%	4.4%	13.6%	14.9%
Hispanic immigrants	20.2%	22.5%	54.3%	58.1%
All immigrants	**15.2%**	**16.9%**	**40.1%**	**43.3%**

	Poverty	In or near poverty
All natives[b, c]	11.4%	28.0%
Hispanic natives[b]	18.2%	41.2%
Non-Hispanic white natives[b]	8.2%	22.7%
Non-Hispanic black natives[b]	24.6%	48.5%
All persons	12.3%	30.5%
Children of immigrants (under 18)[a]	22.6%	53.6%
Children of natives (under 18)[b]	16.0%	35.2%

Note: In or near-poverty defined as income under 200% of the poverty threshold.
[a]Includes U.S.-born children of immigrant fathers under age 18.
[b]Excludes U.S.-born children under age 18 of immigrant fathers.
[c]If the U.S. born children (under 18) of immigrant fathers are included with natives, the share of natives in poverty is 11.9 % and the share in or near poverty is 29.2%. Figures for white and black natives are for those who chose only one race.

SOURCE: Steven A. Camarota, "Table 10. Poverty and Near-Poverty," in *Immigrants in the United States, 2007: A Profile of America's Foreign-born Population*, Center for Immigration Studies, November 2007, http://www.cis.org/articles/2007/back1007.pdf (accessed December 15, 2008)

immigrant poverty rates by country of birth. The 31.2% poverty rate for immigrants from the Dominican Republic and their U.S.-born children was nearly double the 16.9% rate for all immigrants and their U.S.-born children.

IMMIGRANTS WITHOUT HEALTH INSURANCE. Camarota notes that since 1989 the share of the U.S. population without health insurance has grown by 14.6 million people. He explains that immigration has driven most of this growth. He also notes that U.S.-born children of immigrants are eligible for Medicaid, as such the rates of their being uninsured are lower than the rates for their immigrant parents.

Camarota suggests this situation is not likely to improve. Due to their lack of education, many immigrants hold lower-paying jobs that do not offer health insurance. Also, their low incomes prevent them from being able to buy insurance. As

the uninsured population grows, it strains the resources of health care providers. The end result is that the costs of caring for the uninsured are passed along in the form of higher premiums to Americans with insurance and higher taxes for health care services provided through federal, state, and local programs.

IMMIGRANT USE OF GOVERNMENT PROGRAMS. Table 6.2 compares use of welfare programs, the Earned Income Tax Credit (EITC), and the Additional Child Tax Credit (ACTC). Even though the 1996 welfare reforms limited immigrant eligibility for some programs, welfare use among all immigrant households remains higher than use by all native households, except for subsidized housing, which is used equally by 4.1% of both immigrant and native households. Cash assistance includes TANF, state administered general assistance, and SSI for low-income elderly and

TABLE 6.2

Use of welfare programs, EITC, and ACTC native and immigrant households, 2007

			Year of entry[a]			
	Native households	All immigrant households	Pre-1980 immigrant households	1980–89 immigrant households	1990–99 immigrant households	2000–07 immigrant households
Using any welfare program	19.4%	32.7%	24.2%	36.1%	37.9%	33.3%
Cash assistance[b]	4.9%	5.3%	6.0%	6.6%	4.8%	3.1%
Food assistance[c]	10.5%	19.4%	9.7%	21.7%	25.1%	22.4%
Subsidized housing	4.1%	4.1%	4.3%	4.6%	4.1%	3.1%
Medicaid[d]	14.7%	24.4%	19.0%	27.3%	29.2%	21.8%
EITC eligibility	17.8%	31.1%	17.6%	33.5%	37.3%	40.9%
ACTC eligibility	10.9%	22.5%	11.5%	26.7%	28.5%	25.7%

[a]Based on the year the household head said he or she came to the United States.
[b]Anyone in the household using Temporary Assistance for Needy Families (TANF), Supplemental Security Income (SSI), or state general programs.
[c]Anyone in household using food stamps, Women, Infants and Children (WIC) or free school lunch.
[d]Anyone in household using Medicaid.
Note: EITC = Earned Income Tax Credit. ACTC = Additional Child Tax Credit.

SOURCE: Steven A. Camarota, "Table 12. Welfare Programs, EITC, and ACTC, by Households," in *Immigrants in the United States, 2007: A Profile of America's Foreign-born Population*, Center for Immigration Studies, November 2007, http://www.cis.org/articles/2007/back1007.pdf (accessed December 15, 2008)

TABLE 6.3

Socio-economic status of natives and immigrants, by education level, 2006

Education level	Nativity	Median income[a]	Welfare use[b]	In or near poverty (persons 18 & over)[c]	Without health ins. (persons 18 & over)
Overall	Immigrant	$31,074	32.7%	38.7%	33.9%
	Native	$40,344	19.4%	25.7%	14.2%
Less than high school	Immigrant	$21,176	53.8%	60.2%	51.0%
	Native	$24,402	41.3%	53.0%	22.1%
High school only	Immigrant	$26,459	36.1%	41.8%	37.9%
	Native	$31,486	23.4%	31.1%	17.8%
Some college	Immigrant	$35,010	27.8%	28.7%	26.0%
	Native	$37,096	19.0%	22.8%	13.8%
College or graduate degree	Immigrant	$55,582	12.5%	15.5%	13.9%
	Native	$56,583	6.8%	9.5%	12.1%

[a]Persons who worked full-time year-round in 2006.
[b]Based on nativity and education level of household head.
[c]In or near poverty defined as income under 200 percent of the poverty threshold.

SOURCE: Steven A. Camarota, "Table 15. Socio-Economic Status by Education Level," in *Immigrants in the United States, 2007: A Profile of America's Foreign-born Population*, Center for Immigration Studies, November 2007, http://www.cis.org/articles/2007/back1007.pdf (accessed December 15, 2008)

---

disabled people. Food assistance includes food stamps, free school lunch, and WIC. Housing assistance includes both assistance with rent and use of government-owned housing.

Camarota explains that the EITC and ACTC are cash payments to employed people whose income is low enough that they do not owe federal income tax. The EITC is cash assistance based on income and family size. The ACTC is similar but available only to workers with at least one dependent child. The EITC and ACTC are automatically processed by the Internal Revenue Service for qualified people who file a tax return. Illegal aliens are permitted to receive the ACTC and EITC, but to qualify for the latter program they must have a valid Social Security number. The annual costs of these programs exceed $35 billion for the EITC and $14 billion for the ACTC.

COMPARING IMMIGRANT AND NATIVE INCOME.
Table 6.3 compares income (for full-time, year-round workers), welfare use, poverty status, and lack of health insurance by educational levels for immigrant and native populations. In 2006 the $21,176 median (average) annual earnings of immigrants without a high school education was 87% of the $24,202 earned by natives with the same education. For immigrants with at least a college degree, they earned $55,582, or 98% of the $56,583 median annual income of similarly educated natives. Despite this near equality of income at the college-educated level, in 2006 immigrants had nearly double the share of welfare use (12.5%), compared with college-educated natives (6.8%).

Income levels for immigrants differ not only by education but also by where in the United States they live. In

TABLE 6.4

Immigrant and native household size and income, by state of residence, 2006

	Median household income		Number of persons per household		Per-person median household income		Percent native per-person income is higher than immigrant
	Immigrant	Native	Immigrant	Native	Immigrant	Native	
Arizona	$30,590	$51,087	3.2	2.5	$ 9,559	$20,435	114%
Colorado	$35,430	$57,891	3.2	2.5	$11,072	$23,156	109%
Texas	$32,988	$46,332	3.3	2.5	$ 9,996	$18,533	85%
California	$47,292	$60,011	3.4	2.5	$13,909	$24,004	73%
L.A. County	$43,618	$55,087	3.3	2.4	$13,218	$22,953	74%
Massachusetts	$41,634	$59,446	2.9	2.5	$14,357	$23,778	66%
Florida	$41,301	$47,050	3.2	2.3	$12,907	$20,457	58%
Nevada	$46,863	$54,766	3.1	2.4	$15,117	$22,819	51%
Georgia	$49,115	$50,758	3.4	2.4	$14,446	$21,149	46%
New York	$41,212	$51,052	2.8	2.4	$14,719	$21,272	45%
New York City	$38,116	$41,688	2.8	2.2	$13,613	$18,949	39%
Illinois	$48,965	$48,866	3.2	2.4	$15,302	$20,361	33%
North Carolina	$41,230	$39,750	3.3	2.4	$12,494	$16,563	33%
New Jersey	$66,170	$68,988	3.1	2.5	$21,345	$27,595	29%
Maryland	$64,160	$64,273	3.2	2.5	$20,050	$25,709	28%
Virginia	$56,605	$57,536	3.1	2.5	$18,260	$23,014	26%
Nation	**$43,933**	**$49,201**	**3.1**	**2.4**	**$14,172**	**$20,500**	**45%**

SOURCE: Steven A. Camarota, "Table 16. Household Income and Size by State," in *Immigrants in the United States, 2007: A Profile of America's Foreign-born Population*, Center for Immigration Studies, November 2007, http://www.cis.org/articles/2007/back1007.pdf (accessed December 15, 2008)

2006 the average immigrant household in Arizona had an annual income of $30,590, compared with a native household median income of $51,087. (See Table 6.4.) By contrast, in Illinois the median immigrant household income of $48,965 was greater than the average of $48,866 for native households. Nationally, the median native household income of $49,201 was 12% greater than the immigrant household income of $43,933. The income of immigrant households typically supports more people. In 2006, 3.1 people lived in immigrant households, compared with 2.4 people in native households. When the household income is considered by the number of people in the household, the national native income of $20,500 per person was 45% greater than the national immigrant income of $14,172 per person.

FEDERAL SPENDING ON IMMIGRATION

U.S. Department of Homeland Security Budget

In *Homeland Security Budget-in-Brief, Fiscal Year 2009* (2008, http://www.dhs.gov/xlibrary/assets/budget_bib-fy2009.pdf), the U.S. Department of Homeland Security (DHS) states that its budget for FY 2009 was $50.5 billion, a 7% increase over FY 2008. Figure 6.2 shows the distribution of the FY 2009 budget.

The U.S. Customs and Border Patrol (CBP) received the largest share at 22% ($10.9 billion). (See Figure 6.2.) The DHS notes that at the close of FY 2007 the CBP reported 54,868 employees. The new budget request included $442.4 million to hire and train 2,200 new Border Patrol agents. This would bring the total number of agents to 20,000 by September 2009. Another $106.9 million would be used to upgrade infrastructure and technology at land ports of entry for the Western Hemisphere Travel Initiative. The DHS notes that in

FY 2007 "CBP Officers seized more than 820,000 pounds of narcotics, arrested more than 25,000 suspected criminals, turned away more than 170,000 inadmissible aliens at the ports of entry, and conducted approximately 1.5 million agricultural interceptions."

The U.S. Immigration and Customs Enforcement (ICE) received 11% ($5.7 billion) of the DHS budget for FY 2009. (See Figure 6.2.) The DHS states that ICE had 18,965 employees at the close of FY 2007. The new budget request included $46 million for 1,000 additional detention beds, staffing, and associated removal costs. In FY 2007 ICE removed 276,000 illegal aliens from the country (including voluntary removals), a 45% increase from the previous year. ICE also made 1,821 criminal arrests for human smuggling that resulted in 1,209 convictions.

The U.S. Citizenship and Immigration Services (USCIS) had 5% ($2.7 billion) of the total DHS FY 2009 budget. (See Figure 6.2.) According to the DHS, the USCIS had 10,620 employees at the close of FY 2007. The budget included $100 million to expand E-Verify services for employers. Participation in E-Verify doubled from 12,000 employers in FY 2006 to nearly 25,000 employers checking more than 3 million new hires by the end of FY 2007. The USCIS successfully launched the Photo Screening Tool in September 2007, which allows employers to visually compare photo documents presented with Form I-9 with images on documents in USCIS databases.

U.S. Department of State Budget

In "Department of State and Other International Programs" (May 5, 2008, http://www.whitehouse.gov/omb/budget/fy2009/state.html), the Office of Management and

FIGURE 6.2

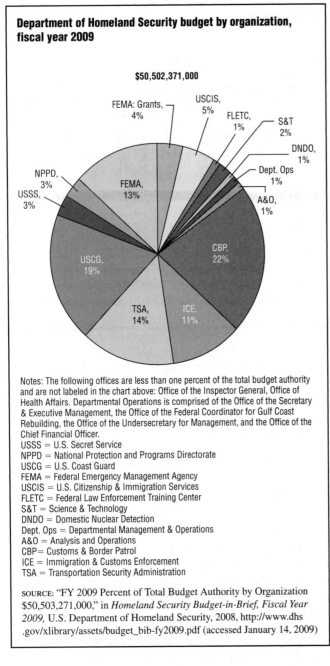

Department of Homeland Security budget by organization, fiscal year 2009

$50,502,371,000

Notes: The following offices are less than one percent of the total budget authority and are not labeled in the chart above: Office of the Inspector General, Office of Health Affairs. Departmental Operations is comprised of the Office of the Secretary & Executive Management, the Office of the Federal Coordinator for Gulf Coast Rebuilding, the Office of the Undersecretary for Management, and the Office of the Chief Financial Officer.

USSS = U.S. Secret Service
NPPD = National Protection and Programs Directorate
USCG = U.S. Coast Guard
FEMA = Federal Emergency Management Agency
USCIS = U.S. Citizenship & Immigration Services
FLETC = Federal Law Enforcement Training Center
S&T = Science & Technology
DNDO = Domestic Nuclear Detection
Dept. Ops = Departmental Management & Operations
A&O = Analysis and Operations
CBP = Customs & Border Patrol
ICE = Immigration & Customs Enforcement
TSA = Transportation Security Administration

SOURCE: "FY 2009 Percent of Total Budget Authority by Organization $50,503,271,000," in *Homeland Security Budget-in-Brief, Fiscal Year 2009*, U.S. Department of Homeland Security, 2008, http://www.dhs.gov/xlibrary/assets/budget_bib-fy2009.pdf (accessed January 14, 2009)

Budget explains that in FY 2009 the U.S. Department of State allocated $522 million for its Educational and Cultural Exchange Programs, which included the new Partnership for Latin American Youth. The partnership will offer thousands of students opportunities to study in the United States. Another $809 million was allocated to the refugee assistance fund, which helps support refugees around the world, many of whom will eventually be resettled in the United States.

Other Government Spending

The Centers for Medicare and Medicaid Services (CMS) explains in "Section 1011: Fact Sheet—Federal Reimbursement of Emergency Health Services Furnished to Undocumented Aliens" (May 19, 2006, http://www.cms.hhs.gov/MLNProducts/downloads/Sect1011_Web05-19-06.pdf) that Section 1011 of the Medicare Prescription Drug, Improvement, and Modernization Act of 2003 provided $250 million annually from FY 2005 to FY 2008 to reimburse eligible hospitals, physicians, and ambulance services for costs incurred from treating unauthorized immigrants. According to the CMS, "two-thirds of the funds are divided among all 50 states and the District of Columbia, based on their relative percentage of undocumented aliens.... One-third of the funds are divided among the six states with the largest number of undocumented aliens for each FY."

In *FY 2008 State Allocations for Section 1011 of the Medicare Modernization Act* (2008, http://www.cms.hhs.gov/UndocAliens/downloads/fy08_state_alloc.pdf), the CMS indicates that in FY 2008 the six states with the largest undocumented populations received $83 million: Arizona ($38 million), California ($19.6 million), Texas ($19.6 million), New Mexico ($4.1 million), Florida ($1.1 million), and New York ($607,000).

IMMIGRANT USE OF TAX-BASED PROGRAMS

According to Robert E. Rector and Christine Kim of the Heritage Foundation, in *The Fiscal Cost of Low-Skill Immigrants to the U.S. Taxpayer* (May 21, 2007, http://www.heritage.org/Research/Immigration/upload/sr_14.pdf), low-skilled immigrant households (defined as households headed by immigrants without high school diplomas) cost U.S. taxpayers $89.1 billion per year. The researchers estimate there were 4.5 million low-skilled immigrant households in the United States in 2004. The 15.9 million people living in these households represented about 5% of the U.S. population.

Based on their research, Rector and Kim calculate that each low-skilled immigrant household received $10,428 in means-tested benefits (welfare) and $4,891 in direct benefits (mainly Social Security and Medicare) in FY 2004. (See Figure 6.3.) These benefits plus the costs of education and population-based services totaled $30,160 per household.

Figure 6.4 details the estimated taxes and revenues paid by these low-skilled immigrant households. Federal, state, and local taxes paid totaled $10,573 in FY 2004. Rector and Kim note that federal and state individual income taxes accounted for only 15% of total taxes paid. On average, low-skilled immigrant households paid $1,815 in state and local sales and consumption taxes. This analysis assumes that a significant portion of property taxes on rental and business properties was passed on to renters and consumers.

The $30,160 in government benefits and services these households received exceeded their $10,573 in taxes paid in FY 2004. (See Figure 6.3 and Figure 6.4.) According to Rector and Kim, these immigrant households received an average of $3 in benefits and services for every $1 they paid in taxes. The estimated government benefits were also greater

FIGURE 6.3

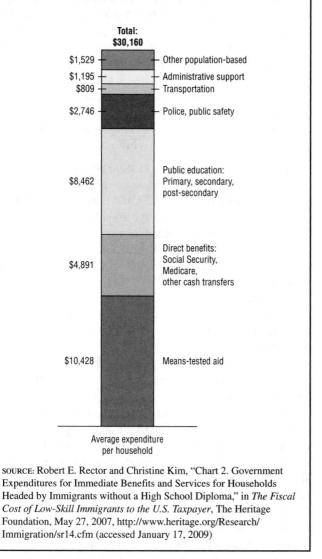

Government expenditures for immediate benefits and services for households headed by immigrants without a high school diploma, fiscal year 2004

Total:
$30,160

$1,529 — Other population-based
$1,195 — Administrative support
$809 — Transportation
$2,746 — Police, public safety
$8,462 — Public education: Primary, secondary, post-secondary
$4,891 — Direct benefits: Social Security, Medicare, other cash transfers
$10,428 — Means-tested aid

Average expenditure per household

SOURCE: Robert E. Rector and Christine Kim, "Chart 2. Government Expenditures for Immediate Benefits and Services for Households Headed by Immigrants without a High School Diploma," in *The Fiscal Cost of Low-Skill Immigrants to the U.S. Taxpayer*, The Heritage Foundation, May 27, 2007, http://www.heritage.org/Research/Immigration/sr14.cfm (accessed January 17, 2009)

FIGURE 6.4

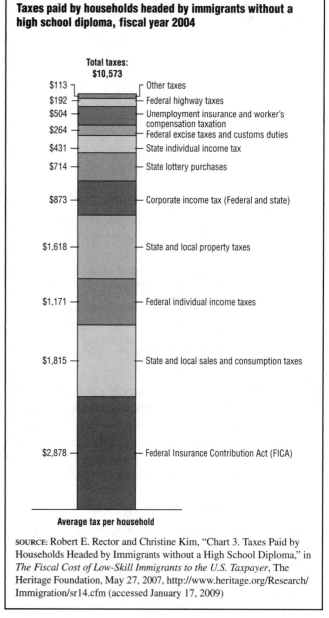

Taxes paid by households headed by immigrants without a high school diploma, fiscal year 2004

Total taxes:
$10,573

$113 — Other taxes
$192 — Federal highway taxes
$504 — Unemployment insurance and worker's compensation taxation
$264 — Federal excise taxes and customs duties
$431 — State individual income tax
$714 — State lottery purchases
$873 — Corporate income tax (Federal and state)
$1,618 — State and local property taxes
$1,171 — Federal individual income taxes
$1,815 — State and local sales and consumption taxes
$2,878 — Federal Insurance Contribution Act (FICA)

Average tax per household

SOURCE: Robert E. Rector and Christine Kim, "Chart 3. Taxes Paid by Households Headed by Immigrants without a High School Diploma," in *The Fiscal Cost of Low-Skill Immigrants to the U.S. Taxpayer*, The Heritage Foundation, May 27, 2007, http://www.heritage.org/Research/Immigration/sr14.cfm (accessed January 17, 2009)

than their average annual earnings of $28,890 per household. On average, low-skilled immigrant households received $30,160 in government benefits and services in FY 2004, and they paid only $10,573 in taxes; thus, the deficit per household was $19,588. (See Figure 6.5.)

Rector and Kim note, "The fiscal cost of low-skill immigrants will be increased in the future by government policies that increase: the number of low-skill immigrants, the immigrants' length of stay in the U.S., or the access of low-skill immigrants to government benefits. Conversely, fiscal costs will be reduced by policies that decrease these variables."

Social Security and Immigrant Earnings

In *A Summary of the 2008 Annual Social Security and Medicare Trust Fund Reports* (April 2, 2008, http://www.ssa.gov/OACT/TRSUM/tr08summary.pdf), the Social Secur-

ity trustees warn that "Social Security's current annual surpluses of tax income over expenditures will begin to decline in 2011 and then turn into rapidly growing deficits as the baby boom generation retires. Medicare's financial status is even worse.... Growing annual deficits are projected to exhaust [Medicare] reserves in 2019 and Social Security reserves in 2041."

Paul N. Van de Water of the Center on Budget and Policy Priorities indicates in "Immigration and Social Security" (November 20, 2008, http://www.cbpp.org/11-20-08 socsec.pdf) that the Social Security trustees and the CBO agree that increases in immigration generally improve Social Security's finances. The immigrant workforce is generally younger than the native workforce; therefore, adding more young workers to the labor force increases current payroll

FIGURE 6.5

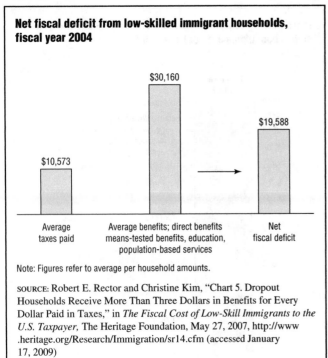

Net fiscal deficit from low-skilled immigrant households, fiscal year 2004

$30,160

$19,588

$10,573

Average
taxes paid

Average benefits; direct benefits
means-tested benefits, education,
population-based services

Net
fiscal deficit

Note: Figures refer to average per household amounts.

SOURCE: Robert E. Rector and Christine Kim, "Chart 5. Dropout Households Receive More Than Three Dollars in Benefits for Every Dollar Paid in Taxes," in *The Fiscal Cost of Low-Skill Immigrants to the U.S. Taxpayer*, The Heritage Foundation, May 27, 2007, http://www.heritage.org/Research/Immigration/sr14.cfm (accessed January 17, 2009)

tax collections. Furthermore, the Social Security benefits for those young workers who are legal immigrants are mostly payable "in the more distant future." According to Van de Water, the Social Security trustees estimate that an increase in net immigration of 300,000 people per year would eliminate about one-tenth of Social Security's 75-year deficit.

Van de Water explains:

> The presence of unauthorized (undocumented) workers in the United States also has a positive effect on the financial status of Social Security. The earnings of unauthorized workers are less likely to be reported for tax purposes than the earnings of the rest of the population and even less likely to result in future benefits, according to Social Security's chief actuary.... [T]he actuary has estimated that unauthorized immigrants paid as much as $13 billion in Social Security payroll taxes in 2007. About $1 billion in benefit payments were made based on unauthorized work (for example, survivor benefits paid to U.S. citizens who were dependents of deceased individuals who had made payments into the Social Security system while performing unauthorized work). Thus, undocumented immigrants improved Social Security's cash flow by an estimated $12 billion in 2007.

Totalization Agreements

Noncitizens who work in the United States for more than five years may recover Social Security taxes paid, if their country has a totalization agreement with the United States. These arrangements also allow U.S. employees of international companies to work abroad and receive credit for that work toward their future Social Security benefits.

Opponents of totalization agreements argue that long-time illegal workers could return to their home country and claim their benefits through totalization. In January 2009 the U.S. House of Representatives proposed greater control of this with the Total Overhaul of Totalization Agreements Law of 2009 (http://thomas.loc.gov/cgi-bin/query/z?c111:H.R.132.IH:). This proposed amendment to Title II of the Social Security Act would "prohibit crediting of individuals under such title with earnings from employment or self-employment in the United States performed while such individuals are not citizens, nationals, or lawful permanent residents of the United States and are not authorized by law to be employed in the United States." As of spring 2009, this bill was still in committee.

EXISTING U.S. TOTALIZATION AGREEMENTS. In 2006 the United States had totalization agreements with 21 countries. (See Table 6.5.) The 127,978 beneficiaries of these agreements received an average monthly U.S. benefit of $188.44. Citizens of the United Kingdom received the highest average monthly benefit at $232.24. Denmark became a totalization agreement participant in 2008 and the agreement between the United States and the Czech Republic became effective January 1, 2009. Agreements with Poland and Mexico were signed in 2004, but as of spring 2009 they were still pending review by Congress and each respective country's legislature.

Reimbursing States for the Cost of Incarcerating Criminal Aliens

The Bureau of Justice Assistance (BJA; October 8, 2008, http://www.ojp.usdoj.gov/BJA/grant/scaap.html) oversees the State Criminal Alien Assistance Program (SCAAP), which "provides federal payments to states and localities that incurred correctional officer salary costs for incarcerating undocumented criminal aliens with at least one felony or two misdemeanor convictions for violations of state or local law, and incarcerated for at least 4 consecutive days during the reporting period." SCAAP covers only a share of corrections staff salaries related to the incarceration of criminal aliens. Other expenses, such as feeding, clothing, and providing medical attention to the prisoners, are not included in this federal reimbursement program.

The BJA reports in "SCAAP 2007" (2008, http://www.ojp.usdoj.gov/BJA/grant/07SCPay.pdf) that SCAAP awarded more than $377 million to the states in FY 2007. Five states—Arizona, California, Florida, New York, and Texas—received $259.3 million (69%) of the funds. California received $151.5 million (40%) of the total SCAAP funds.

COMMUNITIES MUST EDUCATE IMMIGRANT CHILDREN

According to the CBO, in *Impact of Unauthorized Immigrants on the Budgets of State and Local Governments*, "education is the largest single expenditure in state and local budgets. Because state and local governments bear

TABLE 6.5

Totalization agreement countries and U.S. Social Security benefits paid, 2006

	Total	Retired workers	Disabled workers	Spouses	Widow(er)s	Children
Workers	127,978	85,862	2,956	26,495	11,2731	1,392
Avg monthly payment	$188.44	$220.28	$411.64	$78.79	$155.37	$106.01

Top five countries by number of beneficiaries	Total benecifiaries	Average monthly payment	Totalization agreement countries, 2006		
Canada	45,840	$163.02	Australia	Germany	Netherlands
Germany	18,921	$219.64	Austria	Greece	Norway
United Kingdom	15,861	$232.24	Belgium	Ireland	Portugal
Japan	9,587	$199.65	Canada	Italy	Spain
Italy	8,831	$175.99	Chile	Japan	Sweden
			Finland	Korea	Switzerland
			France	Luxebourg	United Kingdom

SOURCE: Adapted from "Table 5.M1. Benefits in Current-Payment Status, International Agreements," in *Annual Statistical Supplement, 2007*, U.S. Social Security Administration, Office of Policy, April 2008, http://www.ssa.gov/policy/docs/statcomps/supplement/2007/5m.html (accessed December 29, 2008)

the primary fiscal and administrative responsibility of providing schooling from kindergarten through grade 12, they incur substantial costs to educate children who are unauthorized immigrants."

Educating immigrant children who do not speak English is not a new issue. It began with the Bilingual Education Act, Title VII of Elementary and Secondary Education Act of 1967. Title VII provides funds to school districts to create and supplement programs to meet the needs of children with limited English proficiency (LEP). A few years later, in *Lau v. Nichols* (414 U.S. 563 [1974]), a case involving Chinese students in San Francisco, California, who were placed in an English-only class, the U.S. Supreme Court ruled that the English-only policy was discriminatory and in violation of the Federal Civil Rights Act of 1964.

The rights of LEP students were clarified in 1974, when Congress adopted the Equal Educational Opportunity Act (EEOA), which stated that "no state shall deny equal educational opportunity to an individual on account of his or her race, color, sex, or national origin, by . . . the failure by an educational agency to take appropriate action to overcome language barriers that impede equal participation by its students in its instructional programs." In 1982 the Supreme Court ruled in *Plyler v. Doe* (457 U.S. 202) that individual states could not exclude children from public education because of their immigration status. Obstacles persisted for school children learning English, with some groups pushing to pass state ballot initiatives to bar bilingual instruction—favoring English "immersion" in the classroom over English instruction. In 1998 California passed Proposition 227, banning bilingual classes.

English Proficiency of Immigrant Children

Table 6.6 profiles characteristics of children aged 5 to 17 with different levels of English language skills. In 2006 there were 53.4 million children in the United States, and 10.8 million (20.3% of the total number of children) spoke a language other than English at home. Of those who spoke a language other than English at home, 2.8 million (5.2%) spoke English with difficulty. Not all children with difficulty speaking English were immigrants; 12,000 were Native American and Alaskan native children.

Among children in Table 6.6 who were not U.S. citizens, 89.9% spoke a language other than English at home and 39.9% spoke English with difficulty. Of these children who were aged 5 to 9, 50.5% had difficulty with English, compared with 35.6% who were aged 10 to 17. This suggests that English language skills improved with age due to time in school learning English.

Cost to the U.S. Department of Education

In *The Biennial Report to Congress on the Implementation of Title III State Formula Grant Program, School Years 2004–06* (June 2008, http://www.ed.gov/about/offices/list/oela/title3biennial0406.pdf), the U.S. Department of Education reports that between 2004 and 2006 there were approximately 4.9 million LEP students in the United States who spoke over 400 different languages. Nearly 80% spoke Spanish.

According to the Education Department, in *English Language Acquisition: Fiscal Year 2009 Budget Request* (2008, http://www.ed.gov/about/overview/budget/budget09/justifications/g-ela.pdf), its budget requests for English language acquisition grew by 76%, from $415 million in 2000 to $730 million in 2009. (See Table 6.7.) These funds were distributed as grants to states under the No Child Left behind Act of 2001. California, which had the largest LEP population, received $169 million (25%) out of the total $669 million in funds in 2007. Minimum grants of $500,000 went to states with the fewest LEP students: Montana, North Dakota, Vermont, West Virginia, and Wyoming.

TABLE 6.6

Selected characteristics of children ages 5–17 who spoke a language other than English at home and who spoke English with difficulty, 2006

[Numbers in thousands]

Characteristic	Total population	Spoke a language other than English at home						
		Number	Percent of total population	Spoke English with difficulty				
				Total		Ages 5–9		Ages 10–17	
				Number	Percent of total population	Number	Percent of population	Number	Percent of population subgroup
Total	**53,406**	**10,845**	**20.3**	**2,758**	**5.2**	**1,372**	**6.9**	**1,386**	**4.1**
Language spoken at home									
Spanish	7,787	7,787	100	2,071	26.6	1,054	35.4	1,018	21.1
Other Indo-European	1,434	1,434	100	277	19.3	121	23.6	156	16.9
Asian/Pacific Islander	1,200	1,200	100	333	27.8	161	36.2	172	22.9
Other	424	424	100	77	18.1	36	21.3	40	15.9
Race/ethnicity									
White	31,154	1,762	5.7	378	1.2	134	1.2	245	1.2
Black	7,870	429	5.5	99	1.3	34	1.2	65	1.3
Hispanic	10,250	7,038	68.7	1,882	18.4	1,011	24.6	870	14.2
Mexican	6,986	4,998	71.5	1,463	20.9	821	28.5	641	15.6
Puerto Rican	936	465	49.7	78	8.3	32	8.9	46	7.9
Cuban	218	149	68.4	24	11	11	13.7	13	9.4
Dominican	274	243	88.6	49	17.9	17	18	32	17.9
Central American	614	510	83.2	137	22.3	69	29.1	68	18
South American	398	314	78.9	58	14.6	25	16.9	33	13.2
Other Hispanic	823	358	43.5	73	8.9	36	11.2	38	7.5
Asian	2,042	1,321	64.7	350	17.1	172	21.7	178	14.2
Pacific Islander	84	25	30	5	6.1	2	7.5	3	5.2
American Indian/Alaska Native	436	85	19.6	12	2.8	5	3.4	7	2.5
More than one race	1,383	116	8.4	18	1.3	7	1.2	11	1.4
Citizenship									
U.S.-born	50,701	8,571	16.9	1,831	3.6	1,044	5.5	787	2.5
Naturalized U.S. citizen	544	331	60.9	66	12.1	18	13.3	48	11.7
Non-U.S. citizen	2,161	1,942	89.9	861	39.9	310	50.5	551	35.6
Poverty status[6]									
Poor	9,083	2,742	30.2	881	9.7	464	12.7	417	7.7
Near-poor	11,002	3,276	29.8	885	8	468	10.9	417	6.2
Nonpoor	32,348	4,661	14.4	937	2.9	411	3.6	526	2.5
Region									
Northeast	9,321	1,869	20.1	409	4.4	180	5.3	229	3.8
Midwest	11,859	1,338	11.3	363	3.1	179	4.1	184	2.5
South	19,401	3,339	17.2	886	4.6	445	6.1	440	3.6
West	12,825	4,299	33.5	1,101	8.6	568	11.9	533	6.6

Note: Detail may not sum to totals because of rounding.

SOURCE: "Table 7-2. Number and Percentage of Children Ages–17 Who Spoke a Language Other Than English at Home and Who Spoke English with Difficulty, by Selected Characteristics: 2006," in *Participation in Education*, U.S. Department of Education, National Center for Educational Statistics, 2008, http://nces.ed.gov/programs/coe/2008/section1/table.asp?tableID=866 (accessed November 19, 2008).

LEP Impact on States

Figure 6.6, Figure 6.7, and Figure 6.8 demonstrate different patterns of LEP enrollment (kindergarten through high school) in three states—Arkansas, Iowa, and Oklahoma—during the academic years 1995–96 through 2005–06.

- At the end of the 10-year period, Arkansas had 6.2% more total enrollment and 361.3% more LEP students. (See Figure 6.6.) These numbers suggest that LEP students coming into the schools replaced students who graduated or left the state.

- In the period 1995–96 to 2003–04, the number of LEP students in Iowa increased and then decreased while the number of total school enrollments dropped. (See Figure 6.7.)

- Oklahoma's pattern of LEP student enrollments had increased 58.9% by 2000–01. (See Figure 6.8.) During the 2001–02 school year LEP students began to leave as rapidly as they had arrived.

These differing patterns of LEP enrollment illustrate the challenges faced by local school administrators, school boards, and state legislatures in terms of staffing and budget planning. For example, concerning the LEP enrollment patterns in Oklahoma, local school districts had to request additional funds to recruit LEP teachers as enrollments increased,

TABLE 6.7

U.S. Department of Education English language appropriations requests, 2001–09

	Budget estimate to Congress	Appropriation
2000	$415,000	$406,000
2001	460,000	460,000
2002	460,000	665,000
2003	665,000	685,515
2003 Supplemental	0	−1,768
2004	665,000	681,215
2005	681,215	675,765
2006	675,765	669,007
2007	669,007	669,007
2008	670,819	700,395
2009	730,000	

SOURCE: Adapted from "English Language Acquisition: Appropriations History," in *English Language Acquisition: Fiscal Year 2009 Budget Request*, U.S. Department of Education, 2008, http://www.ed.gov/about/overview/budget/budget09/justifications/g-ela.pdf (accessed January 9, 2009)

FIGURE 6.6

LEP growth in Arkansas schools, 1995–96 to 2005–06

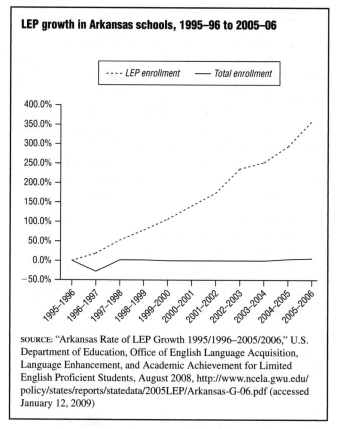

SOURCE: "Arkansas Rate of LEP Growth 1995/1996–2005/2006," U.S. Department of Education, Office of English Language Acquisition, Language Enhancement, and Academic Achievement for Limited English Proficient Students, August 2008, http://www.ncela.gwu.edu/policy/states/reports/statedata/2005LEP/Arkansas-G-06.pdf (accessed January 12, 2009)

FIGURE 6.7

Limited English proficiency (LEP) growth in Iowa schools, 1995–96 to 2005–06

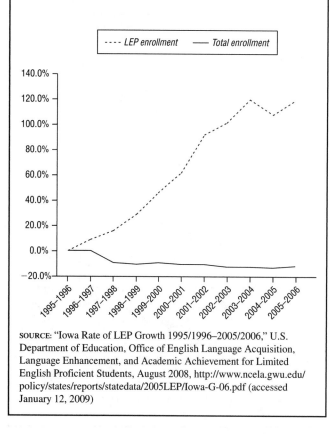

SOURCE: "Iowa Rate of LEP Growth 1995/1996–2005/2006," U.S. Department of Education, Office of English Language Acquisition, Language Enhancement, and Academic Achievement for Limited English Proficient Students, August 2008, http://www.ncela.gwu.edu/policy/states/reports/statedata/2005LEP/Iowa-G-06.pdf (accessed January 12, 2009)

data as of spring 2009 on LEP students and teachers in the nation's public schools. In the 2003–04 academic year 62.9% of all U.S. public schools had LEP students. Nationwide, 10.8% of all public school students were LEP.

Vacancies for English as a second language (ESL) teachers are often difficult to fill. Figure 6.9 reports that 31.4% of public schools nationwide had vacant ESL positions identified as "very difficult" to fill. The only positions more challenging to staff were foreign language teachers in 33.6% of schools. Among all 50 states and the District of Columbia, eight reported more than 50% of schools with difficulty filling vacant ESL teaching positions: Vermont, 70.5%; Delaware, 68.8%; Missouri, 66.9%; Indiana, 59%; Washington, 53.3%; South Dakota, 53.2%; Tennessee, 52.8%; and the District of Columbia, 50.5%.

LEP Students in Iowa

Annual reports of the Iowa Department of Education (2009, http://www.iowa.gov/educate/index.php?option=com_docman&task=cat_view&gid=532&Itemid=55) reveal that total prekindergarten through 12th-grade public school enrollment increased about 2%, from 478,217 in 1992–93 to 487,559 in 2008–09. The share of LEP students increased by 380%, from 4,240 to 20,334 during this same period. Regardless, LEP students represented just 4% of the state's total public school enrollment by the

only to find that many of these teachers were no longer needed when enrollments dropped just as quickly as they rose.

FINDING QUALIFIED ESL TEACHERS. In *Characteristics of Schools, Districts, Teachers, Principals, and School Libraries in the United States: 2003–04 Schools and Staffing Survey* (June 2007, http://nces.ed.gov/pubs2006/2006313.pdf), Gregory A. Strizek et al. offer the most recent national

FIGURE 6.8

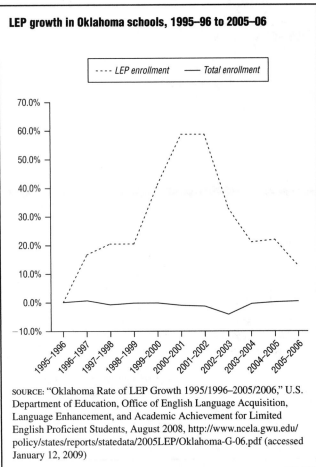

LEP growth in Oklahoma schools, 1995–96 to 2005–06

SOURCE: "Oklahoma Rate of LEP Growth 1995/1996–2005/2006," U.S. Department of Education, Office of English Language Acquisition, Language Enhancement, and Academic Achievement for Limited English Proficient Students, August 2008, http://www.ncela.gwu.edu/policy/states/reports/statedata/2005LEP/Oklahoma-G-06.pdf (accessed January 12, 2009)

2008–09 academic year. Furthermore, the distribution of LEP students was not equal across the state.

In 2008–09 every one of Iowa's public school districts reported having LEP students. Four districts reported LEP students represented more than 25% of their total student populations. Table 6.8 shows that the number of LEP students in the Denison district increased 19.8% in the 10 years from 1992–93 to 2002–03 and then doubled to 39.5% in the 6 years from 2002–03 to 2008–09.

The challenge for Iowa schools was not simply the number of LEP students and the number of languages but also the periodic addition of students who spoke new languages. Table 6.9 shows the addition of new students by language. In the nine years between 1997–98 and 2006–07, an influx of new students arrived in the state who spoke Russian, Serbian, Marshallese, Sudanese, Swahili, Dinka, Somali, Ukrainian, Tagalog, and Sundanese. The schools that received these students had to make quick adaptations to serve the new students.

ADULTS WITH LIMITED ENGLISH PROFICIENCY

Margie McHugh, Julia Gelatt, and Michael Fix state in *Adult English Language Instruction in the United States:*

Determining Need and Investing Wisely (July 2007, http://www.migrationpolicy.org/pubs/NCIIP_English_Instruction073107.pdf) that because the baby-boom generation (people born between 1946 and 1964) is beginning to retire, "the United States cannot afford to have a substantial share of its workforce poorly educated and unable to meet the global economy's escalating demands for high worker productivity. Sustaining productivity and paying health and Social Security bills will require the country's largely younger first- and second-generation immigrant population to succeed in schools and the labor market and be deeply invested in the American community. Investing in an adult English instruction system that can meet the demand for high-quality instruction and allow the nation to meet these challenges is an obvious strategy whose adoption is long overdue."

Even though immigrant children who are enrolled in U.S. schools are taught English, immigrant adults often have more difficulty learning the language. Those who live in communities with other immigrants who speak the same language have less incentive to learn English. In addition, many immigrant adults did not receive basic education in their native country.

The adult literacy organization ProLiteracy notes in *First 100-Day Plan for Adult Literacy in the U.S.* (November 14, 2008, http://www.proliteracy.org/NetCommunity/Document.Doc?id=75), a document that was sent to the transition team of then president-elect Barack Obama (1961–), that 30 million adults have difficulty reading and that another 63 million "have significant gaps in basic literacy skills." The organization suggests that many of the socioeconomic problems in the United States can be linked to "adult low literacy," noting that:

> One-half of the two million immigrants entering the U.S. each year are not literate in their own language. This makes it more difficult for them to gain the English-speaking skills they need to find jobs, advance to better jobs, and maintain safety on the job. Programs that provide these individuals with English-as-a-second-language instruction need support if they are to keep pace with the demand for their services.... Basic literacy, GED preparation, and English-as-a-second-language services are provided by community based organizations (CBOs) and adult basic education (ABE) programs. More than 90 percent of these programs have waiting lists for classroom space or tutors.

English Proficiency Levels of Adult Immigrants

Robert A. Kominski, Hyon B. Shin, and Karen Marotz indicate in *Language Needs of School-Age Children* (2008, http://www.census.gov/population/www/documentation/paa2008/Language-Needs-of-School-Age-Children-PAA-2008.xls) that of adults in the United States who spoke a language other than English at home in 2006, 18.4% spoke English "not well" and 9.9% "not at all." (See Table 6.10.) In *Accessing and Using Language Data from the Census Bureau* (2007, http://www.census.gov/), Deborah H. Grif-

FIGURE 6.9

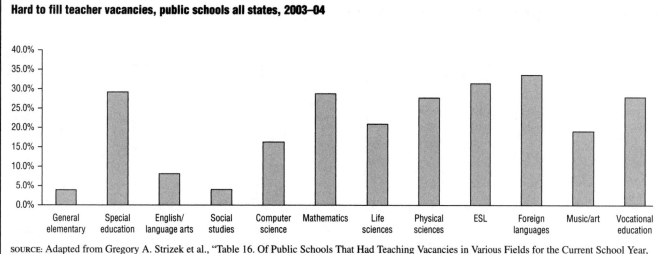

Hard to fill teacher vacancies, public schools all states, 2003–04

SOURCE: Adapted from Gregory A. Strizek et al., "Table 16. Of Public Schools That Had Teaching Vacancies in Various Fields for the Current School Year, Percentage That Found It Very Difficult or Were Not Able to Fill the Vacancies in These Fields, by State: 2003–04," in *Characteristics of Schools, Districts, Teachers, Principals, and School Libraries in the United States: 2003–04 Schools and Staffing Survey,* U.S. Department of Education, National Center for Educational Statistics, 2006, http://nces.ed.gov/surveys/sass/tables/state_2004_16.asp (accessed January 12, 2009)

TABLE 6.8

LEP growth in Iowa public schools and selected districts, 1992–93, 2002–03, and 2008–09

	1992–93	2002–03	2008–09
All public schools	0.9%	3.2%	4.0%
High growth districts			
Postville	0.1%	20.0%	28.3%
Marshalltown	1.6%	21.6%	29.7%
Dension	0.0%	19.8%	39.5%
Storm Lake	13.7%	49.8%	57.1%

SOURCE: Adapted from "1992–1993 Iowa Public School PK–12 Limited English Proficiency (LEP) Students by District and Grade," "2002–2003 Iowa Public School PK–12 Limited English Proficiency (LEP) Students by District and Grade," and "2008–2009 Iowa Public School PK–12 Limited English Proficiency (LEP) Students by District and Grade," Iowa Department of Education, Education Statistics, 2006–08, http://www.iowa.gov/educate/component/option,com_docman/task,cat_view/gid,130/Itemid55/index.php?option=com_docman&task=cat_view&Itemid=99999999&gid=532 (accessed October 9, 2008)

fin and Hyon B. Shin of the Census Bureau note that data on ability to speak English represent the person's own perception about his or her ability to speak the language. Some individuals may feel they get along just fine on limited English or may be embarrassed to admit their limited English language skills. McHugh, Gelatt, and Fix note that individuals may report they speak English well but they cannot read or write in English.

The National Clearing House for English Language Acquisition (April 2006, http://www.ncela.gwu.edu/expert/faq/13adult.html) reports that 1.2 million adults were enrolled in state-administered ESL classes during the 2003–04 academic year. Adult ESL enrollments accounted for 38% of all adult education enrollments in California, 10% in Florida, and 8% in New York. (See Figure 6.10.)

The Cost of Adult ESL

McHugh, Gelatt, and Fix peg the average cost of one hour of language instruction at $10 per immigrant. To bring all current adult legal permanent residents to a level of proficiency needed to pass the naturalization test, the researchers estimate that it would take 277 million hours of English language instruction per year, for six years. An additional 319 million annual hours of instruction, for six years, would be needed to bring all current adult unauthorized immigrants to these levels of English ability.

The Education Department (2008, http://www.ed.gov/about/overview/budget/statetables/09stbyprogram.pdf) notes that Adult Basic and Literacy Education grants to the 50 states, the District of Columbia, American Samoa, Guam, Northern Mariana Islands, Puerto Rico, Virgin Islands, Freely Associated States, and other allocations totaled $496.1 million in 2007 and were estimated at $486.2 million in 2009.

States that experience surges of new immigrants are often challenged to fund adult ESL classes for these new arrivals. For example, the Minnesota Department of Education explains in "Revision to the Minnesota State Plan for Adult Basic Education—2008–2009" (March 25, 2008, http://mnabe.themlc.org/sites/4067033a-d03f-4965-945a-c68493 3b56c4/uploads/State_Plan_revision_3-08_final.doc) that Minnesota has received a large influx of immigrants and refugees from Asia, East Africa, and Mexico. As a result, waiting lists for adult ESL classes have grown. In response to this growth, the Minnesota Department of Education mentions that it was awarded two grants for the 2007–08 school year: $1,250,000 in State ESL Supplemental Aid and $600,000 in the Minnesota Department of Human Services. According to the Education Department, these

TABLE 6.9

Increase in number of languages spoken by students in Iowa schools, 1997–1998, 2006–07 and 2007–08

Language	1997–1998	2006–2007	2007–2008	Percent 2007–2008	Cumulative percent 2007–2008
Spanish	4,885	13,793	14,666	74.2%	74.2%
Vietnamese	776	736	808	4.1	82.4
Bosnian	696	841	804	4.1	78.3
Laotian; Pha Xa Lao	438	456	456	2.3	84.7
Arabic	44	273	317	1.6	86.3
Chinese; Zhongwen	112	214	248	1.3	87.5
Russian	—	190	211	1.1	88.6
Serbian; Srpski	—	193	142	0.7	89.3
Korean; Choson-O	93	118	140	0.7	90.0
Nuer	114	122	139	0.7	90.7
Marshallese	—	78	103	0.5	91.2
German	212	94	87	0.4	91.7
Swahili	—	53	76	0.4	92.1
Dinka	—	46	74	0.4	92.4
Somali	—	66	73	0.4	92.8
Germanic (other)	—	—	71	0.4	93.2
French	20	55	66	0.3	93.5
Ukrainian	—	61	57	0.3	93.8
Tagalog	—	47	54	0.3	94.1
Sundanese	—	50	52	0.3	94.3
Hmong	94	61	—	0.0	94.3
Cambodian; Khmer	108	—	—	0.0	94.3
Thai; Thai Dam	65	—	—	0.0	94.3
Other	425	883	1,120	5.7	100.0
Total	**8,082**	**18,430**	**19,764**	**100.0**	**—**

Note: Table reflects only those languages identified by 50 or more students in a given year.

SOURCE: "Table 6. Iowa's Public and Nonpublic School K–12 English Language Learners' Primary Language, 1997–1998, 2006–2007 and 2007–2008," in *The Annual Condition of Education Report,* Iowa Department of Education, 2008, http://www.iowa.gov/educate/index.php?option=com_docman&task=doc_download&gid=6111 (accessed January 14, 2009)

TABLE 6.10

English speaking ability of population who spoke a language other than English at home, 2006

English speaking ability	Adult population who spoke language other than English at home	Percent of total
Very well	22,803,731	51.3%
Well	9,067,525	20.4%
Not well	8,182,833	18.4%
Not at all	4,421,683	9.9%

Note: Total survey population = 44,475,772.

SOURCE: Adapted from Robert A. Kominski, Hyon B. Shin, and Karen Marotz, "Table 1. Population 5 Years and Older by Language Use and English-Speaking Ability, 2006," in *Language Needs of School-Age Children,* U.S. Census Bureau, 2008, http://www.census.gov/population/www/documentation/paa2008/Language-Needs-of-School-Age-Children-PAA-2008.xls (accessed February 10, 2009)

FIGURE 6.10

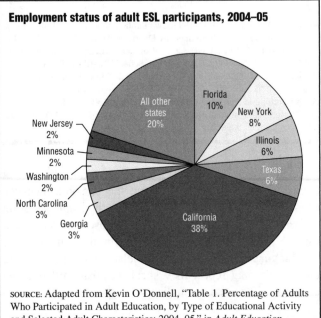

Employment status of adult ESL participants, 2004–05

SOURCE: Adapted from Kevin O'Donnell, "Table 1. Percentage of Adults Who Participated in Adult Education, by Type of Educational Activity and Selected Adult Characteristics: 2004–05," in *Adult Education Participation in 2004–05,* U.S. Department of Education, National Center for Education Statistics, May 2006, http://nces.gov/pubs2006/adulted/tables/table_1.asp (accessed February 10, 2009)

funds were used in conjunction with the $114.6 million federal Adult Basic and Literacy Education grant that Minnesota received in 2007.

COLLEGE TUITION FOR ILLEGAL IMMIGRANTS

According to Eddy Ramírez, in "Should Colleges Enroll Illegal Immigrants?" (*U.S. News and World Report,* August 7, 2008), a proposed federal law—the Development, Relief, and Education for Alien Minors Act (better known as the Dream Act)—would enable undocumented students who have attended U.S. schools and met other conditions to gain legal status and qualify for some college student aid, particularly instate tuition. Typically, the students illegally entered the United States as small children accompanying their parents. The children grew up attending U.S. schools and many excelled. As of March 2009, this act failed to win enough support in Congress, leaving states to cobble together their own policies for handling these students in higher education.

Ramírez notes that "some legal scholars believe the federal government has already made a stand. In 1996, Congress passed [the Illegal Immigration Reform and Immigrant Responsibility Act] barring states from giving unlawful residents 'postsecondary education benefit[s]' that they don't offer to U.S. citizens. But since then, state legislatures in Illinois, Kansas, Nebraska, Utah, and six other states have waived out-of-state tuition fees for illegal immigrant students."

States Deny Tuition to Undocumented Students

Sentiments changed with the declining 2008 economy. Ramírez, indicates that in the summer of 2008, South Carolina became the first state to ban undocumented students from all of its public colleges and universities. In May 2008, North Carolina's community colleges ordered its 58 campuses to stop enrolling undocumented students after the state attorney general said admitting them might violate federal law. Arizona, Colorado, Georgia, and Oklahoma deny instate tuition benefits to illegal immigrants. Supporters of these policies say that scarce education dollars should be spent on making college more affordable for U.S. citizens, not on illegal immigrants.

Martinez v. Regents, the California Case

In 2006 Kris W. Kobach, the senior counsel for the Immigration Law Institute, filed a lawsuit against the University of California, California State University, and the California community college systems on behalf of students paying out-of-state tuition to attend these schools. Their suit alleged that the Illegal Immigration Reform and Immigrant Responsibility Act (IIRIRA) of 1996 prohibits states from favoring illegal immigrants over U.S. citizens. California's tuition rate for out-of-state students is about four times the instate tuition that undocumented students living there are eligible to receive. Testifying before the House Judiciary Committee, Kobach (May 18, 2007, http://judiciary.house .gov/hearings/May2007/Kobach070518.pdf) estimated the cost to California taxpayers at more than $100 million annually to subsidize undocumented students enrolled in the state's public colleges.

Kobach's suit, *Martinez v. Regents* (No. CV 05-2064), claimed violation of the IIRIRA. The plaintiffs argued that U.S. citizens from other states were charged out-of-state tuition, whereas unauthorized immigrant students paid instate tuition. The school's decision to grant instate eligibility to

unauthorized immigrants who lived in the state was initially upheld in an October 2006 decision. In September 2008 the lawsuit was reinstated by a California appeals court and returned to the original court for consideration. A judgment in favor of Kobach and his clients might force California to reimburse out-of-state students and drop its instate tuition policy for illegal immigrants.

REMITTANCES FROM THE UNITED STATES TO LATIN AMERICA

Men and women who leave their homeland for work opportunities in another country often send money home to support family members who remain behind. These funds, called remittances, often support many people. The high volume of remittances have caused organizations such as the Inter-American Development Bank (IDB) to monitor values, survey remittance senders, and publish annual trend reports. In *The Changing Pattern of Remittances: 2008 Survey of Remittances from the United States to Latin America* (April 2008, http://idbdocs.iadb.org/wsdocs/getdocument .aspx?docnum=1418521), the IDB estimates that in 2008, 18.9 million immigrant workers from Latin American countries sent $45.9 billion in remittances and contributed $504.5 billion to the U.S. economy.

Impact on Hispanic Immigrants

According to the IDB, in *Changing Pattern of Remittances*, the economic downturn in the United States caused Hispanic unemployment to rise from 5.2% in 2006 to 7.1% by the first quarter of 2008. In addition, the rising costs of food and fuel cut into remittance funds. The IDB reports that 81% of migrant workers surveyed said finding a good-paying job in 2008 was more difficult than in past years. When asked to describe their financial situation in the United States, 63% of Latin American immigrants said it was good compared with back home.

Decrease in Remittances in 2008

In the press release "Economic Downturns, Inflation Hit Remittances to Latin America" (October 1, 2008, http:// www.iadb.org/news/detail.cfm?language=English&id= 4779), the IDB notes that since 2000 the amount of remittances to Latin America and the Caribbean grew by double digits every year. In fact, these remittances exceeded the amount of overseas development aid and foreign direct investment in the region. However, the IDB indicates these remittances were expected to decrease in value in 2008, attributing this drop to the combined effects of the economic downturn, inflation, and a weaker U.S. dollar.

The IDB estimates in *Changing Pattern of Remittances* that this decline in remittances could drive at least 2 million Latin American families below the poverty level. The impact is projected to be most severe in Mexico and may cause more migrants to leave home in search of work.

FIGURE 6.11

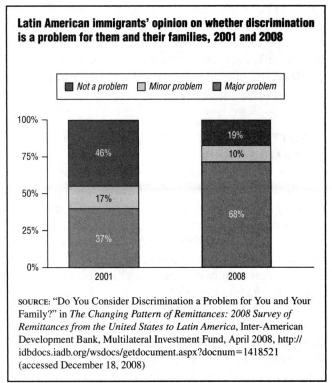

Latin American immigrants' opinion on whether discrimination is a problem for them and their families, 2001 and 2008

SOURCE: "Do You Consider Discrimination a Problem for You and Your Family?" in *The Changing Pattern of Remittances: 2008 Survey of Remittances from the United States to Latin America*, Inter-American Development Bank, Multilateral Investment Fund, April 2008, http://idbdocs.iadb.org/wsdocs/getdocument.aspx?docnum=1418521 (accessed December 18, 2008)

Meanwhile, many immigrant workers in the United States, unable to continue supporting families back home through remittances, considered returning to their home countries. According to the IDB, the problem of declining work opportunities in the United States was compounded by growing anti-immigrant sentiment. The IDB indicates that 68% of migrant workers said discrimination was a major problem for them and their families, compared with 37% in 2001. (See Figure 6.11.) Anti-immigrant sentiment was noted by 51% of those surveyed.

Who Sends Money Home and How Much?

The IDB finds in *Survey of Latin American Immigrants in the United States* (April 30, 2008, http://idbdocs.iadb.org/wsdocs/getdocument.aspx?docnum=1417613) that the average remittance from the United States to Latin America was $325 and that the average immigrant sent money home 15 times per year. In 2008, 50% of immigrants surveyed said they sent money home regularly, compared with 73% in 2006.

According to the IDB, 21% of the remittance senders were U.S. citizens, 32% were legal residents, and 47% were undocumented immigrants. The majority had been in the United States five or more years; only 20% had lived in the United States less than five years. Of employed immigrants surveyed, the greatest share worked in construction (14%). Nearly one out of ten (22%) were homemakers, retired people, or students.

The IDB notes that 56% of migrants lacked a full-time job before coming to the United States. They earned the equivalent of $160 per month in their home countries. Thirty-nine percent of these workers found jobs within two weeks of arriving in the United States. At their first job the migrants earned about $900 per month. This was more than five and a half times what they earned in their home countries.

Table 6.11 shows that immigrants in California sent home the largest dollar volume of remittances in 2008 ($14.6 billion, or 32% of the total remittances sent from the United States). Four states—Virginia, Maryland, Pennsylvania, and Delaware—and the District of Columbia had the highest percentage of remittance senders, at 88%. Close behind were Georgia (85%) and North Carolina (84%), two states that experienced recent surges of new immigrants.

The 2008 economic downturn affected the amount of money immigrants sent home. In *Hispanics and the Economic Downturn: Housing Woes and Remittance Cuts* (January 2009, http://pewhispanic.org/files/reports/100.pdf), a nationwide survey of Hispanics, Mark Hugo Lopez, Gretchen Livingston, and Rakesh Kochhar of the Pew Hispanic Center state that 68% of all Hispanics and 71% of foreign-born Hispanics said they had sent less money home during the past year. (See Figure 6.12.) Even though the amount of money decreased, the share of Hispanic immigrants who said they sent remittances to family back home remained unchanged since 2006.

The Cost of Sending Money Home

Dilip Ratha and William Shaw of the World Bank compare in *South-South Migration and Remittances* (April 2007, http://siteresources.worldbank.org/INTPROSPECTS/Resources/334934-1110315015165/SouthSouthMigrationandRemittances.pdf) the cost of sending a $200 remittance by Western Union, MoneyGram, and other services in various parts of the world. The average cost included a fee plus a percentage of the $200 paid to the sending company and the receiving company. The average cost to send $200 from Los Angeles, California, to Mexico City ranged from $9.49 at Western Union to a low of $5.50 through unidentified other services.

UNDOCUMENTED WORKERS ARE KEY TO BUSINESS CYCLES

In *An Essential Resource: An Analysis of the Economic Impact of Undocumented Workers on Business Activity in the US with Estimated Effects by State and by Industry* (April 2008, http://www.americansforimmigrationreform.com/files/Impact_of_the_Undocumented_Workforce.pdf), the Perryman Group, an economic and financial analysis firm, suggests the United States will suffer $1.8 trillion in lost annual spending and $651.5 billion in lost annual employee output if the undocumented workforce is eliminated. Industries that would suffer include administrative and support services, construction, farming, food services, and manufacturing.

TABLE 6.11

Remittances from the U.S. to Latin America, 2008

[Estimated $ in millions]

State	LAC-born adults (2008, in thousands)	% that send regularly 2006	% that send regularly 2008	Total remittances 2006	Total remittances 2008	Contribution to US economy
California	5,759	63%	52%	13,191	14,599	160,354
Texas	2,799	47%	30%	5,222	4,299	47,220
New York	1,427	77%	53%	3,714	3,933	43,200
Florida	1,354	70%	48%	3,083	3,071	33,732
Illinois	924	73%	58%	2,583	2,813	30,898
New Jersey	704	79%	56%	1,869	1,943	21,342
Georgia	460	85%	53%	1,736	1,443	15,850
Arizona	694	57%	39%	1,378	1,357	14,905
North Carolina	371	84%	59%	1,221	1,243	13,653
Virginia	314	88%	59%	1,110	1,023	11,237
Maryland	261	88%	55%	921	818	8,985
Nevada	311	57%	49%	618	768	8,436
Colorado	325	57%	49%	646	764	8,392
Massachusetts	303	74%	45%	579	654	7,183
Washington	231	70%	44%	504	572	6,283
Connecticut	158	74%	52%	301	434	4,767
Oregon	175	70%	55%	383	431	4,734
Tennessee	139	78%	58%	407	411	4,514
Wisconsin	124	71%	44%	335	399	4,383
Indiana	146	68%	49%	386	389	4,273
Pennsylvania	146	88%	44%	517	370	4,064
New Mexico	186	57%	31%	370	346	3,800
Minnesota	107	71%	58%	292	344	3,778
Michigan	124	71%	49%	337	331	3,636
South Carolina	110	78%	58%	322	325	3,570
Utah	130	57%	31%	258	242	2,658
Alabama	75	78%	57%	219	218	2,394
Oklahoma	114	57%	36%	226	213	2,340
Ohio	79	71%	49%	214	211	2,318
Louisiana	71	78%	57%	208	206	2,263
Rhode Island	68	74%	52%	130	175	1,922
Iowa	52	68%	58%	138	167	1,834
Arkansas	86	78%	46%	253	166	1,823
Kentucky	55	78%	58%	161	163	1,790
Idaho	65	70%	55%	142	160	1,757
Kansas	81	68%	36%	215	152	1,670
Nebraska	58	68%	51%	154	135	1,483
Missouri	63	68%	46%	166	122	1,340
Delaware	44	88%	52%	105	113	1,241
Mississippi	34	78%	57%	100	99	1,087
DC	29	88%	52%	154	75	824
Hawaii	16	70%	49%	34	47	516
Alaska	15	70%	49%	33	44	483
New Hampshire	17	74%	41%	32	40	439
Wyoming	15	70%	51%	33	35	384
Maine	11	74%	41%	22	6	66
South Dakota	9	68%	51%	23	21	231
North Dakota	6	68%	51%	15	14	154
Vermont	5	74%	41%	9	12	132
West Virginia	4	n/a	49%	n/a	11	121
Montana	2	n/a	51%	n/a	5	55
Total 50 states and DC	**18,856**	**73%**	**50%**	**45,276**	**45,932**	**504,513**

Note: LAC = Latin America and the Caribbean.

SOURCE: "Remittances 2008: U.S. To Latin America," in *The Changing Pattern of Remittances: 2008 Survey of Remittances from the United States to Latin America*, Inter-American Development Bank, Multilateral Investment Fund, April 2008, http://idbdocs.iadb.org/wsdocs/getdocument.aspx?docnum=1418521 (accessed December 18, 2008)

Perryman states that "while undocumented workers make up about 5% of the total labor force, short-term undocumented workers account for about 40% of all undocumented workers." Furthermore, Perryman explains that "undocumented immigrants pay sales taxes, property taxes (either explicitly or implicitly through rental outlays) and other types of fiscal levies. On every purchase of taxable goods or services, they are contributing to the fiscal receipts of state and local governments. In states that do not impose a personal income tax (such as Texas, Tennessee, and Florida), these forms of revenue generation are the primary vehicles for obtaining fiscal resources, and undocumented workers are not exempt from payment. Moreover, for many legitimate operations, they are subject to Social Security and other payroll deductions, yet are ineligible for the corresponding benefits."

FIGURE 6.12

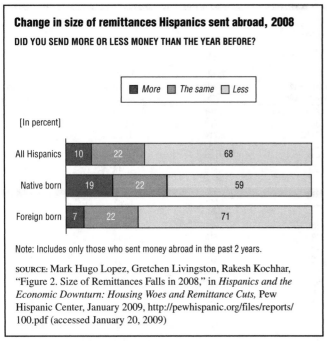

Change in size of remittances Hispanics sent abroad, 2008

DID YOU SEND MORE OR LESS MONEY THAN THE YEAR BEFORE?

Note: Includes only those who sent money abroad in the past 2 years.

SOURCE: Mark Hugo Lopez, Gretchen Livingston, Rakesh Kochhar, "Figure 2. Size of Remittances Falls in 2008," in *Hispanics and the Economic Downturn: Housing Woes and Remittance Cuts,* Pew Hispanic Center, January 2009, http://pewhispanic.org/files/reports/100.pdf (accessed January 20, 2009)

Immigrants, including undocumented workers, have held rallies and marches in major cities across the United States demanding various rights, including the right to stay in America. One such demonstration, the May Day Immigration Rally, has taken place every year since 2006 in New York City. According to Jesse Solomon for CNN.com ("Hundreds Rally in New York for Immigrants' Rights," May 1, 2009, http://www.cnn.com/2009/US/05/01/may .day.rally/index.html?eref=time_us), these immigrants are "calling for workers' rights and a path to citizenship for the country's nearly 12 million undocumented immigrants." Solomon quoted one attendee as saying, "It's about awareness, letting media and America know that we are immigrants and we are the backbone of this country."

Financial Impact of Immigrants in Arkansas

Randy Capps et al. find in *A Profile of Immigrants in Arkansas: Executive Summary* (April 3, 2007, http://www .urban.org/UploadedPDF/411441_Arkansas_complete.pdf) that immigrants generated "a net surplus to the state budget of $19 million—approximately $158 per immigrant." In determining the immigrant population's financial impact on Arkansas, Capps et al. estimate that 123,000 immigrants had about $2.7 billion in after-tax income in 2004. About 20% of this was either sent home as remittances, saved, or used for interest payments. That left $2.9 billion, which the immigrants spent in the state. The costs to the state in education, health services, and law enforcement that related to immigrants totaled an estimated $237 million. Direct and indirect taxes paid by the immigrants amounted to about $257 million. The difference between taxes paid and services received was a $19.4 million surplus to the state.

Capps et al. state that immigrants worked in all major industries, but they were found predominantly in manufacturing and education, health, and social services. The researchers note that educated immigrant workers appeared to earn more than native workers in education, health, and social services. In manufacturing, less-educated immigrants earned less than natives. Mexican and Central American immigrants were less educated than natives, whereas immigrants from Asia, Europe, and other regions (primarily South America and Africa) were more likely than native adults to have high school diplomas.

According to Capps et al., between 1990 and 2000 Arkansas's native-born workforce grew only 15%, whereas the immigrant workforce increased by 201%. The number of native workers in manufacturing decreased by 9,000 (4%) between 1990 and 2000, whereas the number of immigrants rose by 12,000 (294%). The manufacturing sector had been losing jobs since 1995, but immigrants slowed that decline. In 2000 the majority (56%) of immigrants employed in manufacturing worked in poultry or other meat processing. The researchers note that a reported benefit of immigrant workers was the lower cost of their labor, which resulted in lower costs to consumers and aided in the competitiveness of Arkansas's industries.

CHAPTER 7
THE IMPACT OF IMMIGRATION ON THE UNITED STATES IN THE 21ST CENTURY

WHAT WILL THE UNITED STATES LOOK LIKE IN ANOTHER 50 YEARS?

In the press release "An Older and More Diverse Nation by Midcentury" (August 14, 2008, http://www.census.gov/Press-Release/www/releases/archives/population/012496.html), the U.S. Census Bureau states "the nation will be more racially and ethnically diverse, as well as much older, by midcentury.... Minorities, now roughly one-third of the U.S. population, are expected to become the majority in 2042, with the nation projected to be 54 percent minority in 2050." The Census Bureau estimates that the non-Hispanic white population will decrease from 66% of the total U.S. population in 2008 to 46% in 2050. By contrast, the Asian-American population will increase from 5.1% to 9.2% during this same period, as will the African-American population, from 14% to 15%. Hispanics will experience the most growth, however. The Census Bureau projects that the Hispanic population will triple, from 46.7 million in 2008 to 132.8 million in 2050, and that its share of the total population will double, from 15% to 30%. By mid-century, a third of the U.S. population—one out of three U.S. residents—will be Hispanic.

According to Haya El Nasser, in "Counties Feel Impact of Hispanic Immigrants" (*USA Today*, June 29, 2008), Dowell Myers of the University of Southern California said, "For a nation bracing to support 79 million Baby Boomers in their old age, the growing and younger population of Hispanics should be viewed as economic salvation."

LATIN AMERICAN IMPACT

In *Latino Settlement in the New Century* (October 23, 2008, http://pewhispanic.org/files/reports/96.pdf), Richard Fry of the Pew Hispanic Center reports that Latinos account for 50.5% of the U.S. population growth since 2000. Among the top 25 counties with the greatest Hispanic population growth, seven were in Virginia and five in Georgia. (See Table 7.1.) Frederick and Culpepper counties in Virginia

and Paulding County in Georgia experienced greater than 310% growth in Hispanic population between 2000 and 2007. According to Fry, the majority of Hispanic population increase during this period occurred in the South (49%) and the West (35%). The smallest share (6%) of Hispanic growth was in the Northeast.

Fry describes the Latinos in the fastest-growing counties: 35% speak limited English, 38% did not finish high school, and they are "nearly twice as likely as their non-Hispanic neighbors to live in poverty."

Expanding Influence of Spanish Language

The Census Bureau reports in *Statistical Abstract of the United States: 2009* (2008, http://www.census.gov/compendia/statab/2009edition.html) that 54.9 million people living in the United States in 2006 spoke a language other than English at home. Of those who did not speak English at home, 47% spoke Spanish. (See Figure 7.1.) Chinese remained the second most spoken-at-home language (4%).

HISPANIC IMMIGRANTS IN SMALL TOWNS. El Nasser explains that the arrival of Hispanics is revitalizing several small, rural communities that are shrinking because young people are moving away and those who stay behind are getting older and dying. The immigrants are young and their families are growing. In many shrinking towns, Hispanic births now outnumber local deaths. Change does not come without problems, but the immigrants offer hope for the future of many small towns.

The Joint Center for Housing Studies of Harvard University finds in *The State of the Nation's Housing 2008* (2008, http://www.jchs.harvard.edu/publications/markets/son2008/son2008.pdf) that "international migrants are settling in locations where the foreign-born share of the population is relatively low." The center notes that the foreign immigrants fill voids left by young natives who have moved to cities by taking jobs, buying houses, and keeping

TABLE 7.1

U.S. counties with largest Hispanic population growth, 2000–07

County	State	2000 to 2007 Hispanic population growth (in %)	2000 to 2007 Hispanic population growth rank	2007 Hispanic population
Frederick County	Virginia	335	1	4,371
Culpeper County	Virginia	312	2	3,533
Paulding County	Georgia	306	3	5,677
Kendall County	Illinois	279	4	15,466
Henry County	Georgia	243	5	9,240
Fauquier County	Virginia	240	6	3,791
Barrow County	Georgia	239	7	4,946
Luzerne County	Pennsylvania	222	8	11,971
Newton County	Georgia	214	9	3,628
Spotsylvania County	Virginia	208	10	7,800
Stafford County	Virginia	203	11	10,139
Wapello County	Iowa	202	12	2,413
Loudoun County	Virginia	183	13	28,529
Flagler County	Florida	180	14	7,108
Frederick County	Maryland	177	15	12,900
Douglas County	Georgia	174	16	7,235
Berkeley County	West Virginia	171	17	3,127
Lake County	Florida	163	18	31,071
Robertson County	Tennessee	161	19	3,782
Hamilton County	Indiana	158	20	7,518
Delaware County	Ohio	157	21	2,853
Jefferson County	West Virginia	155	22	1,871
Prince William County	Virginia	153	23	69,222
St. Lucie County	Florida	152	24	39,695
Lancaster County	South Carolina	151	25	2,453

Note: Based on the 1,362 counties with at least 1,000 Hispanics in 2007.

SOURCE: Adapted from Richard Fry, "Table 4.25 Counties with Largest Hispanic Population Growth, 2000 to 2007," in *Latino Settlement in the New Century*, Pew Hispanic Center, October 23, 2008, http://pewhispanic.org/files/reports/96.pdf (accessed January 6, 2009)

FIGURE 7.1

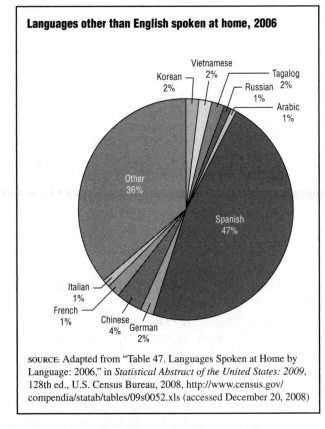

Languages other than English spoken at home, 2006

SOURCE: Adapted from "Table 47. Languages Spoken at Home by Language: 2006," in *Statistical Abstract of the United States: 2009*, 128th ed., U.S. Census Bureau, 2008, http://www.census.gov/compendia/statab/tables/09s0052.xls (accessed December 20, 2008)

up school enrollments. The economically competitive environments and desirable climates of the South and West are projected to continue to attract both international and domestic migrants. According to the center, foreign-born migrants will spread into more housing markets that have been abandoned by young native workers and families.

Like the rest of the country, native-born and immigrant Hispanics who own homes have been affected by the economic downturn that began in 2008. Mark Hugo Lopez, Gretchen Livingston, and Rakesh Kochhar of the Pew Hispanic Center indicate in *Hispanics and the Economic Downturn: Housing Woes and Remittance Cuts* (January 2009, http://pewhispanic.org/files/reports/100.pdf) that in 2008, 15% of native-born Hispanics worried a lot about foreclosure, compared with 39% of foreign-born Hispanics. Sixty-two percent of all Hispanics surveyed reported foreclosures in their neighborhood in the past year. Nine percent reported missing a mortgage payment or making only partial payment and 3% had received a foreclosure notice.

Immigration Energizes the Catholic Church

According to David Rieff, in "Nuevo Catholics" (*New York Times Magazine*, December 24, 2006), Hispanic immigrants are leading a nationwide resurgence of the Catholic Church. He mentions a Catholic church in Smyrna, Georgia, where Hispanic immigration has been a recent phenomenon. The church offers three out of seven Sunday masses in Spanish. Rieff states, "Today, more than 40 percent of the Hispanics residing in the United States, legally and illegally, are foreign-born, and the fate of the American Catholic Church has become inextricably intertwined with the fate of these immigrants and their descendants."

FINDING SPANISH-SPEAKING PRIESTS. The new challenge is finding enough priests. According to Rieff, attendance at Mass dropped from 74% in 1958 to 25% in 2000 among self-identified Catholics. Half of all Catholic high schools had closed by 2002, and the number of seminarians preparing for the priesthood fell from 49,000 in 1965 to 4,700 in 2002.

The Catholic Church has been forced to search outside the United States to find priests, particularly those able to speak Spanish. In "Serving U.S. Parishes, Fathers without Borders" (*New York Times*, December 28, 2008), Laurie Goodstein reports that the 2006 study "International Priests in America" estimated that one out of six priests serving in American dioceses and one-third of students in American Catholic seminaries were foreign born.

In Owensboro, Kentucky, an estimated 10,000 of the 60,000 Catholics in the diocese population spoke Spanish in 2008. Most of those who spoke Spanish were part of an influx of immigrants who came to work at poultry plants or in construction jobs beginning in the late 1990s. With a Spanish-speaking population south of the U.S. border eager to immigrate, recruiting priests would seem to be a simple task. However, the shortage of priests is worse in Mexico and Central and South America. According to Goodstein, those regions "have one priest for about every 7,000 Catholics; the United States has one for every 1,500." As a result, bishops in Mexico and Latin America are rarely willing to give up their priests.

Goodstein profiles Father Darrell Venters, who recruits priests to serve rural churches in the Owensboro region. In recent years Father Venters has turned to Africa and Asia to supply his pulpits. Between March 2006 and June 2007 he welcomed six priests from India. He also has had success bringing priests from Kenya, Nigeria, and Uganda.

ATTRACTING FOREIGN PRIESTS. Some dioceses pay foreign priests less than American priests, but in Owensboro they all receive the same $1,350 per month base salary. They can earn additional income for special request Masses, weddings, and baptisms. The pay exceeds anything the priests could earn in their home countries and helps support their families back home.

In *Catholic Ministry Formation Enrollments: Statistical Overview for 2007–2008* (April 2008, http://cara.georgetown.edu/Overview0708.pdf), Mary L. Gautier of the Center for Applied Research in the Apostolate (CARA) notes that in 2008 about four out of ten seminary students in the United States were part of a minority group. (See Figure 7.2.) Fifteen percent were Hispanic/Latino, 12% Asian-American, and 5%

African-American. In the 2007–08 academic year, 27% of students in Catholic seminaries were foreign born, compared with 23% in 2005–06.

CHALLENGES IN THE IMMIGRATION MICROCOSM: NEW YORK CITY

The New York City Department of City Planning states in *Proposed Consolidated Plan, Annual Performance Report 2007* (March 12, 2008, http://home2.nyc.gov/html/dcp/pdf/pub/affh2007.pdf) that with more than 3 million foreign-born residents, "New York City has the largest immigrant population of any city in the United States." In 2006, 37% of the city's population was foreign born and represented approximately 200 ethnic groups.

The Department of City Planning notes that in 2006 nearly 1.6 million of the city's 3 million foreign-born people were naturalized citizens. Furthermore, the immigrants tended to be younger than the general population. According to the department, "The median age for recent immigrants to New York City in the 2000–2006 period was 30 years, well below the figure of 36 years for the general population reported in the 2006 American Community Survey.... Eighteen percent of immigrants were 18 to 24 years of age compared to 9 percent for the general population of the city. Forty-seven percent of all immigrants to the city were 25 to 44 years of age compared to 31 percent for the general population."

New immigrant arrivals were more likely to work in the service industry (35%), compared with 22% of all city workers. By contrast, 35% of all city workers were employed in management and professional occupations, compared with 19% of immigrants.

Communicating in Many Languages

In *Proposed Consolidated Plan*, the Department of City Planning suggests that one measure of the impact of immigrant communities is how many of its residents speak a language other than English at home. Over 3.7 million people in New York City (45% of the entire city population aged five and older) spoke a language other than English at home in 2006. Nearly half (1.8 million) were not proficient in English. Among all people who spoke a language other than English at home, 1.9 million spoke Spanish and 515,000 spoke an Asian or Pacific Island language. The most frequent languages into which New York City documents were translated were Spanish, Chinese, Russian, French, Haitian Creole, Korean, Polish, and Urdu.

Bangladesh was the top country of origin for New York City immigrants followed by the former Soviet Union. The department cites growing numbers of immigrants from Nigeria, Ghana, and Mexico and refugees from Serbia and Montenegro.

FIGURE 7.2

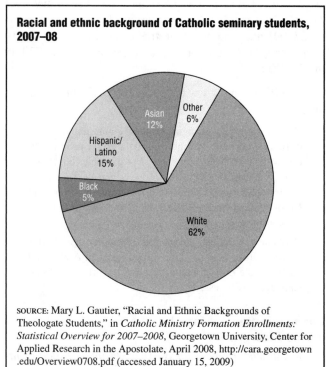

Racial and ethnic background of Catholic seminary students, 2007–08

Asian 12%
Other 6%
Hispanic/Latino 15%
Black 5%
White 62%

SOURCE: Mary L. Gautier, "Racial and Ethnic Backgrounds of Theologate Students," in *Catholic Ministry Formation Enrollments: Statistical Overview for 2007–2008*, Georgetown University, Center for Applied Research in the Apostolate, April 2008, http://cara.georgetown.edu/Overview0708.pdf (accessed January 15, 2009)

Learning the Ways of a New Culture

Immigrants face challenges beyond language barriers in adjusting to the culture of their new country. They can become victims of discrimination and exploitation because they do not understand U.S. laws and standards. Immigrants often do not seek help because they feel unwelcome outside their own community or, based on experiences in their homeland, do not trust government officials. New York City attempts to address these problems in a variety of ways.

For example, the Mayor's Office of Immigrant Affairs (2009, http://www.nyc.gov/html/imm/html/about/about.shtml) "promotes the well-being of immigrant communities by recommending policies and programs that facilitate successful integration of immigrant New Yorkers into the civic, economic, and cultural life of the City."

The New York City Commission on Human Rights offers extensive education programs for immigrants regarding fair housing—the right of people to housing opportunity without regard to their sex, religion, age, or familial status (according to federal law); or to marital status, citizenship status, sexual orientation, or lawful occupation (according to the New York City Human Rights Law). The Neighborhood Human Rights Program works to foster positive relations among residents of diverse racial, ethnic, and religious backgrounds. It offers mediation and conflict resolution services through community service centers.

Language Barriers in Health Care

In September 2006 the New York State Department of Health implemented new regulations requiring all hospitals to provide a language assistance program for all patients. Larry Tung reports in "Language Barrier Begins to Fall at City Hospitals" (July 2008, http://www.gothamgazette.com/article/immigrants/20080722/11/2589) that the regulations require language assistance within 10 minutes of a request for emergency patients and within 20 minutes for other patients. Hospitals must "provide translations and transcriptions of important hospital forms and instructions in any language spoken by more than 1 percent of people in the medical center's service area." According to Tung, Stefanie Tice of the Office of Culturally and Linguistically Appropriate Services described the challenge that New York City hospitals face: "Last year we had requests for interpretation in 118 languages."

The Equitable and Effective Government Initiative (EEGI) of New York City evaluated the effects of the new language assistance requirements in 10 city hospitals and reported the findings in *Now We're Talking: A Study on Language Assistance Services at Ten New York City Public and Private Hospitals* (April 2008, http://www.maketheroad.org/pix_reports/Now%20Were%20Talking%20Report%20Final.pdf). The EEGI indicates that it surveyed 617 patients whose primary language was Spanish or Korean and who were identified as limited English proficient. In a 2004–06 study, 29% of patients surveyed "reported they were able to communicate in their primary language with their doctor or staff." In 2008, 79% of patients surveyed in the same hospitals said they "received hospital-based interpretation by a bilingual doctor, nurse, staff interpreter and/or telephonic interpretation."

The EEGI finds that hospitals were better prepared to assist Spanish-speaking patients than those who spoke other languages. Two hospitals were evaluated in the borough of Queens, where 3% of the population was Korean. Patient surveys revealed that 65% of Spanish-speaking patients "received some form of hospital-based interpretation service," compared with 25% of Korean-speaking patients. According to the EEGI, more forms were available in Spanish than in Korean but there were still many not available in Spanish. Only 13% of all limited-English-proficient patients in the survey signed hospital forms written in their own language.

IMMIGRATION SPAWNS MULTILINGUAL JOB OPPORTUNITIES

The Bureau of Labor Statistics (BLS; December 18, 2007, http://www.bls.gov/oco/ocos175.htm) projects that jobs for translators and interpreters (sign language for people who are deaf or hard of hearing) will increase 24% between 2006 and 2016. According to the BLS, growth in jobs for translators and interpreters will be driven partly by a strong demand in health care and homeland security. The increasing number of foreign-language speakers in the United States, because of tourism and international business and political conferences, will also require more translators. In 2006, 33% of interpreters and translators were employed in public and private education. (See Figure 7.3.) The BLS (April 3, 2008, http://www.bls.gov/oes/current/oes273091.htm) reports that the mean (average) hourly wage for salaried interpreters and translators was $20.05 in May 2007.

The BLS (http://www.bls.gov/oco/ocos175.htm) explains that:

> Current events and changing political environments, often difficult to foresee, will increase the need for people who can work with other languages. For example, homeland security needs are expected to drive increasing demand for interpreters and translators of Middle Eastern and North African languages, primarily in Federal Government agencies.
>
> Demand will remain strong for translators of . . . Portuguese, French, Italian, German, and Spanish; Arabic and other Middle Eastern languages; and the principal Asian languages—Chinese, Japanese, and Korean.

Communicating in Many Languages during Emergencies

In *Disaster Preparedness in Urban Immigration Communities: Lessons Learned from Recent Catastrophic Events*

FIGURE 7.3

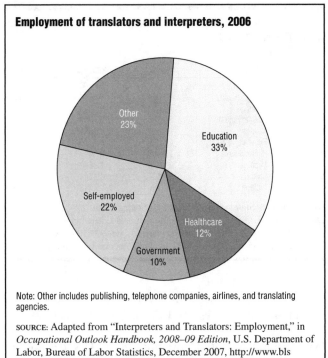

Employment of translators and interpreters, 2006

Other 23%
Education 33%
Self-employed 22%
Healthcare 12%
Government 10%

Note: Other includes publishing, telephone companies, airlines, and translating agencies.

SOURCE: Adapted from "Interpreters and Translators: Employment," in *Occupational Outlook Handbook, 2008–09 Edition*, U.S. Department of Labor, Bureau of Labor Statistics, December 2007, http://www.bls .gov/oco/ocos175.htm (accessed January 7, 2008)

and Their Relevance to Latino and Asian Communities in Southern California (June 2008, http://demographics.apalc .org/wp-content/uploads/2008/07/disaster-report_final.pdf), Ann Bessie Mathew and Kimiko Kelly focus on the Los Angeles area of Southern California, another region with diverse populations speaking many languages. Mathew and Kelly indicate that little has been done to ensure that large populations of immigrants with limited English proficiency have access to information on how to prepare for and survive a major disaster. Information for their study was gathered using Hispanic and Asian focus groups. Mathew and Kelly find that:

- Most local government and nonprofit relief organizations fail to offer "culturally sensitive disaster preparedness education in languages that reflect the demographics of the populations being served."

- Ability to provide emergency information in diverse languages is lacking. Latino, Chinese, and Vietnamese focus groups said they rely on native language radio stations for emergency information. Plans to communicate press releases in various languages other than in English have not been established.

- First responders (police, firefighters, and medical personnel) and nonprofit relief agencies often rely on bilingual bystanders or children in emergency response rather than on translators.

- No mechanisms are in place to ensure both legal and undocumented immigrants that immigration status is not considered when providing emergency services in a disaster.

The Centers for Disease Control and Prevention, however, took measures to disseminate information and instruction to non-English speakers during the spring 2009 outbreak of the H1N1 flu virus (swine flu), providing information in Spanish on how to manage the virus via its Web site ("Influenza H1N1," May 4, 2009, http://www.cdc.gov/ h1n1flu/espanol/).

IMMIGRANT ENTREPRENEURS CONTRIBUTE TO THE U.S. ECONOMY

In *America's New Immigrant Entrepreneurs: Part I* (January 4, 2007, http://www.kauffman.org/uploadedfiles/ entrep_immigrants_1_61207.pdf), Vivek Wadhwa et al. note that immigrants were among the key founders of "25.3% of all engineering and technology companies established in the U.S. between 1995 and 2005." These companies employed roughly 450,000 people and generated $52 billion in sales.

In a similar study, Wadhwa et al. find in *Education, Entrepreneurship, and Immigration: America's New Immigrant Entrepreneurs, Part II* (June 11, 2007, http://www .kauffman.org/uploadedfiles/entrep_immigrants_2_61207 .pdf) that "52.3 percent of immigrant founders initially came to the United States primarily for higher education [and] 39.8 percent entered the country because of a job opportunity."

The article "The World's Billionaires" (Forbes.com, March 11, 2009) offers examples of immigrant entrepreneurs:

- The German-born Andreas von Bechtolsheim (1955–) and the Indian-born Vinod Khosla (1955–) were among the four founders of Sun Microsystems. They built the company using "Bechtolsheim's computer networking technology. Today, Sun employs 34,600 people worldwide and reported $13 billion in revenues [in 2008]."

- Liz Claiborne (1929–2007) was a dressmaker from Belgium who designed clothes for working women and built a business with over 40 brands. In 2009 her company was worth nearly $5 billion.

- Jerry Yang (1968–) immigrated from Taiwan, studied at Stanford University, and cofounded Yahoo!, which was worth $43 billion in 2009.

U.S. SCHOOLS EDUCATING FOREIGN STUDENTS

The Institute of International Education (IIE) notes in *Open Doors 2008 "Fast Facts"* (November 17, 2008, http:// www.opendoors.iienetwork.org/) that enrollments of international students at U.S. colleges and universities increased steadily over the past 54 years from 30,000 students in the 1953–54 academic year to 623,805 students in 2007–08. (See Figure 7.4.)

According to the IIE, the University of Southern California attracted the most international students with 7,189

FIGURE 7.4

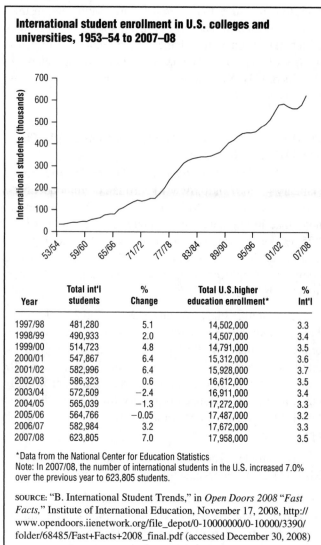

International student enrollment in U.S. colleges and universities, 1953–54 to 2007–08

Year	Total int'l students	% Change	Total U.S.higher education enrollment*	% Int'l
1997/98	481,280	5.1	14,502,000	3.3
1998/99	490,933	2.0	14,507,000	3.4
1999/00	514,723	4.8	14,791,000	3.5
2000/01	547,867	6.4	15,312,000	3.6
2001/02	582,996	6.4	15,928,000	3.7
2002/03	586,323	0.6	16,612,000	3.5
2003/04	572,509	−2.4	16,911,000	3.4
2004/05	565,039	−1.3	17,272,000	3.3
2005/06	564,766	−0.05	17,487,000	3.2
2006/07	582,984	3.2	17,672,000	3.3
2007/08	623,805	7.0	17,958,000	3.5

*Data from the National Center for Education Statistics
Note: In 2007/08, the number of international students in the U.S. increased 7.0% over the previous year to 623,805 students.

SOURCE: "B. International Student Trends," in *Open Doors 2008 "Fast Facts,"* Institute of International Education, November 17, 2008, http://www.opendoors.iienetwork.org/file_depot/0-10000000/0-10000/3390/folder/68485/Fast+Facts+2008_final.pdf (accessed December 30, 2008)

TABLE 7.2

States with the most international college and university students, 2006–07 and 2007–08

Rank	U.S. state	2006/07	2007/08	% change
1	California	77,987	84,800	8.7
2	New York	65,884	69,844	6.0
3	Texas	49,081	51,824	5.6
4	Massachusetts	28,680	31,817	10.9
5	Illinois	25,594	28,804	12.5
6	Florida	26,875	26,739	−0.5
7	Pennsylvania	23,182	26,090	12.5
8	Michigan	21,143	22,857	8.1
9	Ohio	18,607	19,343	4.0
10	Indiana	14,450	15,548	7.6

SOURCE: "F. U.S. States with the Most Int'l Students, 2007/08," in *Open Doors 2008 "Fast Facts,"* Institute of International Education, November 17, 2008, http://www.opendoors.iienetwork.org/file_depot/0-10000000/0-10000/3390/folder/68485/Fast+Facts+2008_final.pdf (accessed December 30, 2008)

physical sciences (9.6%), whereas U.S. students went abroad to study social sciences (21.4%) and humanities (13.2%).

Do Foreign Students Contribute to the U.S. Economy?

The IIE reports in "Economic Impact of International Students" (November 17, 2008, http://opendoors.iienetwork.org/file_depot/0-10000000/0-10000/3390/folder/77606/Economic+Impact.pdf) that international students contributed $15.5 billion to the U.S. economy in 2007–08. This figure included $10.6 billion in tuition and fees paid by the students, plus $10.9 billion in living expenses the students paid for themselves and their dependents. Funding provided by universities or other U.S. sources represented a 30% deduction from the total amount foreign students spent on their education in the United States.

David North of the Center for Immigration Studies disputes this IIE assessment. In *Who Pays? Foreign Students Do Not Help with the Balance of Payments* (June 2008, http://www.cis.org/articles/2008/back608.pdf), he argues that the IIE information is gathered, not directly from students, but from university advisers who offer estimates related to the foreign student population.

North suggests a more accurate study is *Doctorate Recipients from United States Universities: Summary Report 2006* (2007, http://www.norc.org/NR/rdonlyres/C22A3F40-0BA2-4993-A6D3-5E65939EEDC3/0/06SRRevised.pdf) by Thomas B. Hoffer et al. of the National Opinion Research Center. This report is based on a survey of all doctoral recipients in a given year. Table 7.4 compares the results of Hoffer et al.'s survey with the IIE's 2006–07 survey. Hoffer et al. find (Section A of Table 7.4) that U.S. citizens paid 30% of their own doctoral educational costs and their universities funded 64.4% of the expense. Permanent Resident Aliens paid 15.9% of educational expenses and received 82.8% of funding from the university. Temporary Visa Aliens paid just 5.3% of their own educational expenses. The IIE reports (Section B of Table 7.4) that

enrolled for the 2007–08 academic year. California hosted a total of 84,800 students from other countries. New York ranked second with 69,844 international students. The largest growth in foreign students occurred in Illinois and Pennsylvania, which both experienced a 12.5% increase over their 2006–07 enrollments. (See Table 7.2.) The top four countries of birth for international students in the United States were India, China, South Korea, and Japan. Students from these countries represented 45% of all foreign college students studying in the United States in 2007–08.

The number of U.S. students studying abroad grew at a similar pace to that of foreign students studying in the United States. (See Figure 7.5 and Figure 7.4.) However, the number of U.S. students studying abroad (241,791) in 2006–07 was less than half the 582,984 international students studying in the United States during the same academic year. Business and management programs attracted nearly equal shares of international students (19.2%) and U.S. students studying abroad (19.1%). (See Table 7.3.) International students were more likely to enroll in engineering (16.5%) and

FIGURE 7.5

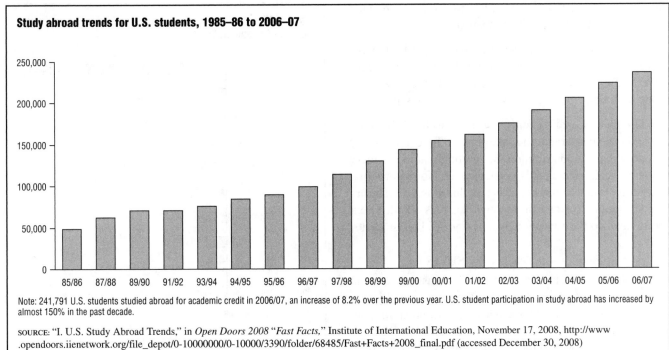

Study abroad trends for U.S. students, 1985–86 to 2006–07

Note: 241,791 U.S. students studied abroad for academic credit in 2006/07, an increase of 8.2% over the previous year. U.S. student participation in study abroad has increased by almost 150% in the past decade.

SOURCE: "I. U.S. Study Abroad Trends," in *Open Doors 2008 "Fast Facts,"* Institute of International Education, November 17, 2008, http://www.opendoors.iienetwork.org/file_depot/0-10000000/0-10000/3390/folder/68485/Fast+Facts+2008_final.pdf (accessed December 30, 2008)

TABLE 7.3

Top fields of study for international students enrolled in U.S. colleges and universities, 2006–07

Top fields of study of international students in the U.S., 2006/07	Percent of total 06/07
Business & management	19.2%
Engineering	16.5%
Physical & life sciences	9.6%
Social sciences	9.1%
Math & computer sciences	8.5%
Fine & applied arts	5.5%
Health professions	5.2%
Intensive English language	4.2%
Education	3.1%
Humanities	3.0%
Agriculture	1.4%
Other	11.0%
Undeclared	3.4%
Top fields of study of U.S. students studying abroad, 2006/07	
Social sciences	21.4%
Business & management	19.1%
Humanities	13.2%
Fine & applied arts	7.7%
Physical & life sciences	7.3%
Foreign languages	7.2%
Education	4.2%
Health sciences	4.1%
Engineering	3.1%
Math & computer sciences	1.5%
Agriculture	1.5%
Other	6.6%
Undeclared	3.1%

Note: Students enrolled in other fields of study and students without declared majors are not reported.

SOURCE: Adapted from "G. Top Fields of Study of Currently Enrolled International Students, 2006/07 and 2007/08," and "L. Fields of Study of U.S. Study Abroad Students, 2005/06 and 2006/07," in *Open Doors 2008 "Fast Facts,"* Institute of International Education, November 17, 2008, http://www.opendoors.iienetwork.org/file_depot/0-10000000/0-10000/3390/folder/68485/Fast+Facts+2008_final.pdf (accessed December 30, 2008)

TABLE 7.4

Primary source of funding for foreign and domestic university students in the United States, 2006

A. Doctoral recipients

Civil status and numbers	U.S. citizens (25,301)	Permanent resident aliens (1,688)	Temporary visa aliens (13,164)
Primary source of support			
Own resources	30.0%	15.9%	5.3%
U.S. university	64.4%	82.8 %	90.7%
Other and unclassified	5.6%	1.3%	4.0%

Surveyed population	Individuals receiving U.S. doctorates, 2006
Nature of data	First-hand estimates of the individuals' own finances
Response rate	88.3% in 2006

B. International students generally

Civil status and numbers	Doctoral candidates (341,971)	All others (240,648)
Primary source of support		
Personal, family, and other overseas	55.2%	83.5%
U.S. sources	43.5%	16.4%
Other	13%	0.1 %

Surveyed population	International student advisers at U.S. universities
Nature of data	Second-hand estimates of the finances of International at their Institutions made by the advisers
Response rate	52.5% in 2006–2007, lower in earlier years

SOURCE: David North, "Exhibit 1. Primary Source of Financial Support for Various Groups of University Students (Foreign & Domestic) in the U.S.," in *Who Pays? Foreign Students Do Not Help with the Balance of Payments,* Center for Immigration Studies, June 2008, http://www.cis.org/foreign_students.html (accessed December 30, 2008). Data from T.B. Hoffer, M. Hess, V. Welch, and K. Williams, *Doctorate Recipients from United States Universities: Summary Report, 2006,* National Opinion Research Center, 2007.

---

international doctoral candidates paid 55.2% of their own educational costs, whereas international students in other college programs paid 83.5% of their own expenses.

Besides the lack of specific data obtained by the IIE survey method, North states that the IIE study overlooks government subsidies to state schools and endowments made by foundations and individuals to private schools.

Do international students contribute to the U.S. economy? Those who remain to take jobs in the United States certainly make a contribution. Suggesting that the primary value of foreign students is noneconomic, North notes that educating future foreign leaders builds positive international relationships and that foreign students add different worldviews to the educational experience of U.S. students.

Foreign Student Visas Tracked by SEVIS

Within the U.S. Immigration and Customs Enforcement (ICE) the Student and Exchange Visitor Information System (SEVIS) monitors the status and activities of nonimmigrant students and exchange visitors who enter the United States. ICE uses SEVIS to monitor foreign students who have been issued visas to attend U.S. schools. ICE notes in *Student and Exchange Visitor Information System, General Summary Quarterly Review* (January 15, 2008, http://www.ice.gov/doclib/sevis/pdf/quarterly_report_jan08.pdf) that for the quarter ending December 31, 2007, SEVIS reported 673,761 active students with F (academic) and M (vocational) visas enrolled in approved schools. The majority (69%) of these students were enrolled in college-level programs. The 271 students enrolled in high schools, the 25,027 in secondary schools, and the 4,627 in primary (elementary) schools represented just 4% of total F and M visa students. (See Figure 7.6.) SEVIS tracking includes students attending flight training schools (4,612) and other vocational programs (2,872).

The numbers of students reported by SEVIS differ from those reported by the IIE in *Open Doors 2008*. The SEVIS report tallies only students with F and M visas attending schools that have been approved for foreign students. Colleges and universities also admit students holding J (exchange visitor) visas and other visa categories. For example, a person with a work visa might enroll for part-time education. This person would be counted by the IIE but not by SEVIS.

National Foundation for American Policy Studies Technology Jobs

According to the National Foundation for American Policy (NFAP), in *H-1B Visas and Job Creation* (March 2008, http://www.nfap.com/pdf/080311h1b.pdf), "for every H-1B position requested, U.S. technology companies increase their employment by 5 workers." As described in Chapter 3, the H1B program allows employers to temporarily employ foreign workers on a nonimmigrant basis in a specialty occupation or as a model of distinguished merit

FIGURE 7.6

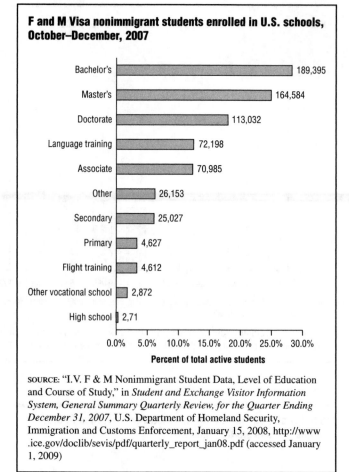

F and M Visa nonimmigrant students enrolled in U.S. schools, October–December, 2007

SOURCE: "I.V. F & M Nonimmigrant Student Data, Level of Education and Course of Study," in *Student and Exchange Visitor Information System, General Summary Quarterly Review, for the Quarter Ending December 31, 2007*, U.S. Department of Homeland Security, Immigration and Customs Enforcement, January 15, 2008, http://www.ice.gov/doclib/sevis/pdf/quarterly_report_jan08.pdf (accessed January 1, 2009)

and ability. The NFAP notes that critics of the H1B program allege companies fire U.S. employees to replace them with cheaper H1B workers, a concern that was heightened in the economic downturn in the United States in 2008 and 2009. However, the federal government requires that H1B workers receive "the *higher* of the prevailing wage or the actual wage paid to similarly employed Americans." In addition, employers pay an estimated $6,000 in legal and government fees per H1B worker. The NFAP indicates that employer costs could increase as much as $12,000 to sponsor the employee for permanent residence.

BRING WORKERS TO THE UNITED STATES OR SEND WORK OUT OF THE COUNTRY? The NFAP reports in *H-1B Visas and Job Creation* that the low annual limit on available H1B visas could cause U.S. companies to send work to other countries, either by contract or by opening offshore facilities. Seventy-four percent of companies responding to the survey said a lack of H1B workers might affect the company's international competitiveness.

The NFAP cites Google as an example of a technology company that needs H1B workers. In 2008 about 8% of the company's U.S. workforce consisted of H1B workers who came from over 80 countries. Laszlo Bock (June 6, 2007, http://judiciary.house.gov/hearings/printers/110th/35858.PDF), the Google vice president for people operations, testified before the House Judiciary Immigration Subcommittee on Immigration, Citizenship, Refugees, Border Security, and International Law in 2007. He discussed the need for hiring foreign nationals and particularly foreign students who gain their education in the United States, and said, "Simply put, if U.S. employers are unable to hire those who are graduating from our universities, foreign competitors will. The U.S. scientific, engineering, and tech communities cannot hope to maintain their present position of international leadership if they are unable to hire and retain highly educated foreign talent. We also cannot hope to grow our economy and create more jobs if we are ceding leadership in innovation to other nations."

U.S. COMPETITIVENESS IN SCIENCE AND TECHNOLOGY

Titus Galama and James Hosek explain in *U.S. Competitiveness in Science and Technology* (2008, http://www.rand.org/pubs/monographs/2008/RAND_MG674.pdf):

The United States accounts for 40 percent of total world [research and development] spending and 38 percent of patented new technology inventions by the industrialized nations of the Organisation for Economic Co-operation and Development (OECD), employs 37 percent (1.3 million) of OECD researchers (FTE), produces 35 percent, 49 percent, and 63 percent, respectively, of total world publications, citations, and highly cited publications, employs 70 percent of the world's Nobel Prize winners and 66 percent of its most-cited individuals, and is the home to 75 percent of both the world's top 20 and top 40 universities and 58 percent of the top 100.

The researchers conclude:

Our assessment of the measures we have examined indicates that the U.S. S&T [science and technology] enterprise is performing well. We find that the United States leads the world in S&T and has kept pace or grown faster than the rest of the world in many measures of S&T. Although developing nations such as China, India, and South Korea showed rapid growth in S&T, these nations still account for a small share of world innovation and scientific output. Furthermore, we find that the consequences of the globalization of S&T and the rise of S&T capability in other nations are more likely to be economically beneficial to the United States than harmful. We also find that the United States has continued to invest in its S&T infrastructure and that the S&E [science and engineering] workforce has managed to keep up with the demand for highly skilled S&E workers through immigration.

Will U.S. Students Fill the United States' Future Jobs?

Galama and Hosek offer a key observation: "However, there are potential weaknesses in the persistent underperformance of older K–12 students in math and science, in the limited attractiveness of S&E careers to U.S. students, and in the heavy focus of federal research funding on the life sciences, and we do not yet fully understand the consequences of an increasing reliance on foreign-born workers in S&E."

U.S. RELIANCE ON FOREIGN-BORN WORKERS IN SCIENCE AND ENGINEERING

In "Workforce Competitiveness in a Global Economy" (December 11, 2007, http://montevideo.usembassy.gov/usaweb/2007/07-513bEN.shtml), a speech before the Chamber of Commerce in Uruguay, the former U.S. secretary of labor Elaine Chao (1953–) projects the United States' needs in high-growth jobs for the coming decade: "Between 2006 and 2016...our country will need 2.8 million healthcare professionals, and over 950,000 engineers, including aerospace, biomedical, civil, computer software, and environmental engineers. The United States will also need workers in other high growth industries including nanotechnology, geospatial technology, and the life sciences, to name a few."

The U.S. Department of Labor (DOL) reports in *Foreign Labor Certification: International Talent Helping Meet Employer Demand* (September 2007, http://www.foreignlaborcert.doleta.gov/pdf/FY2007_OFLCPerformanceRpt.pdf) that health care, financial services, information technology, advanced manufacturing, and hospitality are five of the fourteen industry sectors that are anticipated to grow in coming years. "These areas represent the top five high-growth industry sectors" requesting certification for foreign workers in fiscal year (FY) 2007.

The DOL is required to conduct two important functions during the labor certification process: determine the "the availability of able, willing, and qualified domestic workers" for specific jobs and guarantee that the hiring of foreign workers for specific positions will not have an "adverse effect on the wages and working conditions of similarly employed U.S. workers." U.S. employers recruit foreign workers when there are not enough qualified U.S. workers available and when U.S. workers are unwilling to work for the wages offered.

In July 2007 the DOL tightened regulations related to permanent labor certifications for foreign workers. These changes came about after U.S. Department of Justice investigations and prosecutions revealed fraudulent practices, in that the name of a different worker could be substituted after the DOL issued a certification. The DOL states that labor certifications had become "commodities that were being sold by unscrupulous employers, attorneys, or agents to those seeking permanent residence. The ability to sell labor certifications was greatly enhanced by their open-ended validity, providing a lengthy period during which a certification could be marketed. For many of these certifications, the job was fictitious. For others, the job in question existed but was never truly open to U.S. workers. Rather, the job was steered to a specific alien in return for a substantial fee, or kickback."

Employer Demand for Permanent Labor Certification Grows

In *Foreign Labor Certification*, the DOL explains that permanent labor certifications increased 6%, from 80,029 in FY 2006 to 85,112 in FY 2007. The 28,000 certifications in professional, scientific, and technical services represented 33% of all permanent certifications and a one-year increase of 3,000 positions in this job sector.

In FY 2007 California received 20,222 certifications, or 24% of the total 85,112 positions certified. New York received 8,843, or 10% of total certified positions, and gained about 1,000 certifications over its FY 2006 total. By contrast, Oregon's 494 FY 2007 certifications were half of its 856 certifications in FY 2006.

High-Growth Industries

According to the DOL, in *Foreign Labor Certification*, high-growth industries received approximately 60,000 permanent certifications in FY 2007. Table 7.5 identifies the projected high-growth industries and the top three growth occupations in each. Information technology received 25% of FY 2007 certifications to hire foreign workers. (PERM in the graphic is the DOL's abbreviation for its Permanent Labor Certification Program.) The jobs identified in these high-growth industries were diverse in the type of education and training required: computer software and applications engineers, medical equipment repairers, home health aids, and amusement and recreation attendants.

TABLE 7.5

Projected occupation growth in top five high-growth industries

High-growth industry sector	Top three occupations with projected growth	Percent of PERM certifications
Information technology	• Network systems and data communications analysts • Computer software and applications engineers • Computer systems analysts	25%
Advanced manufacturing	• Environmental science and protection technicians, including health • Environmental scientists and specialists, including health • Medical equipment repairers	14%
Financial services	• Personal financial advisors • Financial analysts • Customer service representatives	6%
Healthcare	• Personal and home care aides • Home health aides • Medical assistants	6%
Hospitality	• Amusement and recreation attendants • Gaming dealers • Counter and rental clerks	6%

SOURCE: "Projected Occupation Growth in Top Five High-Growth Industries," in *Foreign Labor Certification: International Talent Helping Meet Employer Demand. Performance Report October 1, 2006–September 30, 2007*, U.S. Department of Labor, Employment and Training Administration, Office of Foreign Labor Certification, January 2009, http://www.foreignlaborcert .doleta.gov/pdf/FY2007_OFLCPerformanceRpt.pdf (accessed January 19, 2009)

Table 7.6 reveals the number of certificates issued in FY 2007 for foreign workers in the high-growth industries by the top 10 states. California received the most certificates in four of the five high-growth industries: information technology, advanced manufacturing, health care, and hospitality.

More than half (51%) of certified positions were filled by workers from India, China, Mexico, and South Korea. (See Table 7.7.) The types of workers coming from India and Mexico are vastly different in skills and pay rates received in the United States.

Table 7.8 shows the top 10 jobs filled by permanent labor certification from India. The greatest number (7,319) were computer software applications engineers. The highest average wage went to the 1,342 computer and information systems managers at an average annual salary of $91,409. The DOL indicates that among the top employers for workers from India were Microsoft Corporation (which had the most certified positions—613), Oracle USA, Cisco Systems, and Marlabs (which had the highest average pay rate of $94,014). Ninety-six percent of the workers from India had bachelor degrees or higher and 88% were eligible for H1B visas.

Table 7.9 shows the top 10 jobs filled by permanent labor certification from Mexico. The greatest number (815) were restaurant cooks. The highest average wage ($40,571) went to 232 elementary school teachers. The DOL notes that among the top employers for workers from Mexico were Eddy Packing Company, the Dallas Independent School District, Billy Cook Harness and Saddle Manufacturing, and Microsoft Corporation (which had the highest average pay rate of $80,698). One-fourth of the workers from Mexico had bachelor degrees or higher, and 16% were eligible for H1B visas.

Jobs American Workers Are Unwilling or Unable to Perform

Workers in agriculture and service jobs arrive with H2B visas (see Chapter 3 for a description of the H2 visa program). According to the DOL, in *Foreign Labor Certification*, the top positions filled with certified H2B visas were 62,442 landscapers and 22,347 housekeepers. The average hourly wage for landscapers was $8.00, and housekeepers were paid an average of $7.75 per hour. The top employers for H2B housekeepers were Ambassador Hospitality Solutions, Anchor Building Services, and Marriott International.

The DOL shares Galama and Hosek's concerns that the United States is not developing its own students to fill future employment needs, particularly in science and technology jobs. It also indicates that in 2003 it established the High Growth Job Training Initiative, which "engages business, education and the workforce investment system to work together to develop solutions to the workforce challenges facing high-growth industries."

TABLE 7.6

Number of Department of Labor (DOL) certifications in the top ten states for high-growth industries, 2007

State	Information technology	Advanced manufacturing	Financial services	Healthcare	Hospitality	Total positions in high-growth industries
California	4,672	4,399	944	1,725	948	12,688
New Jersey	3,115	606	314	113	387	4,535
New York	885	733	1,440	372	721	4,151
Texas	1,400	1,155	198	229	217	3,199
Illinois	1,318	559	278	197	197	2,549
Washington	1,892	151	52	94	47	2,236
Florida	492	453	413	279	309	1,946
Virginia	1,085	292	216	77	255	1,925
Massachusetts	969	416	187	153	190	1,915
Pennsylvania	873	231	102	222	136	1,564
Industry total in top 10 states	16,701	8,995	4,144	3,461	3,407	36,708

SOURCE: "Number of Certifications in the Top Ten States for High-Growth Industries," in *Foreign Labor Certification: International Talent Helping Meet Employer Demand. Performance Report October 1, 2006–September 30, 2007*, U.S. Department of Labor, Employment and Training Administration, Office of Foreign Labor Certification, January 2009, http://www.foreignlaborcert.doleta.gov/pdf/FY2007_OFLCPerformanceRpt.pdf (accessed January 19, 2009)

TABLE 7.7

Countries of origin with more than 800 DOL certified positions, 2007

Country of citizenship	Positions certified	Percent of total	Average annual salary*
India	24,573	29%	$72,643
China	6,846	8%	$62,053
Mexico	6,442	8%	$34,738
South Korea	5,159	6%	$50,056
Canada	4,837	6%	$72,483
Philippines	4,821	6%	$43,483
United Kingdom	1,811	2%	$70,345
Taiwan	1,503	2%	$60,306
Pakistan	1,486	2%	$61,082
Colombia	1,482	2%	$52,063
Brazil	1,460	2%	$48,411
Ecuador	1,411	2%	$37,584
Japan	1,258	1%	$56,499
Venezuela	1,150	1%	$57,013
Poland	1,035	1%	$43,821
Turkey	893	1%	$63,218
Peru	837	1%	$48,207
Israel	836	1%	$64,155
Germany	829	1%	$67,314

*The average wage is weighted per worker. DOL = Department of Labor

SOURCE: "Countries of Alien Origination with More Than 800 Certified Positions," in *Foreign Labor Certification: International Talent Helping Meet Employer Demand. Performance Report October 1, 2006–September 30, 2007*, U.S. Department of Labor, Employment and Training Administration, Office of Foreign Labor Certification, January 2009, http://www.foreignlaborcert.doleta.gov/pdf/FY2007_OFLCPerformanceRpt.pdf (accessed January 19, 2009)

TABLE 7.8

Top 10 U.S. occupations filled by workers from India, 2007

No	Occupation	Apps certified	Avg wage offer
1	Computer software engineers, applications	7,319	$76,717
2	Computer software engineers, systems software	3,233	$82,643
3	Computer systems analysts	2,905	$68,613
4	Computer and information systems managers	1,342	$91,409
5	Computer programmers	868	$63,911
6	Electronics engineers, except computer	739	$82,159
7	Electrical engineers	510	$71,001
8	Database administrators	436	$72,282
9	Mechanical engineers	416	$67,572
10	Network and computer systems administrators	372	$69,867

SOURCE: "Country Profile: India, Fiscal Year 2007 Summary Statistics: Top 10 Occupations," in *Foreign Labor Certification: International Talent Helping Meet Employer Demand. Performance Report October 1, 2006–September 30, 2007*, U.S. Department of Labor, Employment and Training Administration, Office of Foreign Labor Certification, January 2009, http://www.foreignlaborcert.doleta.gov/pdf/FY2007_OFLCPerformanceRpt.pdf (accessed January 19, 2009)

AMERICAN VIEWS ON IMMIGRATION

Immigration was the hot topic of debate in 2007, but by the middle of 2008 it was overshadowed by the economy. In a March 12–15, 2009, poll (http://www.pollingreport.com/prioriti.htm), CNN/Opinion Research Corporation found that 63% of respondents said the economy was the most important issue facing the country. Immigration was not cited as one of the important issues. However, a December 19–21, 2008, CNN/Opinion Research poll found that 5% of respondents said illegal immigration was the most important. Immigration held similar rankings in a variety of other polls taken in the summer and fall of 2008.

In *An Even More Partisan Agenda for 2008* (January 24, 2008, http://people-press.org/report/388/), the Pew Research Center for the People and the Press reports on its annual survey of the U.S. public's policy agenda. Respondents were asked to name the most important problem facing the nation. Among Republicans, Democrats, and Independents, an average of 34% said economic problems were the top issue. (See Table 7.10.) Just 6% of all respondents named immigration as the most important problem.

TABLE 7.9

Top 10 U.S. occupations filled by workers from Mexico, 2007

No	Occupation	Apps certified	Avg wage offer
1	Cooks, restaurant	815	$22,431
2	Farmworkers, farm and ranch animals	340	$17,840
3	Landscaping and groundskeeping workers	247	$22,473
4	Elementary school teachers, except special education	232	$40,571
5	Slaughterers and meat packers	199	$16,630
6	Chefs and head cooks	170	$30,019
7	Agricultural equipment operators	141	$14,688
8	Construction laborers	117	$23,413
9	Cement masons and concrete finishers	114	$26,841
10	First-line supervisors/managers of production and operating workers	82	$39,247

SOURCE: "Country Profile: Mexico, Fiscal Year 2007 Summary Statistics: Top 10 Occupations," in *Foreign Labor Certification: International Talent Helping Meet Employer Demand. Performance Report October 1, 2006–September 30, 2007,* U.S. Department of Labor, Employment and Training Administration, Office of Foreign Labor Certification, January 2009, http://www.foreignlaborcert.doleta.gov/pdf/FY2007_OFLCPerformanceRpt.pdf (accessed January 19, 2009)

TABLE 7.10

Public opinion on most important problem facing the nation, January 2008

	Total %	Rep %	Dem %	Ind %
Economic problems (net)	34	27	39	35
Economy	20	17	22	21
Unemployment	5	2	8	5
Energy/gas prices	3	2	5	3
Inflation/cost of living	3	2	4	3
Iraq	27	21	36	25
Health care	10	6	10	11
Immigration	6	10	3	6
Dissatisfaction w/govt	6	7	5	6
Education	4	3	4	4
Terrorism	3	7	1	2
Defense/security	3	7	*	2

Note: Based on open-ended question, multiple responses allowed.

SOURCE: "Most Important Problem Facing the Nation," in *An Even More Partisan Agenda for 2008,* The Pew Research Center for the People & the Press, January 24, 2008, http://people-press.org/report/388/ (accessed January 6, 2009)

FIGURE 7.7

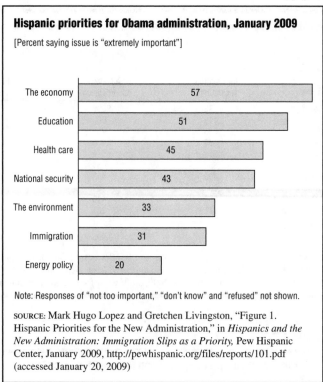

Hispanic priorities for Obama administration, January 2009

[Percent saying issue is "extremely important"]

The economy — 57
Education — 51
Health care — 45
National security — 43
The environment — 33
Immigration — 31
Energy policy — 20

Note: Responses of "not too important," "don't know" and "refused" not shown.

SOURCE: Mark Hugo Lopez and Gretchen Livingston, "Figure 1. Hispanic Priorities for the New Administration," in *Hispanics and the New Administration: Immigration Slips as a Priority,* Pew Hispanic Center, January 2009, http://pewhispanic.org/files/reports/101.pdf (accessed January 20, 2009)

with immigration, 50% of Democrats and 28% of Republicans said, "Allow illegal immigrants to stay." Concerning the option to "enforce law & cause [illegal immigrants] to leave," 56% of Republicans and 37% of Democrats said this was the best solution.

According to Jeffrey M. Jones of Gallup, in *Fewer Americans Favor Cutting Back Immigration* (July 10, 2008, http://www.gallup.com/poll/108748/Fewer-Americans-Favor-Cutting-Back-Immigration.aspx), 64% of Americans said in 2008 that immigration is good for the country. Regarding the level of immigration, 39% believed it should be kept at its present level, another 39% favored a decrease, and 18% wanted an increase in immigration.

In *Hispanics and the New Administration: Immigration Slips as a Priority* (January 15, 2009, http://pewhispanic.org/files/reports/101.pdf), Mark Hugo Lopez and Gretchen Livingston of the Pew Hispanic Center find that in 2008, 31% Hispanics rated immigration as "extremely important." (See Figure 7.7.) Among Hispanics, immigration ranked sixth in a list of priority issues for the newly elected Obama administration.

The Center for Immigration Studies surveyed people who voted in a 2008 primary or caucus, and the results were reported by Steven A. Camarota in "Poll: Voters Unaware of Candidates' Immigration Positions; McCain Supporters Farthest off the Mark" (March 2008, http://www.cis.org/node/13). When asked in 2008 about the best way to deal

CHAPTER 8
THE UNITED STATES NEEDS MORE TOLERANT IMMIGRATION LAWS

STATEMENT OF JOHN PEARSON, DIRECTOR OF THE BECHTEL INTERNATIONAL CENTER AT STANFORD UNIVERSITY, BEFORE THE SUBCOMMITTEE ON IMMIGRATION, CITIZENSHIP, REFUGEES, BORDER SECURITY, AND INTERNATIONAL LAW, COMMITTEE OF THE JUDICIARY, U.S. HOUSE OF REPRESENTATIVES, HEARING ON THE NEED FOR GREEN CARDS FOR HIGHLY SKILLED WORKERS, JUNE 12, 2008

My name is John Pearson, and I am director of the Bechtel International Center at Stanford University. I am testifying today on behalf of my professional association, NAFSA, the Association of International Educators. NAFSA is the world's largest professional association dedicated to the promotion and advancement of international education and exchange. I am also testifying with support from Stanford [University].

My remarks today will focus on the broad challenges the United States now faces in attracting and retaining international students. Of specific interest, of course, is the current law capping the number of green cards issued annually, even to those who graduate from U.S. colleges and universities with higher degrees.

The United States is in a global competition for international students and scholars. That may seem like an unremarkable statement, but often U.S. law and policy does not always reflect an understanding of this reality.

Though the U.S. is renowned and still renowned for being home to the majority of the top colleges and universities in the world, the international student market is being transformed in this century. There are many new players in the game, acting much more purposefully and strategically than ever before.

Competitor countries have implemented strategies for capturing a greater share of this market. Their governments are acting to create more streamlined visa and entry processes and more welcoming environments and are setting goals for international student recruitment.

Our neighbor, Canada, recently changed its employment policy to allow international graduates to work for up to 3 years after graduation, and, in fact, Canada does recruit international students on our own campuses, including my own. They have visited Stanford three times in the last few years to talk to students about opportunities in Canada.

At Stanford, we have been recently dealing with the homeland security extension on practical training for STEM [science, technology, engineering, and mathematics] students. A broader context is that France, Germany, the United Kingdom, and Canada have all made similar changes to the possibilities for international students remaining in those countries and working after graduation.

New competitors will also enter the market for international students. Primary among them is the European higher education area which compromises the signatories to the Bologna Declaration. This goal is to create a seamless higher education system in Europe by 2010 with credits entirely transferrable among their higher education institutions and often instruction in English. The European Union is also considering a blue card, similar to our green card, to be more competitive for non-European talent.

Other countries are recognizing the value of educating the next generation of leaders and attracting the world's scientific, technological, and intellectual elite. U.S. immigration law and policy has not yet effectively been adapted to this era of globalization. My own institution has been witness to this, as we also offer services to hire foreign-born faculty and researchers.

But even so, many of the best and the brightest around the world still wish to come here and study. We should welcome them by creating a clearer path to green card status for them that is not tied to these low caps on the green cards available annually.

In a global job market, employers look for the talent they need wherever they can find it, and students and highly talented workers look for the places to study and work that offer them the most opportunity. This means the options for employment after graduation are integral to attracting bright and talented international students.

Employment prospects are often a part of their calculus in deciding where to study, work, and live. Not all students who arrive in the U.S. wish to remain. Some have commitments to their home country. But others discover their potential in the environment of U.S. higher education and their career and life goals are changed. Google, Hotmail, Yahoo are some examples in Stanford's own backyard of former students who have remained in the United States.

I do not think it is a secret that U.S. immigration law often makes it difficult for international students to work after graduating, even from the most prestigious U.S. higher education institutions. The annual H-1B cap lottery is reported internationally, highlighting that the entire annual allotment is depleted in a day or two.

In conclusion, what better way to capture the world's best and brightest who want to become part of our Nation than to make it easier for them to remain to contribute to American economic and scientific leadership after they graduate from U.S. universities? (http://judiciary.house.gov/hearings/printers/110th/42851.PDF)

STATEMENT OF LEE COLBY, ELECTRICAL ENGINEER, LEE COLBY & ASSOCIATES, PAST CHAIR OF THE INSTITUTE OF ELECTRICAL AND ELECTRONICS ENGINEERS (IEEE), SANTA CLARA VALLEY SECTION, BEFORE THE SUBCOMMITTEE ON IMMIGRATION, CITIZENSHIP, REFUGEES, BORDER SECURITY, AND INTERNATIONAL LAW, COMMITTEE OF THE JUDICIARY, U.S. HOUSE OF REPRESENTATIVES, HEARING ON THE NEED FOR GREEN CARDS FOR HIGHLY SKILLED WORKERS, JUNE 12, 2008

My name is Lee Colby, and I am testifying today on behalf of IEEE-USA, which represents a group of engineers 215,000 strong in the United States, of which 22 percent are foreign-born Americans.

I have been a professional electrical engineer for over 50 years in Santa Clara Valley. In fact, I was in the Valley when it was called the Valley of Hearts Delight. For my first 36 years of my career, I worked at Hewlett-Packard as an electrical engineer.

I left HP in 1997 and started Lee Colby and Associates[,] which consults on circuit and system designs for some of the world's leading technology firms. In 2000, I decided to try my hand in a technology startup, O'LE Communications, as chief technical officer.

It was at O'LE that I had my most direct experience with our immigration system. We employed about 24 employees, half in Taiwan and half in the United States. During the dot.com boom, we had trouble finding American workers, so we turned to the H-1B program. When the dot.com boom burst, those workers were unable to transfer to another company and so had to leave. H-1B workers are effectively tied to their employer, creating a dependency that is both unjust and harmful.

In 2005, I chaired, as Chairwoman Lofgren said, the IEEE Santa Clara Valley section, representing over 13,000 electrical and electronics engineers in the San Jose area. I also, though, volunteer as a math and science teacher assistant at the Sunnyvale Middle School and teach a class in fuel cells and solar cells for advanced high school children at San Jose State University.

In other words, I know both ends of the technology sector inside and out. For almost 50 years, I have been deeply involved with cutting-edge technology and the men and women who developed it. I understand the problems faced by engineers and employers, and I believe the approach to high-skill immigration reform being offered by Chairman Lofgren is a good one for all parties.

Earlier this year, the House Immigration Subcommittee, Chair Zoe Lofgren, and a bipartisan team of legislators introduced three important proposals. We support all three bills, as noted in the record. I am especially pleased to see that H.R. 6039 would allow graduate students to move quickly from a student visa to a green card.

Remember it is not a question of whether the talented graduates of our schools get jobs but only where those jobs would be located, and if we force them to leave, the jobs created by the world's most talented people will not be in our country, but rather in whatever nation had the foresight to accept them.

Today, my neighborhood is filled with workers on H-1B visas. In the evening, while walking Heidi, my miniature schnauzer, they tell me what they will do once they become American citizens. They plan to start their own companies, create exciting and profitable new products— entirely new industries, in some cases. Why are we making them leave?

On the plane coming over, I met James Stubbs, chief science officer of Cianna, a small 35-person medical company. They make a cutting-edge device for treating breast cancer. They employ two H-1Bs. One is from Costa Rica and is in their advanced research R&D. The other is from India and does field research. Both of these H-1Bs are integral to the success of their company. Do you want the company to be successful for 6 years or 30 years?

Temporary visas like H-1B do nothing to enhance America's long-term competitiveness. They are a short-term fix that will weaken us in the long run. The H-1B visa is a great way to train our overseas competition but is an awful way to build our workforce.

Innovative companies do not need innovative people for 6 years. They need them for 30. Moreover, H-1B visa engineers are easy to exploit, harming both American and foreign engineers. America does not need skilled temporary workers. We need skilled Americans, and citizenship requires at least an EB visa.

In conclusion, IEEE-USA members share the belief that making foreign nationals with the knowledge, skills, and determination citizens has always served America's best interests. We urge Congress to reform the Nation's permanent employment-based admissions system. An integration policy based on the concept of green cards, not guest workers, will help America create jobs, maintain its technological competitiveness, and ensure our success.

The goal of U.S. immigration policy should be to facilitate the entry of talented people, including potential inventors, innovators, and entrepreneurs from other countries. Congress should grant them legal permanent resident status and put them on a path to full-fledged American citizenship (http://judiciary.house.gov/hearings/printers/110th/42851.PDF).

TESTIMONY OF JOHN TRASVIÑA, PRESIDENT AND GENERAL COUNSEL, MEXICAN AMERICAN LEGAL DEFENSE AND EDUCATIONAL FUND, LOS ANGELES, CALIFORNIA, BEFORE THE SUBCOMMITTEE ON SOCIAL SECURITY, HOUSE COMMITTEE ON WAYS AND MEANS, U.S. HOUSE OF REPRESENTATIVES, MAY 6, 2008

I am John Trasviña, President and General Counsel of the Mexican American Legal Defense and Educational Fund (MALDEF). Thank you for this opportunity to testify on Employment Eligibility Verification Systems (EEVS or E-Verify) and the Potential Impacts on American Workers.

For forty years, MALDEF has served as the law firm for the Latino community. Today, immigration affects every family, business and community across the nation. Immigration policy and enforcement practices are uppermost in MALDEF's litigation and policy agendas as they affect both newcomer and native-born Latinos.

There are a number of bills addressing EEVS currently under consideration in Congress. The "SAVE Act of 2007," H.R. 4088, and the "New EEVS Act of 2008," H.R. 5515, are among them. At the core of these two bills is the expanded application of EEVS, a deeply flawed system which would threaten the jobs of nearly 13 million

native-born U.S. citizens and increase discrimination against Latinos and other national origin minorities.

According to U.S. Citizenship and Immigration Services (USCIS) the E-Verify program goals are as follows: 1. Reduce unauthorized employment; 2. Minimize verification-related discrimination; 3. Be quick and non-burdensome to employers; and 4. Protect civil liberties and employee privacy. In fact, none of these program goals can be met, regardless of the vehicle used, under EEVS as currently constructed.

Worksite enforcement is a necessary component of comprehensive immigration reform, but it must be done with accurate records and through a better process. The notion that we can simply, cheaply, or easily turn over verification to computers without adequately managing or safeguarding the data weakens both the effectiveness of the verification system and jeopardizes the mission of the Social Security Administration relied upon by all Americans.

I. EEVS Creates a Flawed No-work List

Applying a flawed EEVS system will harm American workers creating an official "no-work list" requiring millions of U.S. citizens and other authorized workers to bear the burden of proving their legal status and seek an unseen government computer's permission to work. Moreover, EEVS will create a new market for fraudulent documentation and drive unauthorized workers further into an underground labor market.

A. EEVS CREATES A NO-WORK LIST. Mandatory EEVS will adversely affect American workers at an economically fragile time for our country. The Social Security Administration (SSA) Office of Inspector General estimates that 17.8 million (or 4.1 percent) of its records contain errors, and that 12.7 million (about 70 percent) of those records with errors belong to native-born U.S. citizens. According to the Cato Institute, a mandatory EEVS would result in 11,000 workers per day, or just over 25 people per congressional district per working day, who would receive a tentative non-confirmation (TNC) throughout a given year (based on an average of 55 million new hires per year).

It is a bedrock principle of employee rights in this country to be free from discrimination based on race, color, religion, sex, or national origin. But EEVS database errors have a disproportionate impact on foreign-born U.S. citizens, with almost 10 percent initially being told that they are not authorized to work (versus 0.1 percent for native-born U.S. citizens). From October 2006 to March 2007, about 3,200 foreign-born U.S. citizens were initially erroneously disqualified from working by EEVS. This is a major concern because disparate impacts on certain U.S. workers may violate Title VII of the Civil Rights Act of 1964 (Title VII).

Myriad reasons account for errors in the SSA database, including clerical errors made by agency employees unbeknownst to employers or workers, and an employer's or a worker's own errors when completing government forms. Errors are more likely for a worker who has a hyphenated name or different surname when applying for a Social Security card than when he or she did when applying for a job. Moreover, an error may stem from a name change due to marriage, divorce, or naturalization. Finally, an error may come from the misuse of an SSN by an unauthorized worker.

In December of last year, Abel Pacheco of Arizona, a naturalized U.S. citizen for eight years, lost his job as a truck driver in a troubled economy. He applied with eight different companies, but not one called him back. Finally, he found work but his new employer notified him that it had received a tentative non-confirmation of his employment eligibility. This turned out to be due to an error in the SSA database. However, by the time Pacheco cleared up the problem by presenting his citizenship certificate at his local SSA office, the few weeks without an income had forced his family into financial trouble.

Juan Carlos Ochoa, also a naturalized U.S. citizen from Arizona, is a car salesman who quit his job at the end of last year and took another at a Dodge dealership two months later. Unfortunately for Ochoa, a father of two, days after starting his new job his employer informed him that E-Verify classified him as a possible illegal immigrant. Having only days to convince SSA that he was a U.S. citizen, he took his U.S. passport, Social Security card, drivers license and Arizona voter identification card to the local SSA office. He was then informed he would have to request new paperwork from DHS, which may take 10 months. In the meantime, Mr. Ochoa, a U.S. citizen will be unable to find legitimate work and support his family.

B. EEVS INCREASES A MARKET FOR FRAUDULENT DOCUMENTS. In 1986, when Congress adopted employer sanctions as a means to keep unauthorized workers from being hired, MALDEF predicted that document fraud would render sanctions ineffective. We were correct. Fraudulent use of valid documents will similarly undermine the EEVS system contemplated by the pending legislation.

Even if EEVS may appear effective at ending the employment of individuals who receive final non-confirmations, it may simply drive many employers and workers to rely upon fraudulent documents when SSN combinations do match in order to achieve the appearance of a valid authorized worker status. The foreseeable consequence is a significant increase in the demand for valid identities, which can only be met by an expanded market for identity theft. The social cost of this effect will be hardest upon citizens, work-authorized immigrants and their minor children.

The cost of a fraudulent document market goes beyond the financial cost. A victim of identity theft, in a mandatory

EEVS scenario, would stand falsely accused of violating immigration law and committing identity fraud each time a worker seeks employment. While this will have overwhelming financial obstacles for those U.S. citizens unable to work, the results could be even more devastating for work authorized immigrants. To remain in the United States and be eligible for various immigration related benefits, immigrants must comply with a number of document requirements under the Immigration and Nationality Act (INA). Under the INA, a person who uses, acquires, or produces fraudulent documents for immigration-related purposes may be subjected to civil penalties and denied certain immigration benefits, including the ability to enter or remain in the United States. Further, certain fraudulent actions may carry criminal penalties under both the INA and the United States Criminal Code. Thus, if a work-authorized immigrant becomes a victim of identity theft, he or she may be wrongly subject to civil penalties and deportation, irrespective of any involvement or culpability in the misuse and theft of his or her valid documents by another person far away.

U.S. citizens and work-authorized immigrants will bear the burden of proving their identities to the government's satisfaction and it is they, not unauthorized workers, who will suffer the most. The financial impact will be on their ability to receive income through work and they could face threats of eviction, repossession, or default.

C. EEVS UNINTENTIONALLY ENDORSES THE UNDERGROUND ECONOMY. The real beneficiaries of EEVS are unscrupulous employers. Under EEVS employers are intended to be deprived of significant numbers of unauthorized individuals currently in their employ or in the workforce. Employment verification, properly done, must be combined with a process to adjust the status of existing workers in order to ameliorate the economic impact costs of verification. This impact will not be felt by unscrupulous employers. They will continue to employ unauthorized workers knowing they are more susceptible than ever before to exploitation and intimidation, and they are effectively bereft of labor organizing rights or the ability to complain about illegally dangerous worksite conditions. Their authorized co-workers and companies facing unfair competition of unscrupulous employers are also harmed in this situation.

Unscrupulous employers will also be free to avoid payroll taxes, unemployment and workers compensation and other withholding requirements. The Congressional Budget Office and the Joint Committee on Taxation recently estimated that a bill requiring employers to use the government's E-Verify system would reduce tax collections by about $770 million per year once fully implemented, because unauthorized workers would enter the underground economy.

II. EEVS Increases Verification-Related Discrimination

EEVS fails to prevent discrimination or address the increased levels of discrimination it causes. Moreover, it lacks provisions to safeguard employees from employer abuse of the system. There is a significant risk that more employers will opt to play it "safe" and fire workers who may look or sound "illegal" regardless of citizenship or work-authorization status.

A 2007 assessment of Basic Pilot/E-Verify concluded that the rate of noncompliance with the system is "substantial" and that employers engaged in prohibited employment practices including pre-employment screening, adverse employment action based on a tentative non-confirmation, and failure to inform workers of their rights under the program. Abel Pacheco, the Arizona truck driver, is a prime example of someone who was prescreened and never informed of the adverse results from [E-Verify].

Mandatory EEVS without protection for workers is a disastrous proposition. Currently, the U.S. Department of Justice Office of Special Counsel (OSC) for Immigration Related Unfair Employment Practices does not have the necessary resources to make the public aware of what is and what is not permissible under EEVS. During fiscal year 2006, OSC received 346 charges of alleged discrimination, handling approximately 7,500 calls, and resolving 85 investigations. For OSC, the prospect of a mandatory EEVS, educating the more than 7.5 million American businesses and their workers of their rights and obligations, will be overwhelming without the necessary resources. If only 1 percent of these employers call OSC about just one hiring question during the year, it will mean a tenfold increase in OSC work.

In 1997, a month after I was confirmed by the Senate to a four-year term as Special Counsel for Immigration Related Unfair Employment Practices, Immigration and Naturalization Service officials took me to Chicago to observe newly trained employers using one of the Basic Pilot systems. As you know, the OSC is the federal government's only office devoted solely to immigrant workplace rights. OSC has the dual role of educating employers about their responsibilities under IRCA not to discriminate against qualified U.S. workers and enforcing the anti-discrimination provisions.

Each recently trained employer whose premises I visited with INS got it wrong. In different but critical ways, their application of the computer verification system failed to follow the training or the law. One employer used it only for foreign-born workers. Another employer failed to tell employees who received a tentative non-conformation that they could address discrepancies with SSA or INS. The third employer told us that they used it only on those employees who "needed" it. When I inquired how he made that determination, the employer stated that it was for employees who had an accent or looked "illegal."

Simply stated, even if the training is understandable and actually understood, the federal government is hard pressed to ensure that millions of employers—even those who want to do the right thing—will do it correctly. Similarly, employers will have difficulty when there is a turn over in their human resources staff to an individual who is not trained. And there is very little done to ensure that an employee may not utilize the system selectively or overuse it to check other people's status. Expanding EEVS prematurely, without proper training and monitoring of employers, educating the working public, or strengthening the federal government's capacity to respond to problems and enforce anti-discrimination protections will cause undue hardship on U.S. citizens and legally authorized workers and do nothing to reduce unauthorized hiring.

III. EEVS Will Burden Employers

Because EEVS is not well understood by the nation's employers, it will significantly disrupt our [national] economy. Where it has been mandated it has been controversial and disastrous. In Arizona, where E-Verify is mandatory under state law, only 15 percent of the 145,000 state employers (or 25,000) had registered for the program as of April 2008. Factors driving the slow enrollment rates range from employer uncertainty of the legal requirements, the confusion of how to register for the program, the lack of resources such as high-speed internet, and the fact that there has been little need to hire new workers, and a slowdown in the economy and new hiring.

Businesses and workers that have used the system have been openly critical. Ken Nagel, a restaurant owner in Phoenix, recently hired one of his daughters, processed her information with E-Verify and received a tentative non confirmation of her eligibility to work in the United States. Mr. Nagel, whose 19-year-old daughter is a native-born U.S. citizen, "scoffs at the E-Verify system."

American businesses, currently struggling in this economy, are faced with unforeseen burdens and problems because of the new law. Typical situations include lack of human resource personnel to navigate a program which is not user-friendly; upgrading operating costs to subscribe to high-speed internet; purchasing or upgrading computers suitable for the program; and being targeted by companies alleging to facilitate the process as their "designated agents" at high costs.

IV. Protecting Civil Liberties

Both H.R. 4088 and H.R. 5515 require that DHS and SSA exchange confidential information, including social security numbers (SSN). It is alarming that the information-sharing provisions in H.R. 4088 are broad and do not require independent review, privacy protections, or notice to workers that their private information has been disclosed. H.R. 5515 is equally troubling as it would give DHS primary authority to determine whether SSA can credit work history to non-U.S. citizens. This however would require that SSA share its data with DHS regarding all persons who have been identified as non-citizens. H.R. 5515 would also create a privately run ID verification system to collect biometrics such as fingerprints and retinal scans.

Given the error rates previously mentioned, nearly 13 million U.S. citizens, and according to the SSA Office of Inspector General, at least 3.3 million persons whose data records [contain] incorrect citizenship status codes, would become vulnerable to this information sharing between DHS and SSA. Increasing the number of times data, including names, SSNs, date and place of birth, are exchanged will increase the opportunity for error and for opportunistic individuals seeking to steal valid identification by hacking into a system without adequate privacy protections.

V. EEVS Will Harm SSA

EEVS stands to cripple an SSA already overburdened under its current workload trying to carry out the purpose for which the agency was created. Last year, the president of the National Council of Social Security Management Associations, Inc. stated that a mandatory EEVS could not only "cripple SSA's service capabilities," it could also negate progress in addressing the backlog of applications for disability benefits. SSA estimates that the average wait time for more than 750,000 cases awaiting a hearing decision on just disability cases is 499 days. SSA field offices receive over 60 million phone calls each year, over half of the callers receive busy signals. Mara Mayor, member of the Board of Directors for AARP, recently told this committee that SSA's workload is about to increase with the "long-anticipated" retirement of the Baby Boom generation. Director Mayor explained that . . . this "challenge . . . will add nearly 80 million new beneficiaries to the Social Security rolls—nearly 13 million in the next 10 years alone, and upwards of 16,000 per working day." And this does not even account for the backlog of disability cases. As of early 2008, there are 1.4 million people waiting for a decision on their initial claim or appeal for Social Security or Supplemental Security Income (SSI).

A mandatory EEVS will have a devastating impact on the Social Security Administration, authorized U.S. workers, and SSA beneficiaries. Without SSA hiring new employees to take on the EEVS fallout and addressing the system errors, existing services will continue to deteriorate. As our nation finds itself in a recession and Americans are struggling to make ends meet, U.S. workers and SSA beneficiaries will have a difficult time understanding the government's decision to further exacerbate their situation with a mandatory EEVS . . . .

MALDEF strongly supports fixing this nation's broken immigration system, but forcing a deeply flawed system upon an unstable economy is not the answer. A mandatory EEVS will not only impose unnecessary financial burdens upon U.S. businesses, it will lead to unnecessary and unlawful terminations when employers receive tentative non-confirmation reports from the government and they or their employees do not complete the process. Further, EEVS will result in discrimination by employers who choose to not comply with the program. Additionally, a mandatory EEVS will drive the undocumented into an underground labor force without legal protections which will affect all U.S. workers and harm businesses that comply with the law. Recognizing the dangers that come with a mandatory EEVS which will increase discrimination against Latinos and other national origin minorities, present burdensome costs to businesses, and threaten the jobs of nearly 13 million native-born U.S. citizens, Congress should reject the pending legislation (http://waysandmeans .house.gov/hearings.asp?formmode=view&id=6897).

TESTIMONY OF KIM GANDY, PRESIDENT, NATIONAL ORGANIZATION FOR WOMEN (NOW) FOUNDATION, BEFORE THE SUBCOMMITTEE ON IMMIGRATION, CITIZENSHIP, REFUGEES, BORDER SECURITY, AND INTERNATIONAL LAW, COMMITTEE OF THE JUDICIARY, U.S. HOUSE OF REPRESENTATIVES, ON HEARING TO EXAMINE H.R. 750, THE "SAVE AMERICA COMPREHENSIVE IMMIGRATION ACT OF 2007," NOVEMBER 8, 2007

Today we are here because there is a drumbeat of anger across this nation aimed at immigrant workers and their families, with little regard for the truths about the lives and livelihoods of millions of people living and working here among us. As our nation, and this Congress, works to clarify our residency and citizenship laws, improve our security and safeguard our communities, we must not forget the needs and rights of immigrant women and children, whose concerns are too often overlooked and under-played.

Last year, we took a leadership role in convening the National Coalition for Immigrant Women's Rights, and gathered together grassroots and advocacy organizations nationwide with the goal of defending and promoting equality for immigrant women and their families living and working in the United States.

We integrate human rights principles into our work and believe that immigrant women's rights are both civil rights and women's rights. We believe that comprehensive immigration reform must include fair and non-discriminatory implementation of our immigration and enforcement policies, and that must include economic, legal and social justice for immigrant women.

Equality for immigrant women can only be attained when immigrant women can live free from discrimination, oppression and violence in all their forms. It is imperative that policies promoting comprehensive immigration reform also support fair and just policies that protect the rights of immigrant women. Millions of immigrant women's lives are at stake and we hope that this hearing is the beginning of a national dialogue that brings immigrant women's concerns out in the open and up for discussion.

For the record, there are 14.2 million foreign born women in the United States. Five and a half million are naturalized citizens, another five and a half million are documented and 3.2 million are undocumented. Women make up over 30% of the over 10 million undocumented immigrants in the United States today. Another 1.6 million are children under 18. And HALF of all undocumented immigrants originally came here with legitimate paperwork or visas and they have simply overstayed their time and are now undocumented, many lined up to renew their paperwork while they work at our colleges, in our businesses and pay taxes in our communities.

Each year, half of all immigrants entering the United States are female—women and girls. However, public policies regarding immigrants do not reflect the impact that being female has on immigrants' lives in the United States. This applies to both documented and undocumented women.

The economic issues affecting undocumented immigrant women are basic: their work is not valued or counted. That is why NOW strongly supports the inclusion of provisions in any immigration reform legislation that would offer a path to residency and citizenship for the undocumented living in the United States. Undocumented women will benefit significantly economically, and be less subject to exploitation, if they can come out of hiding, apply for residency and seek employment in the general labor market, earn at least the federal minimum hourly wage and be eligible to contribute to and receive social security and unemployment benefits as other workers do.

The economic reality of immigrant women and children today is disheartening. According to the Pew Hispanic Center, 31% of family households headed by foreign-born women live in poverty today as compared to 27% of native born women-led households. [Sixteen percent] of all those who are foreign born live in poverty compared to 11.8% of the native born. One of the reasons for the higher number of foreign-born women in poverty is the fact that foreign-born women who are full time workers make less than their native born counterparts. For example, the median income for foreign-born women age 16 and over who are year-round, full time workers is $22,106 while the median income for native born women is $26,640.

Among the factors affecting low wages is the high percentage of immigrant women, both documented and undocumented, working in the service industry, primarily in domestic work. Forty-two percent of private household services are provided by immigrants under arrangements that are often informal, prone to abuse and exploitation. Domestic workers are the lowest paid of all major occupational groups tracked by the US Census. The true numbers are unknown for the most part due to the fact that many of these workers are not reported by employers, are not on anyone's official payroll, and are paid "under the table."

Protections for domestic workers must be included in any immigration reform legislation. Domestic workers, in particular undocumented immigrant women, are faced with extremely low wages, working 60–70 hours per week or more for as little as $200 per week. This is exploitation, sometimes amounting to servitude or even slavery, under the most hostile conditions.

And yet, domestic service, in particular for those living in private households, remains excluded from and unregulated by our country's employment protections and labor laws. These women do not have the right to organize, strike or bargain for wages. The protections against sexual harassment in the workplace (through Title VII which applies to employers of 15 or more employees) are not available to domestic workers. They are similarly excluded from the Fair Labor Standards Act overtime provisions and from the Occupational Safety and Health Act. These omissions must be corrected through comprehensive immigration reform legislation. Domestic service is a category of work that must be addressed, not ignored and excluded from labor standards and protections afforded to other workers.

H.R. 750's alternatives to detention programs, exempting certain individuals based on age, health, children, victims of trafficking and sexual abuse is a good step towards bringing some humanity to what is undeniably an unjust and reckless approach to resolving the issue of illegal immigration.

On the whole, as you discuss H.R. 750 and other proposed immigration reform, we urge you to consider the following:

- An end to discriminatory, militaristic and inhumane immigration enforcement practices that destroy the families, homes and communities of immigrant women.

- Freeing immigrant women from mental, physical and emotional violence at the hands of traffickers, smugglers, intimate partners, employers, family members and others who exploit immigrant women's legal and economic vulnerability. Our immigration and criminal justice systems must ensure that immigrant women and their children are protected from gender-based violence, and must not perpetuate the cycle of violence by failing to provide adequate remedial measures that promote their safety and physical integrity.

- A responsible path to citizenship, which must allow immigrant women to obtain work permits, to travel internationally and access higher education and federal financial aid. Immigrant women must have viable options that will permit them to be full contributors to the U.S. economic and societal landscape. We can no longer afford to lose these valuable contributions.

- Protections for all immigrant women workers from exploitation and abuse in the workplace by providing fair wages and safe working conditions.

- Acknowledgement of the need for public awareness, education, and understanding of the fundamental and pivotal role immigrant women play in the familial, cultural and social spheres of the United States.

- The elimination of all forms of human trafficking through a survivor-centered advocacy model that opposes all forms of exploitation (http://judiciary.house.gov/hearings/pdf/Gandy071108.pdf).

TESTIMONY OF CHRISTOPHER NUGENT, SENIOR COUNSEL, HOLLAND & KNIGHT LLP, BEFORE THE SUBCOMMITTEE ON IMMIGRATION, CITIZENSHIP, REFUGEES, BORDER SECURITY, AND INTERNATIONAL LAW, COMMITTEE OF THE JUDICIARY, U.S. HOUSE OF REPRESENTATIVES, ON HEARING TO EXAMINE H.R. 750, THE "SAVE AMERICA COMPREHENSIVE IMMIGRATION ACT OF 2007," NOVEMBER 8, 2007

I am a full-time... Senior Counsel who works exclusively on domestic and international immigration law and policy issues and individual client cases with the international law firm of Holland & Knight LLP. I have two decades of experience in immigration law.... In my current capacity, I am privileged to act as counsel to many non-governmental immigration and refugee organizations (NGOs) working for positive changes in governmental policy and practices in the area of immigration proceedings and detention involving vulnerable populations including but not limited to the Women's Commission for Refugee Women and Children, the Rights Working Group and the National Immigration Law Center. The statements, opinions, and views expressed today however are my own....

IN FY 2007, United States taxpayers funded the Department of Homeland Security (DHS) at a record 945 million dollars to detain a daily average population of 27,500 aliens at more than 325 facilities nationwide. The annual DHS detainee population exceeds 261,000. While this detention is intended to be civil and not punitive since the detainees are being held for civil immigration removal proceedings, the vast majority of detainees, including non-criminal asylum-seekers, are detained in actual prisons and thus unfortunately commingled with America's finest

criminal convicts. In this regard, DHS only owns and operates 9 civilian detention facilities. Thus, the vast majority of private prisons contracted by DHS operate for profit, as well as state and county jails, given that DHS' per diem cost is higher than their actual cost of detention. Average DHS daily detention cost per detainee is $95 per day or $34,765 annualized (which would apply to asylum-seekers and others in DHS custody)....

Sec. 621 of the Save America Act would mandate that the Office of Civil Rights and [Civil] Liberties (OCRCL) monitor *all* facilities that are being used to hold detainees for more than 72 hours including evaluating whether the facilities are in compliance with the Detention Standards. This innovation is welcome and salutary considering that the OCRCL has only been sporadically engaged [in] detention oversight issues on either an as needed or ad hoc basis given their currently limited staffing and competing demands. Engaging OCRCL is essential to reinforcing reform of conditions of confinement for detainees whether OCRCL reports are ultimately made available to the public or not—the preference being within DHS that OCRCL resolves problems internally albeit without any public or Congressional oversight.

As regards Sec. 622(b) of the Save America Act concerning secure alternatives to detention, this provision provides necessary reform to a detention system which to date has failed to provide any national binding criteria and guidance prosecutorial discretion as to who needs to be detained.... [It] prioritizes the most vulnerable in detention for eligibility including alien parents detained with their children; aliens with serious medical or mental health needs; aliens who are mentally retarded or autistics; pregnant alien women; elderly aliens who are over the age of 65; and aliens placed in expedited removal proceedings after being rescued from trafficking or criminal operations by Government authorities....

[It] will promote optimal efficiency and effectiveness of the federal government in its detention capacity to enforce the United States border. The Department currently lacks adequate or sufficient facilities to hold *all* aliens subject to expedited removal until removal is effectuated. Sec. 622(b) of the Save America Act provides a safety valve to allow people who have every safeguard in place to comply with removal orders be released pending their actual removal so that Customs and Border Protection (CBP) can continue to arrest and detain the maximum numbers of immigration violators at the border. Otherwise, CBP has scant incentive to arrest *all* aliens if Immigration and Customs Enforcement (ICE) lacks bed-space to house them. Sec. 622(b) provides the teeth for DHS' catch and remove approach. Additionally, most notably, Sec. 622(b) does not create any independent right or legal review of the implementation of the program exception through a report to Congress which is Congress' preeminent and essential prerogative in exercising its oversight function of executive branch agencies.

Sec. 622(b) will be particularly instrumental if and when expedited removal is to be invoked system-wide including the interior under Section 235(b) of the Immigration and Nationality Act (INA) and not only within 100 miles of land borders of the United States as under current policy....

... Through this program, the Department will thereby have a range of humane and more cost-effective alternatives besides prisons and jails to ensure an alien's appearance before immigration officials for their removal. This program is based on the best practices utilized by the Appearance Assistance Program of the Vera Institute and DHS' Intensive Supervision Appearance Program which have achieved remarkably high compliance rates for aliens including a 94 percent appearance rate at final removal hearings. Additionally, the program will be implemented by NGOs in order to achieve a cost-savings for DHS. With this provision, catch and detain can truly become catch and remove with the most vulnerable in safe and secure situations pending removal.

By focusing on DHS' arrest and detention capacity constraints and prioritizing key vulnerable populations, Sec. 622(b) differs materially from Sec. 177 of the STRIVE Act of 2007 (H.R. 1645). Sec. 177 of the Strive Act establishes a secure alternatives program for aliens without specifying rigorous criteria for participation such as vulnerable populations who pose no flight risk or danger to the community and triggered by detention capacity constraints. Sec. 177 further does not designate as extensive options of alternatives under Sec. 622(b) including, for example, facilities under armed guard at the perimeter. Given the chronic state of deplorable conditions of confinement for immigration detainees under DHS mismanagement, immigration detainees obviously would prefer *any* non-penal facility run by a reputable non-governmental organization as a preferable and viable alternative to detention—even if there were a guard posted at the perimeter for security purposes. The STRIVE Act would benefit from incorporating these pragmatic considerations from the Save America Act into its provision concerning secure alternatives to detention.

Turning to Secs. 1201 and 1202 of the Save America Act, under current law, children of refugees or asylees are eligible for derivative status when their parents are granted asylum or refugee status. If, however, the child is over age 21 at the time of the parent's approval, the child is no longer [considered] a "child" for immigration purposes under the INA and is not eligible for the derivative status. The Child Status Protection Act (CSPA), Pub.L. 107-208 (Aug. 6, 2002), provided age-out protection for children included on parents' applications filed before the child has attained age 21. CSPA however failed to address the

unique and compelling predicament of children over age 21 who have aged out of protection but are mentally disabled and dependent on their parents as caregivers despite their chronological age. Secs. 1201 and 1202 would correct this injustice by facilitating the admission of refugee and asylee children who are severely impaired by mental retardation, autism, or some other disability of that type who have aged out of classification as a "child." While this may appear to be a small class, it is among the most vulnerable of asylees and refugees and warrants redress through this legislation.

I personally recall meeting an unaccompanied refugee child in a camp in Guinea suffering from severe mental retardation. The camp had no specialized services to offer him and he remains in Guinea now as an adult with no prospect for any future besides becoming a beggar. Secs. 1201 and 1202 protection will allow such vulnerable children to reunify with the parents or legal guardians as refugees or asylees in the United States to receive the care they need and deserve to become productive, contributing members of the United States (http://judiciary.house.gov /hearings/pdf/Nugent071108.pdf).

TESTIMONY OF WILLIAM E. SPRIGGS, CHAIR OF THE DEPARTMENT OF ECONOMICS, HOWARD UNIVERSITY, BEFORE THE SUBCOMMITTEE ON IMMIGRATION, CITIZENSHIP, REFUGEES, BORDER SECURITY, AND INTERNATIONAL LAW, COMMITTEE OF THE JUDICIARY, U.S. HOUSE OF REPRESENTATIVES, ON HEARING TO EXAMINE H.R. 750, THE "SAVE AMERICA COMPREHENSIVE IMMIGRATION ACT OF 2007," NOVEMBER 8, 2007

The views I express are my own, and do not necessarily reflect those of my employer, Howard University.... I will direct my comments on the legislation towards its implication for the labor market. I think it is important that the legislation has specific policy recommendations for the labor market. Economists do not have a consensus on the labor market effects of immigration on the native work force. A basic disagreement exists between economists on how to measure the impacts of immigration on the native work force, whether the effects can be seen by comparing labor markets in cities with different rates of immigration or looking at the national labor market over time. There is also disagreement on identifying which workers are most likely to have their labor market outcomes affected by immigration.

There is some agreement however, that a sizable group of native and immigrant low-wage workers do have similar occupations.... I want to concentrate on the agreement that there is similarity in the occupations of immigrant and native workers to underscore the importance of including specific policies aimed at insuring an efficient labor market. In particular, I want to commend the legislation for calling on employers to make extensive searches for workers, and to require documentation of the employers' efforts to look for workers....

Economists are more keenly aware of the importance of job networks—the informal exchange of information on job openings and job recommendations among workers—as important to getting workers access to jobs. Economists however have fewer consensuses on whether job networks can boost the wages of individual workers, and have less information on the impact of such networks on wage levels in general. I think the evidence leans toward the networks making the labor market less efficient by lowering the amount of information that employers and potential employees have. I think the growing occupational segregation suggests that employers may be limiting their search for workers.

So, I think the legislation is correct when it calls for extensive search methods by employers. I think the legislation might go further in requiring all employers looking for workers with less education to centrally post their job openings. The legislation then might consider using that data as stronger evidence of the existence, or absence, of available workers.

Congress has already taken some steps to improve the general low wage labor market by increasing the federal minimum wage. This was a very important step in improving the functioning of the low wage labor market. Increasing the flow of information on job openings and making job matches happen faster is another; and this legislation takes the steps to move in that direction.

The legislation is also on target in calling for increased funding for job training. While the wage gap between high school educated and high school drop-outs has remained fairly flat over the last twenty-years, there is a growing gap between workers with high school education and those who have some post-secondary education. Increasing the skills of less educated native workers will, of course, reduce the supply of less educated workers in the work force and help offset any effects of the increase in the supply of less educated workers through immigration (http://judiciary .house.gov/hearings/pdf/Spriggs071108.pdf).

CHAPTER 9
THE UNITED STATES NEEDS TOUGHER IMMIGRATION LAWS

STATEMENT OF MARK KRIKORIAN, EXECUTIVE DIRECTOR, CENTER FOR IMMIGRATION STUDIES, BEFORE THE SUBCOMMITTEE ON IMMIGRATION, CITIZENSHIP, REFUGEES, BORDER SECURITY, AND INTERNATIONAL LAW, COMMITTEE OF THE JUDICIARY, U.S. HOUSE OF REPRESENTATIVES, HEARING ON THE NEED FOR GREEN CARDS FOR HIGHLY SKILLED WORKERS, JUNE 12, 2008

The public is assured that employment-based immigration categories in our law is Einstein immigration. Even many of those concerned about the harmful impacts of low-skilled immigration often take for granted that higher skilled workers are needed.

But like everything else in immigration policy, skills-based immigration is not what it seems. Once we peel away the misconceptions, we find that the highly skilled workers in question often really are not that highly skilled, and the need for them is really more an employer need for cheaper labor.

First, a couple of numbers. Last year, 162,000 or so foreigners were granted legal permanent residence in the five employment based categories. More than half of them were in the third category, EB-3, which is for skilled workers and professionals, though a majority of those were really for family members, and this is the category that is at the center of the discussion about the supposed need for high-skilled workers.

Research shows that, contrary to the claims of lobbyists, these workers are not necessarily the best and brightest. Dr. Norman Matloff, professor of computer science at UC-Davis, has found that there is no premium paid to foreign workers in science, technology, engineering, and mathematics whose employers are petitioning for green cards. In a market economy, if these foreign workers were indeed the outstanding talents we are told they are, they would be paid accordingly with wages far above the prevailing wage, and they are not.

What is more, Dr. Matloff has found that the large majority of these foreign workers are hired in the two lowest levels of ability, according to the Labor Department's classifications and thus unlikely to be contributing much to innovation. In fact, most of the large tech firms had only a handful of workers in the highest skill level category where the innovations are most likely to be found. As he summed up, "The vast majority of the foreign workers, including those at most major tech firms, are people of just ordinary talent doing ordinary work. They are not the innovators the industry lobbyists portray them to be."

And we see a similar situation looking at H-1B visas that are the supposedly temporary visas that serve as a stepping stone to much of employment-based immigration, with software expert John Miano finding the overwhelming majority of them are not highly skilled for their occupations and are paid well below the median for comparable American workers.

So what should our skills-based immigration program look like? The first thing to keep in mind is that in today's America "skilled" does not mean what it did a century ago in the Ellis Island era. Then a high school graduate anywhere in the United States was unusual and a college graduate was rare indeed.

Today, with Americans having attained dramatically higher levels of education, any foreigner asking to be admitted based on exceptional skills would need to demonstrate even greater levels of accomplishment acquired abroad without subsidies from the American taxpayer, and every foreign student is subsidized to the tune of thousands of dollars by the taxpayer to justify admission.

And another very important point is that the admission of large numbers of technical workers or other skilled workers would have a perverse long-term effect by decoupling

American business from the fate of the American educational system, since companies could simply import their workers from abroad. Business is the country's single most important interest group, and if it is true that American students are not being adequately trained for the technical jobs of tomorrow, mass skilled immigration actually frees American firms from the need to pressure lawmakers and schools for whatever educational reforms might be needed to address the problem.

For instance, if hospitals and other firms had easy access to foreign nurses,... then the incentive to build those new nursing skills and the other things that Congressman [John] Conyers referred to is simply not there or is dramatically reduced.

There is really no reason any employer should be permitted to make an end-run around our flexible dynamic labor force of 150 million people unless the prospective immigrant in question has unique, remarkable abilities. One way to do that would be simply to give green cards to anybody who scores 140 on an English language IQ test. It certainly would be preferable than this H-1B business that Dr. [Yongjie] Yang rightly criticized.

Another way to do that, maybe a more practical way, would be to use the current system but limit it to the genuinely best and brightest category, EB1-1 and EB1-2. Those are the aliens of extraordinary ability and outstanding professors and researchers.

Congress, in fact, in the legislative history of the immigration law specifically said, "that that visa is intended for the small percentage of individuals who have risen to the very top of their field of endeavor." That is Einstein immigration, if you will, and those are the only foreign citizens who should be granted special immigration rights based on their skills.

Last year, we gave about 11,000 green cards to people in that category, including family members, and, you know, we could easily cap that at 15,000 or not have any cap at all if the standards were high enough because, after all, if we are talking about the immigration of geniuses, how many geniuses really are there in the world? (http://judiciary.house.gov/hearings/printers/110th/42851.PDF)

TESTIMONY OF STEVEN FRANCY, EXECUTIVE DIRECTOR, RNS WORKING TOGETHER, AFL-CIO, BEFORE THE SUBCOMMITTEE ON IMMIGRATION, CITIZENSHIP, REFUGEES, BORDER SECURITY, AND INTERNATIONAL LAW, COMMITTEE OF THE JUDICIARY, U.S. HOUSE OF REPRESENTATIVES, HEARING ON THE NEED FOR GREEN CARDS FOR HIGHLY SKILLED WORKERS, JUNE 12, 2008

First of all, the continuing shortage of Registered Nurses is a problem that virtually everyone acknowledges.

If you were to walk the halls of America's hospitals and asked a nurse what is the number one problem that they face, they would probably say, "We do not have enough staff to deliver quality care."

While we appreciate everyone's efforts in trying to address this crisis, we do not believe that relying upon thousands of additional foreign nurses to deliver health care in the United States is an appropriate solution to the nursing shortage.

There are many factors that contribute to the nursing shortage. Two of the major factors that I would like to draw your attention to today is our inability to train enough Americans to become registered nurses and the difficult working conditions that nurses face. To resolve these and other factors that contribute to the nursing shortage will require a focused, comprehensive strategy.

First, we do not have the capacity to train enough nurses. Last year alone, approximately 150,000 qualified applicants for nursing schools were turned away because there were not enough seats available. Our inability to train these applicants is due to a shortage of RN faculty who are often paid less than practicing nurses.

Congress needs to pass legislation that will increase the capacity of nursing schools to train nurses. This would include incentives to attract nurse faculty as well as to actively recruit and provide financial assistance to those Americans who would like to become nurses.

In addition, it is estimated there are about 2.9 million licensed RNs in the United States, but only 2.4 million are providing care to patients. Hundreds of thousands of licensed nurses have left the bedside in favor of the many other job options now available from outpatient care, computer jobs, pharmaceutical jobs, or leaving nursing entirely.

A key reason for this migration away from the bedside is that chronic understaffing and unmanageable workloads are a day-to-day reality. While increasing the number of visas may seem like an easy solution, in reality, it does nothing to retain nurses that are already trained, skilled professionals.

Stopping this leakage of nurses will require Congress to direct their attention to this issue and pass legislation that will directly improve working conditions. Examples include prohibiting mandatory overtime, passing minimum staffing ratios, and safe patient care to reduce injuries of nurses.

We are confident by taking these steps, many of those nurses who have left the profession and are now thinking about leaving the profession will come back and care for America's sick.

As you know, America is not the only country facing a nursing shortage. Indeed, there is a worldwide shortage of registered nurses. Thus, the use of immigration policies that allegedly benefit one country in the short run can be devastating to a developing country's ability to deliver health care to their citizens.

Some countries have even a greater shortage of nurses, and any loss of the nurses they have trained can undermine their government's efforts to staff their own hospitals and clinics. In 1 year alone, Ghana lost more than 500 nurses, more than double the number of its new graduates. In the Philippines, not only are they losing more nurses than graduate from nursing school, now even doctors...are training to become nurses in the hope that they will find employment in the United States. In Zimbabwe, it has been estimated that the nurse-to-patient ratio is one nurse to every 700 patients.

Obviously, nurses in developing countries will find coming to America for a job very attractive because of the increase in their income, but expanding nurse visas simply outsources nurse training to developing countries and robs them of many of the nurses they have trained.

In sum, taking nurses from poor countries will have a small short-run impact on the U.S. while increasing the short- and long-term misery of poor and developing countries.

Again, I understand that increasing the number of work visas seems like an easy solution. However, we believe that developing a comprehensive long-term strategy that addresses the factors contributing to the nurse shortage in our country, such as increasing our capacity to educate new nurses and improving working conditions, is a more productive use of time and resources and is the only real way in which America can solve this long-term issue (http://judiciary.house.gov/hearings/printers/110th/42851.PDF).

LETTER FROM THE AMERICAN COUNCIL ON INTERNATIONAL PERSONNEL, THE COLLEGE AND UNIVERSITY PROFESSIONAL ASSOCIATION FOR HUMAN RESOURCES, THE NATIONAL ASSOCIATION OF HOME BUILDERS, THE NATIONAL ASSOCIATION OF MANUFACTURERS, AND THE SOCIETY FOR HUMAN RESOURCES MANAGEMENT, SENT TO THE CHAIRMAN OF THE HOUSE WAYS AND MEANS COMMITTEE, U.S. HOUSE OF REPRESENTATIVES, COMMENTING ON THE EMPLOYMENT ELIGIBILITY VERIFICATION SYSTEMS (E-VERIFY) AND IN SUPPORT OF NEW EMPLOYEE VERIFICATION ACT, MAY 6, 2008

We believe the New Employee Verification Act (NEVA) (HR 5515) represents the next generation of electronic verification. NEVA builds upon the lessons learned from the pilot project but changes some fundamental aspects to ensure that any mandatory system meets the needs of both the government and employers. The following are the reasons we believe NEVA is a superior solution over simple mandatory expansion of E-Verify.

NEVA Builds upon Existing Programs in Which 90% of Employers Are Already Enrolled

According to the Department of Homeland Security (DHS), only 62,000 of the nation's approximately 7 million employers are enrolled in E-Verify. DHS notes that 2,000 employers are enrolling every week. These statistics belie the grave challenges in enrolling all U.S. employers. With less than 1% of employers currently enrolled, even at a rate of 5,000 employers per week, it would take over *25 years* to enroll all current U.S. employers! The problem of enrolling employers is illustrated in Arizona, which mandated E-Verify use by all employers as of January 1, 2008. Despite the fact that businesses can lose their license for failing to use E-Verify, fewer than 15% of employers have enrolled.

NEVA avoids the tremendous burden of enrolling virtually all employers in a new system by building upon an existing system that has proven its effectiveness—the National Directory of New Hires. Over 90% of employers currently report new hires to this system which is used to check for child support enforcement. While modifying the National Directory of New Hires for this new purpose would admittedly require resources, the burden would be much less than expanding the current E-Verify pilot program. Resources could be devoted to improving the databases instead of educating employers on enrollment. Employers have been participating in their states "new hire" database since 1986 and are already familiar with the processes and procedures for reporting necessary information. NEVA would utilize information in the new hire database to determine if a new employee's information is consistent with information maintained by [the Social Security Administration (SSA)] or by DHS.

NEVA Provides the Resources to Fix the Database Problems That Hamper E-Verify

Our associations represent thousands of employers who desire a reliable system for determining who is authorized to work in the United States. Mistakes and delays in this process could prove to be costly for a number of employers and employees who are caught in the system. The current system, if mandatory, could prove to be unreliable in terms of providing employers with an effective and efficient electronic employment verification system.

In 2006, SSA's Inspector General issued a report estimating that there are discrepancies in approximately 17.8 million (4.1 percent) of the 435 million social security records. These errors include incorrect social security numbers, names, dates of birth and citizenship status. A recent report compiled by the CATO Institute, and using the estimates from SSA's Inspector General, determined that a mandatory electronic employment verification system would result in 11,000 workers per day receiving a tentative non-confirmation throughout a given year (based on an average of 55 million hew hires per year).

Furthermore, according to a [U.S.] Government Accountability Office (GAO) report released last year, "resolving some DHS non-confirmations can take several days, or in a few cases even weeks." As more employers enroll, this timeframe is likely to get longer. As GAO noted, the expansion of E-Verify will "affect the capacity of the system because of the increased number of employer queries."

NEVA takes several steps to resolve these database errors so that employers and employees will have fewer tentative non-confirmations to resolve. First, NEVA provides for advanced appropriated funds and staffing to clean up the databases. This will benefit not only work authorization, but also the other government programs that rely on these databases for information. Second, NEVA requires SSA and DHS to certify the accuracy of the system in advance of full implementation and annually thereafter. Finally, NEVA requires the GAO to evaluate the accuracy, efficiency and impact of the employment verification system. These checks in the system will ensure that employers are not hamstrung by a system that does not enable them to hire U.S. citizens and other legal workers with ease and certainty.

NEVA Is Truly "Electronic"

There is a great deal of misunderstanding about our current "electronic" pilot program which is really not an all "electronic" system. While E-Verify requires employers to submit an inquiry via the internet to confirm work authorization, an employer can submit this only after it has completed the Form I-9 and examined one or more of 24 paper-based documents to establish identity and work authorization. Employers must retain two sets of records—the electronic one and the Form I-9 (which can be maintained in paper, on microfiche or electronically). Some proposals would expand this dual-recordkeeping by requiring employers to keep photocopies of the documents examined and to record the electronic approval or denial number on the Form I-9. All of these steps cost employers time and money and open the possibility for recordkeeping mistakes.

NEVA brings recordkeeping into the twenty-first century by creating a truly "electronic" verification system that eliminates the Form I-9 (known as the Electronic Employment Verifications System [EEVS]). In addition, NEVA provides flexibility and easy accessibility for all employers by allowing electronic inquiries over the internet and telephone and builds upon a database that is already used by many employers.

NEVA Protects against Identity Theft

One of the acknowledged weaknesses of E-Verify is that it cannot detect stolen identities. Thus, if an undocumented

worker presents legitimate but stolen or forged documents that contain the identity of a U.S. citizen, the worker will appear to be work-authorized, duping the employer into hiring and training someone who may ultimately be deported.

NEVA addresses this problem by allowing employers to elect to participate in a program that makes identity theft extremely difficult. The Secure Electronic Employment Verification System (SEEVS) enables employers to send newly hired employees to government certified private companies that will authenticate their identities through the use of publicly available databases. An employee's identity is temporarily "locked" with a biometric tool until work authorization is verified by the government. Many employers are willing to pay for this additional assurance, particularly where it builds upon other background screening they are already doing.

Individuals could also benefit from this more secure system. Under EEVS or SEEVS, employees could choose to "lock" their identity and their social security number, thus making it very difficult for anyone to steal their information.

SEEVS is a more advanced system than the photo screening tool currently piloted by DHS. It does not require employers to make subjective determinations by visually comparing a scanned photo to a paper document. Furthermore, it does not require integration with state driver's license or federal passport databases. The photo tool is currently limited to verifying the authenticity of Lawful Permanent Residents or individuals with Employment Authorization Documents that contain a photo which comprise a very small percentage of the workforce. Efforts to expand this tool to driver's licenses and passports will take years.

NEVA Preempts the Patchwork of State Employment Verification Laws

Frustrated with Congressional inaction on immigration reform, a growing number of states are mandating the use of E-Verify for employers or contractors, and the list continues to grow. The expanding patchwork of state employment verification laws is causing many problems for human resource managers and employers struggling to maintain consistent and compliant practices across the country. Federal relief is needed.

Many states are exploiting the current [Immigration and Nationality Act] provisions under 8 USCA § 1324 (a)(h)(2) on employment practices. While the language preempts "any State or local law imposing civil or criminal sanctions (other than through licensing and similar laws) upon those who employ, or recruit or refer for a fee for employment, unauthorized aliens," states like Arizona have been using the "licensing exception" language to mandate the use of the E-Verify system—a system that is not ready for large-scale expansion. NEVA clarifies that immigration is solely the purview of the Federal Government by establishing a clearer preemption standard that protects both employers and employees from a patchwork of state laws.

Our organizations strongly support a uniform national policy towards employment verification. The employers we represent want an efficient, effective, and powerful electronic tool to prevent unauthorized employment. We need strong reform that is realistic and workable. That is why we, the listed associations, support HR 5515, the New Employee Verification Act (NEVA) (http://waysandmeans .house.gov/hearings.asp?formmode=view&id=7209).

TESTIMONY OF CONGRESSMAN DENNIS MOORE (D-KS, 3RD DISTRICT), BEFORE THE SUBCOMMITTEE ON SOCIAL SECURITY OF THE HOUSE COMMITTEE ON WAYS AND MEANS, U.S. HOUSE OF REPRESENTATIVES, MAY 6, 2008

Today, I testify before your committee as not only a Member deeply concerned about the current efficiency of the Social Security Administration, but also a Member who hears from countless constituents demanding that the federal government do *something* to put an end to illegal immigration. Especially since the tragedy of September 11, 2001, with the thousands of Americans that died from the senseless acts of terrorism, our citizens have demanded that our government regain full, operational control of our borders. We are putting our citizens' safety at risk if we do not know who is coming into our country.

. . . In 2001, our country had an estimated 6–7 million illegal aliens. With little enforcement of our current immigration laws at either the workplace or the border, that population has ballooned to an estimated 11–12 million illegal aliens, approximately doubling the number of illegal aliens who reside in the United States.

Additionally, in 1999, there were 417 employers that were fined for hiring illegal immigrants. That number dropped to only three employers that received fines for employing illegal aliens in 2004. Even more troubling, the [U.S. Government Accountability Office (GAO)] reported that approximately 20,000 criminals successfully gained entry into the United States just in 2006. Why? Because of staffing shortages at airports and other border entry points. This record is not acceptable to the American people, and it is unacceptable to me.

I am proud that the 110th Congress has decided to act. I voted for H.R. 2399, the Alien Smuggling and Terrorism Prevention Act sponsored by Congressman Baron Hill. The bill would increase penalties for knowingly bringing an illegal immigrant into our country, or harboring an illegal immigrant, and was approved by a vote of 412–0 in the House. Pursuant to H.Res. 1126, the text of H.R. 2399, as approved by the House, was added as Division B to H.R. 2830, the Coast Guard Authorization Act, as approved by

the House on April 24, 2008. The combined bill has been sent to the Senate for consideration.

I also voted for H.R. 2764, the fiscal year (FY) 2008 omnibus appropriations measure which President [George W.] Bush signed into law (P.L. 110-161). The funding measure included $3 billion of emergency border security and immigration enforcement funds that I strongly supported, and those funds are helping our border patrol agents regain operational control of our borders and enforce the laws already on our books.

But that is not enough. A number of my constituents have expressed concern about our border security, but they also point out that immigrants break our laws to earn a better living for them and their families. I do not begrudge anyone who wants to work hard to provide for their families, but as a former District Attorney for twelve years, I understand that if the government turns a blind eye to illegal behavior, our rule of law will be undermined and chaos will ensue. If the prospects of a job attract individuals to illegally cross our borders or overstay their visa, part of our immigration enforcement approach should include verifying who is and who isn't authorized to legally work in our country.

. . . NEVA focuses on improving worksite enforcement, improving the implementation of current law which prohibits the hiring of any illegal immigrant or individual unauthorized to work in the United States. The only government employment eligibility verification system that employers can use is the voluntary E-Verify program . . . that is operated by the Department of Homeland Security (DHS). In 12 years of operation as a pilot program, E-Verify is currently utilized by fewer than one percent of American employers. NEVA would replace E-Verify with the state "new hire" reporting process which most employers already use to check for child support enforcement purposes.

Employers are legally responsible for ensuring a legal workforce, yet today's paper document verification system is unable to prevent document fraud and identity theft. An improved employment verification system that enables employers to effectively identify unauthorized workers and that allows Americans to protect their identities would help prevent identity theft and illegal employment.

H.R. 5515 would also create a voluntary biometrics option that employers could choose to use in the verification process. This Secure Electronic Employment Verification System (SEEVS) would include a standard background check and the collection of a biometric characteristic—a thumb print, for example—to secure an employee's identity and prevent the illegal use of a Social Security number, stolen drivers' license, or the altered identification documents of legitimate citizens and legal residents. A biometric employment verification system is supported by most Americans. A study conducted by Greenberg Quinlan Rosner Research and Public Opinion Strategies this year showed that 79% of Americans surveyed support the use of a biometric employment verification system.

When it comes to worksite enforcement, I believe the federal government needs to work with the business community to develop sound, reasonable policies that will not overtly infringe on the work of legitimate, responsible employers while weeding out the bad employers that exploit illegal immigrants and game the system. NEVA is currently supported by the Society for Human Resource Management (SHRM), the National Association of Home Builders, the National Federation of Independent Business (NFIB), National Franchisee Association, National Association of Manufacturers, Food Marketing Institute, HR Policy Association and other business groups.

It is also important to note that NEVA would preempt any state law with regard to employer fines, sanctions for federal immigration law violations, or with verifying work status and authorizations. Currently, businesses are faced with a confusing patchwork of state and local immigration laws despite the fact that the Constitution gives jurisdiction of immigration matters to the federal government. We should only ask American businesses to comply with one clear and easy to understand employment eligibility verification federal law. Also, NEVA would apply only to employers' newly hired employees and would not require employers to re-verify all existing employees. Employers would be responsible only for the hiring decisions of their own employees, and not be held liable for their subcontractors.

Finally, NEVA would take steps to protect the mission of the Social Security Administration (SSA) and the responsibilities it already maintains. Most experts agree that no matter how mandatory employment verification is implemented, SSA will play a major role based on the identity database it maintains. Unless Congress is willing to create an entirely new, separate and costly identification database, any mandatory employment verification system will require the use of SSA's database, thus requiring SSA's involvement. It is only logical to give SSA as much control and authority as possible over its own database.

Given this context, NEVA would require SSA to act only to the extent that funds are appropriated *in advance* to cover the agencies costs. In other words, the normal administrative budget for SSA's work would not be needed to implement NEVA's requirements. The SSA's Inspector General issued a report in 2006 that estimated the discrepancies in approximately 4.1 percent of agency records could result in incorrect feedback when submitted for employment eligibility verification. Through advance funding, NEVA would provide the resources SSA needs to help clean up its databases, increasing the accuracy and efficiency for all services SSA provides to Americans.

To reiterate, NEVA ensures a legal work force, safeguards workers' identities and protects Social Security as summarized here—

1. Ensures a legal work force

- Strengthens enforcement through enhanced employer penalties.

- Provides a superior, user-friendly employment verification system by replacing the current paper-based, error-prone, I-9 work status verification process with a paperless, reliable Electronic Employment Verification System (EEVS).

- Allows employers to enter EEVS data through an electronic portal they already use to enhance child support enforcement, their State's new hire reporting program.

- Requires the Social Security Administration (SSA) and the Department [of] Homeland Security to certify the accuracy of the system in advance of full implementation, and annually thereafter. Also requires the Government Accountability Office to evaluate the accuracy, efficiency and impact of the EEVS.

- Provides for the verification of U.S. citizens only by the SSA.

- Avoids a "big brother" law enforcement agency building new databases on law abiding citizens.

2. Safeguards workers' identities

- Creates an alternate, voluntary Secure Electronic Employment Verification System (SEEVS) to verify employees' identity and work eligibility and to "lock" that identity once verified.

- Establishes a network of private sector government-certified companies to authenticate new employees' identities utilizing existing background check and document screening tools.

- Ensures each employee's identity is safeguarded through the use of a biometric identifier (such as a thumbprint). The employee would then present their identifier to their employer to confirm their identity and work authorization.

- Curtails the creation of new government bureaucracies to administer the employment verification system and does not require any new national or state identification cards to facilitate the process, thus [saving] billions of dollars as well as preventing another opportunity for identity fraud.

3. Protects Social Security

- Prevents wages earned through future unauthorized work from being used to determine benefits.

- Protects the SSA's primary mission and trust funds by authorizing employment verification only through advanced appropriated funds.

It is clear to me that Congress needs to replace our out-of-date and ineffective immigration laws with strong reforms that will improve our border security and make our immigration policies more realistic, enforceable, and complimentary to the global economy we live in. I appreciate many of the ways NEVA attempts to address these complicated issues.

We must secure our borders. We must strictly enforce our current laws. We must crack down on employers who knowingly hire and exploit illegal immigrants (http://way sandmeans.house.gov/hearings.asp?formmode=printfriendly &id=6891).

TESTIMONY OF CONGRESSWOMAN NANCY BOYDA (D-KS, 2ND DISTRICT), BEFORE THE SUBCOMMITTEE ON IMMIGRATION, CITIZENSHIP, REFUGEES, BORDER SECURITY, AND INTERNATIONAL LAW, COMMITTEE OF THE JUDICIARY, U.S. HOUSE OF REPRESENTATIVES, IN OPPOSITION TO H.R. 750, THE "SAVE AMERICA COMPREHENSIVE IMMIGRATION ACT OF 2007," NOVEMBER 8, 2007

We are at a crisis. The lack of enforcement of our immigration laws has led to increased illegal immigration. This is unacceptable to the people of the Second District of Kansas.

In addition to my concerns about the flood of illegal immigrants, I am concerned about where the immigration conversation is going in our country. We are losing control, not only of our borders, but also of the conversation on illegal immigration and how to fix the problem. The longer we delay action, the worse the rhetoric is going to get. At this time we are able to have a conversation that discusses how we move forward securing our borders, verifying employment and enforcing our laws. If we do not address the immigration crisis soon, we will no longer be able to have a conversation about how we fix the problem—it will instead be a yelling match with heated rhetoric against immigrants and immigration. That would be a conversation about hatred. That is not a conversation that represents America at its finest and it is not a conversation that we need to have.

I believe that there are three steps to stopping the flow of illegal immigrants—secure our borders, require employers to verify employment eligibility and enforce immigration laws. Congress can and must demonstrate to the American people that we are willing and able to protect our nation's borders.

We are a nation of laws—and they must be enforced. Those violating these laws cannot be rewarded. Enforcement of immigration laws would substantially reduce illegal immigration and greatly increase border security. This is why I have serious concerns about some of the provisions of H.R. 750, the Save America Comprehensive Immigration Act of 2007. I believe that several provisions reward those who have broken our laws. And all that does is encourage others to do the same . . . .

. . . H.R. 750 has some worthwhile provisions. It increases the number of border patrol agents by significant numbers and it contains much needed provisions to retain those agents with loan repayments, easing of the regulations on recruitment and retention bonuses, and the repeal of the DHS Human Resources Management System which has been the cause of much of the career dissatisfaction in this vitally important agency.

H.R. 750 also pays particular attention to addressing concerns about sex offenders abusing our already dysfunctional immigration system.

We are at a turning point, the longer we delay action, the more the rhetoric will get out of hand. If that happens, we will not be able to solve this problem.

The solution is clear—secure our borders, eliminate the jobs magnet and enforce our laws (http://judiciary .house.gov/hearings/pdf/Boyda071108.pdf).

TESTIMONY OF JULIE KIRCHNER, GOVERNMENT RELATIONS DIRECTOR, FEDERATION FOR AMERICAN, IMMIGRATION REFORM (FAIR), BEFORE THE SUBCOMMITTEE ON IMMIGRATION, CITIZENSHIP, REFUGEES, BORDER SECURITY, AND INTERNATIONAL LAW, COMMITTEE OF THE JUDICIARY, U.S. HOUSE OF REPRESENTATIVES, IN OPPOSITION TO H.R. 750, THE "SAVE AMERICA COMPREHENSIVE IMMIGRATION ACT OF 2007," NOVEMBER 8, 2007

My name is Julie Kirchner, and I am the Executive Director at FAIR. FAIR is a public interest organization advocating a just immigration policy guided by the national interest and the interests of American citizens. Our organization has over 300,000 members and activists in 49 states and works with over 50 organizations across the country. FAIR does not receive any federal grants, contracts or subcontracts.

. . . For two years, supporters of amnesty have tried to pass so-called "comprehensive immigration reform." They have tried both under a Republican Congress and under the current Democratic Congress. They have tried both "comprehensive" bills and piecemeal approaches. Each time, however, they have failed.

...The American public rejects immigration reform proposals that do not respect the rule of law and only further strain our immigration system. For years, the American people have watched the borders violated *en masse*, the illegal alien population skyrocket out of control, and employment prospects and wages erode as employers hire illegal alien workers to increase their profit margin. The American people are frustrated with our immigration system and want meaningful change, not disregard for the rule of law.

Public opinion polls confirm that Americans have rejected all types of amnesty.... Americans do not oppose immigration, but they want it to come through a system that operates with integrity and at a rate America can absorb.

The Save America Comprehensive Immigration Reform Act [H.R. 750] has several major components that impact legal immigration, illegal immigration, border security and interior enforcement. The impact of these provisions would indeed be severe and continue for generations to come. Below, I will briefly summarize the provisions of this legislation and set forth FAIR's objections to them.

Legal Immigration

The first and obvious change the Save America Act makes to our immigration system is a dramatic expansion of family-based immigration to the United States. It does this by doubling the annual number of family-based immigrant visas from 480,000 to 960,000.... The preferences for *extended* family members built into our immigration laws have created the problem of chain migration, by which extended family members enter the country and are then able to petition for the entry of *their* extended family members, and the cycle repeats itself. Immigration thus grows at an ever-increasing pace and the ability of Congress and the American people to set annual caps or limits is effectively eliminated.

Furthermore, as chain migration grows, it inevitably leads to backlogs and pressure builds to continue raising the visa caps, as this bill demonstrates. This process means immigration runs on auto-pilot. It is the immigrants themselves who decide who comes, not the American people. Indeed, the very nature of chain migration forecloses our ability as a people to select immigrants based on skill, diversity, or other factors that serve the nation's interests. Ultimately, the problem of chain migration will have no end unless Congress is disciplined. By doubling the number of family-based immigrant visas, the Save America Act simply ignores the need for discipline and instead takes the very steps that will exacerbate this problem.

The United States currently admits approximately 1.2 million legal immigrants each year—equivalent to a city the size of Dallas. All told, the Save America Act would expand this number by at least 535,000, leading to an annual admissions rate of 1.8 million. This is almost the population of Dallas and Fort Worth combined.

Border Security

...This legislation would increase the number of border patrol agents by 15,000 over the next five years. It would also provide border agents with improved technology to apprehend illegal border crossers. It would also add 1,000 new inspectors at airports and land crossings each year between 2008 and 2012. And, the number of detention beds would be increased by 100,000, so that those aliens who the Border Patrol apprehends entering the country illegally or who Immigration and Customs Enforcement (ICE) find illegally present in the country can be detained and processed appropriately. Finally, it gives the governors of border states the authority to bring 1,000 border patrol agents to bear on particular areas where there are "international border security emergencies."

Interior Enforcement

Unfortunately, these border security provisions are overshadowed by the complete failure of the legislation to support the interior enforcement of our immigration laws. For example, Section 1402(b) of the Save America Comprehensive Immigration Act repeals one of our most effective and popular enforcement tools, the 287(g) program. The 287(g) program was created in 1996 when Congress passed the Illegal Immigration Reform and Immigrant Responsibility Act...adding Section 287(g) to the Immigration and Nationality Act (INA). This section authorizes the Department of Homeland Security (DHS) to enter into immigration enforcement agreements with state and local law enforcement agencies. These agreements allow designated officers to perform immigration law enforcement functions, pursuant to a Memorandum of Agreement (MOA), provided that the local law enforcement officers receive appropriate training and function under the supervision [of] Immigration and Customs Enforcement (ICE) officers.

...This program has shown tremendous potential and its popularity is growing rapidly. As of September 2007, ICE had entered into 287(g) agreements with 28 cities and had trained 484 police officers who were responsible for over 25,000 arrests. In addition, there are currently 74 jurisdictions that have applications pending, 18 of which are in North Carolina alone. It is ironic...that the Save America Act would place one of the few immigration programs the federal government is running effectively on the chopping block—and would do so in the name of "reform."

In addition to this step backwards, the Save America Comprehensive Immigration Reform Act does nothing to advance worksite enforcement. There is no mandatory use of the E-Verify Program...and there is no increase in employer sanctions for illegal employment practices. This is a gaping hole in any immigration bill that calls itself "comprehensive." Even the Bush-Kennedy Amnesty Bill (S.1639) debated in the Senate this summer contained such provisions.

Amnesty

...On top of all this, the Save America Act effectively contains four amnesty provisions. The first such program is the "Earned Access to Legalization Program," described in Section 501 of the bill. Under this program, an illegal alien would receive lawful permanent resident status if he or she has: been physically present in the United States for five years; good moral character; never been convicted of a crime; completed a course on reading, writing and speaking English; accepted the values and cultural life of the United States; and completed 40 hours of community service. The program waives various grounds of admissibility for participation in the program. These include waivers for illegal aliens who have engaged in document fraud.

The second amnesty program is a modification of the failed DREAM Act that would legalize "children" who have met certain educational requirements. This program is a rolling amnesty, allowing not only an uncapped number of children currently in the country to obtain amnesty, but also granting amnesty to children who enter the U.S. in future years.

The third amnesty can be found in Section 503 of the Save America Act, which makes changes to the Registry Statute. The Registry Statute, found in INA § 249, lets the government create a record of legal status for aliens who have been in the United States for a lengthy period of time, but for whom there is no record of lawful entry. Currently, this remedial "house-cleaning" statute lets the Secretary of Homeland Security create a record of lawful entry for any person who entered before 1972, and is generally neither a terrorist or engaged in criminal activity. The Save America Act would move the date of entry up to 1986, letting those who could not qualify for the amnesty granted under the Immigration Reform and Control Act to obtain amnesty twenty-one years later. It is hard to see why we should permit people who could not qualify for amnesty the first time to receive it now.

The fourth amnesty can be found in Section 805 of the Save America Act, which restores Section 245(i) of the INA. Section 245(i) allowed illegal aliens to become legal residents without leaving the country if they married a U.S. citizen or resident. This provision was clearly incompatible with the intent of Congress in 1996 to penalize those who violated our immigration laws by imposing on them a penalty of foreign residence before they would be eligible to return to the United States as legal residents. Section 245(i) was phased out in 2002 because it encouraged widespread marriage fraud and rewarded illegal aliens with amnesty. During the several years that this provision was in force as an exceptional measure, hundreds of thousands of illegal aliens took advantage of it to gain legal status and remain here. It became the avenue of last resort by an alien facing deportation. Restoring this provision would only encourage more fraud and more illegal immigration.

Policy Considerations

...Granting amnesty to illegal aliens will not solve our immigration crisis—it simply motivates more illegal aliens to come here seeking amnesty. The American people are looking to Congress to break the cycle of this flawed approach, one which is sadly becoming our de facto American immigration policy. Amnesty sends a message to people worldwide that America no longer cares about the enforcement of its laws. Moreover it sends a terrible message to *legal aliens* that their respect for our laws is irrelevant to how they will be treated. Consider the difference in how the Save America Act would treat aliens who have committed social security fraud. If this legislation were passed, a *legal* alien who had committed social security fraud would be charged, prosecuted, tried, convicted, would receive a criminal record, and would be deported. Meanwhile an *illegal* alien who had committed social security fraud would not be charged, not be tried, not be prosecuted, not be convicted, would not receive a criminal record, would be allowed to stay in the U.S. *and* would be issued a valid social security number....There is no justice in this outcome.

In addition to the inherent unfairness of amnesty, the Save America Act further strains our immigration system by encouraging more chain migration. In 1995, the United States Commission on Immigration Reform, headed by Representative Barbara Jordan, recommended that Congress prioritize immediate family members over extended family and limit family-sponsored immigration to only the spouse and minor children of U.S. citizens and legal permanent residents and to the parents of U.S. citizens. These categories, the Commission said, should have a cap of 400,000 per year. It also recommended eliminating preferences for extended family members. The Save [America] Act ignores these recommendations and takes U.S. immigration policy in the exact opposite direction.

...The United States population is currently growing at a rate of over 2.8 million each year, forty percent of whom are legal immigrants. As the rate of immigration grows without limit, so does development and the impact on our environment. America simply cannot sustain perpetual growth in finite places with limited resources. Our immigration policy must recognize this truth. The Save America Act does not (http://judiciary.house.gov/hearings/pdf/Kirchner071108.pdf).

TESTIMONY OF CONGRESSMAN SILVESTRE REYES (D-TX, 16TH DISTRICT), BEFORE THE SUBCOMMITTEE ON IMMIGRATION, CITIZENSHIP, REFUGEES, BORDER SECURITY, AND INTERNATIONAL LAW, COMMITTEE OF THE JUDICIARY, U.S. HOUSE OF REPRESENTATIVES, NOVEMBER 8, 2007

Before coming to Congress, I served for 26 ½ years in the U.S. Border Patrol where I began as an agent and was fortunate enough to be chief in two different locations for the last thirteen of those years. As the only Member of Congress with a background in border enforcement, I have first-hand knowledge of what we need to do in order to reduce illegal immigration while keeping our borders and the nation safe.

During my tenure, I not only oversaw long stretches of terrain between the ports of entry, but for four years, I also worked at the international bridges. I have a broad understanding of what it takes in order to secure the many components [of] our nation's borders.

... I have always said that we need a comprehensive immigration reform plan with three main components: strengthened border security; earned legalization for those who qualify; and a guest worker program with tough employer sanctions. Comprehensive reform is like a three-legged stool. Without one leg, the stool topples.

Our nation's current immigration system is broken and is in desperate need of repair. For the past few years, Congress and the Administration have been very concerned with cracking down on illegal immigration and have focused much of their energy on security-only legislation. While I certainly agree that we need to focus on assuring everyone enters our country legally, we must also remember not to put all of our attention and resources on one particular agency or leg of the stool.

... While the number of United States Border Patrol agents has risen dramatically, the other agencies that assist in the security effort have been neglected. When the average person thinks about the men and women overseeing our nation's borders the first group that comes to mind is the men and women in green. People often forget about the men and women in blue, the Customs and Border Protection Officers (CBOs), those who, for instance in my district, saw more than 28.5 million individuals traveling by car over this past fiscal year alone.

Our international bridges are suffering because attention has not been placed on them. Over the last several months, constituents in my district and across the nation have faced increased wait times, and recent reports state that times have escalated upwards from two to three hours. This problem must be stopped and help must be directed in order to keep security high while allowing for the free flow of trade and commerce.

I would like to take a moment and talk specifically to a section in [Sheila] Jackson-Lee's bill, H.R. 750, the Save America Comprehensive Immigration Act. Section 639 would increase the number of inspectors at our air and land ports of entry. While 1,000 additional officers is an increase, we need to do more. In El Paso alone, four international bridges are in need of a total of more than 150 Custom and Border Protection Officers. We must look at the current state of our nation's ports of entry and commit to properly funding staffing levels adequate enough to provide security for our nation. Being under-staffed and underfunded is unacceptable.

We must also remember all the agencies securing the border along with Border Patrol. We must increase the number of United States Attorneys, Immigration and Customs Enforcement inspectors, immigration judges, federal judges, U.S. Marshals, as well as Bureau of Prison personnel.

Immigration reform must continue to move forward, and we must take a holistic approach to ensure we encompass all relevant agencies (http://judiciary.house .gov/hearings/pdf/Reyes071108.pdf).

POTENTIAL DISCRIMINATION AGAINST IMMIGRANTS BASED ON NATIONAL ORIGIN

This brochure, which was issued in October 2000 and is reprinted virtually in its entirety below, is available on the U.S. Department of Justice Web site (updated July 25, 2008, http://www.usdoj.gov/crt/legalinfo/nordwg_brochure.html). The brochure is published in Arabic, Cambodian, Chinese, English, Farsi, French, Haitian Creole, Hindi, Hmong, Korean, Laotian, Punjabi, Russian, Spanish, Tagalog, Urdu, and Vietnamese.

INTRODUCTION

Federal laws prohibit discrimination based on a person's national origin, race, color, religion, disability, sex, and familial status. Laws prohibiting national origin discrimination make it illegal to discriminate because of a person's birthplace, ancestry, culture or language. This means people cannot be denied equal opportunity because they or their family are from another country, because they have a name or accent associated with a national origin group, because they participate in certain customs associated with a national origin group, or because they are married to or associate with people of a certain national origin.

The Department of Justice's Civil Rights Division is concerned that national origin discrimination may go unreported in the United States because victims of discrimination do not know their legal rights, or may be afraid to complain to the government. To address this problem, the Civil Rights Division has established a National Origin Working Group to help citizens and immigrants better understand and exercise their legal rights....

CRIMINAL VIOLATIONS OF CIVIL RIGHTS

- A young man of South Asian descent is assaulted as he leaves a concert at a nightclub. The assailant, a member of a skinhead group, yells racial epithets as he beats the victim unconscious in the club's parking lot with fists and a pipe.

- At Ku Klux Klan meetings, a Klansman tells other members that Mexicans and Puerto Ricans should go "back where they came from." They burn a cross in the front yard of a young Hispanic couple in order to frighten them and force them to leave the neighborhood. Before burning the cross, the defendant displays a gun and gives one of his friends another gun in case the victims try to stop them.

- An American company recruits workers in a small Mexican town, promising them good work at high pay. The company smuggles the Mexicans to the United States in an empty tanker truck. When they finally arrive in the U.S., the workers are threatened, told that if they attempt to leave their factory they will be killed.

The Criminal Section of the Civil Rights Division prosecutes people who are accused of using force or violence to interfere with a person's federally protected rights because of that person's national origin. These rights include areas such as housing, employment, education, or use of public facilities. You can reach the Criminal Section at (202) 514-3204....

DISABILITY RIGHTS

- An HMO that enrolls Medicaid patients tells a Mexican American woman with cerebral palsy to come back another day for an appointment while it provides immediate assistance to others.

This example may be a violation of federal laws that prohibit discrimination because of disability as well as laws that prohibit discrimination because of national origin. If you believe you have been discriminated against because you have a disability you may contact the Disability Rights Section at (800) 514-0301 (voice) or 800-514-0383 (TTY)....

EDUCATION

- A child has difficulty speaking English, but her school does not provide her with the necessary assistance to help her learn English and other subjects.

- A majority Haitian school does not offer honors classes. Other schools in the district that do not have many Haitian students offer both honors and advanced placement courses.

These examples may be violations of federal law, which prohibits discrimination in education because of a person's national origin. The Division's Educational Opportunities Section enforces these laws in elementary and secondary schools as well as public colleges and universities. The Education Section's work addresses discrimination in all aspects of education, including assignment of students to schools and classes, transportation of students, hiring and placement of faculty and administrators, distribution of school resources, and provision of educational programs that assist limited English speaking students in learning English.

To file a complaint or for more information, contact the Education Section at (202) 514-4092....

EMPLOYMENT

- A transit worker's supervisor makes frequent racial epithets against the worker because his family is from Iran. Last week, the boss put up a fake sign on the bulletin board telling everyone not to trust the worker because he is a terrorist.

- A woman who immigrated from Russia applies for a job as an accountant. The employer turns her down because she speaks with an accent even though she is able to perform the job requirements.

- A food processing company requires applicants who appear or sound foreign to show work authorization documents before allowing them to complete an employment application while native born Caucasian applicants are not required to show any documents before completing employment applications. Moreover, the documents of the ethnic employees are more closely scrutinized and more often rejected than the same types of documents shown by native born Caucasian employees.

These examples may be violations of the law that prohibits discrimination against an employee or job applicant because of his or her national origin. This means an employer cannot discipline, harass, fire, refuse to hire or promote a person because of his or her national origin.

If you believe an employer, labor organization or employment agency has discriminated against you because of your national origin, contact:

Equal Employment Opportunity Commission

(800) 669-4000

(Employers with 15 or more employees)

Office of Special Counsel

(800) 255-7688

(Employers with 4 to 14 employees)

Employment Litigation Section

(202) 514-3831

(State or local government employer with a pattern or practice of illegal discrimination)

In addition, an employer may violate federal law by requiring specific work authorization documents, such as a green card, or rejecting such documents only from applicants of certain national origins. For more information or to file a charge, contact the Division's Office of Special Counsel at the above address or toll-free number.

HOUSING

- A Native Hawaiian family is looking for an apartment. They are told by the rental agent that no apartments are available, even though apartments are available and are shown to white applicants.

- A realtor shows a Latino family houses only in Latino neighborhoods and refuses to show the family houses in white neighborhoods.

These examples may be violations of the federal Fair Housing Act. That law prohibits discrimination because of national origin, race, color, sex, religion, disability, or familial status (presence of children under 18) in housing. Individual complaints of discrimination may be reported to the Department of Housing and Urban Development (HUD) at (800) 669-9777. If you believe there is a pattern or practice of discrimination, contact the Division's Housing and Civil Enforcement Section at (202) 514-4713.

LENDING

- A Latina woman is charged a higher interest rate and fees than white male customers who have similar financial histories and apply for the same type of loan.

This example may be a violation of federal laws that prohibit discrimination in lending because of national origin, race, color, sex, religion, disability and marital status or because any of a person's income comes from public assistance. If you believe you have been denied a loan because of your national origin or other protected reason, you may ask the lender for an explanation in writing of why your application was denied.

If the loan is for a home mortgage, home improvement, or other housing-related reasons, you may file a complaint with the Department of Housing and Urban Development at (800) 669-9777. If the loan is for purposes other than housing (such as a car loan), you may file a complaint either with the Division's Housing and Civil Enforcement Section or with the lender's regulatory agency. If your experience was part of a pattern or practice of discrimination you may also call the Housing and Civil Enforcement Section at (202) 514-4713, to obtain more information about your rights or to file a complaint.

PUBLIC ACCOMMODATIONS

- In a restaurant, a group of Asian Americans waits for over an hour to be served, while white and Latino customers receive prompt service.

- Haitian American visitors to a hotel are told they must pay in cash rather than by credit card, are charged higher rates than other customers, and are not provided with the same amenities, such as towels and soap.

These examples may be violations of federal laws that prohibit discrimination because of national origin, race, color, or religion in places of public accommodation. Public accommodations include hotels, restaurants, and places of entertainment. If you believe you have been denied access to or equal enjoyment of a public accommodation where there is a pattern or practice of discrimination, contact the Housing and Civil Enforcement Section at (202) 514-4713....

POLICE MISCONDUCT

- Police officers constantly pull over cars driven by Latinos, for certain traffic violations, but rarely pull over white drivers for the same violations.

- A police officer questioning a man of Vietnamese origin on the street gets angry when the man is unable to answer his questions because he does not speak English. The Officer arrests the man for disorderly conduct.

These examples may be violations of the Equal Protection Clause of the United States Constitution. They may also be violations of the Omnibus Crime Control and Safe Streets Act of 1968. That law prohibits discrimination because of national origin, race, color, religion, or sex by a police department that gets federal funds through the U.S. Department of Justice. They may also violate Title VI of the Civil Rights Act of 1964, which prohibits discrimination by law enforcement agencies that receive any federal financial assistance, including asset forfeiture property.

Complaints of individual discrimination can be filed with the Coordination and Review Section...at 1-888-848-5306.

Complaints of individual discrimination may also be filed with the Office of Justice Programs...at (202) 307-0690.

The Special Litigation Section investigates and litigates complaints that a police department has a pattern or practice of discriminating on the basis of national origin. To file a complaint, contact the Special Litigation Section at (202) 514-6255....

CIVIL RIGHTS OF INSTITUTIONALIZED PERSONS

- A jail will not translate disciplinary hearings for detainees who do not speak English.

- A state's psychiatric hospital has no means of providing treatment for people who do not speak English.

These examples may be violations of the Equal Protection Clause of the United States Constitution. The Special Litigation Section enforces the constitutional rights of people held in state or local government institutions, such as prisons, jails, juvenile correctional facilities, mental health facilities, developmental disability or mental retardation facilities, and nursing homes. If you are a resident of any such facility and you believe there is a pattern or practice of discrimination based on your national origin, contact the Special Litigation Section at (202) 514-6255....

FEDERALLY ASSISTED PROGRAMS

- A local social services agency does not provide information or job training in Korean even though one quarter of local residents speak only Korean.

- A hospital near the Texas/Mexico border dresses its security officers in clothes that look like INS uniforms to scare Latinos away from the emergency room. Latino patients are told to bring their own translators before they can see a doctor.

These examples may be violations of federal laws that prohibit discrimination because of national origin, race or color by recipients of federal funds. If you believe you have been discriminated against by a state or local government agency or an organization that receives funds from the federal government, you may file a complaint with the Division's Coordination and Review Section at (888) 848-5306.... The Coordination and Review Section will refer the complaint to the federal funding agency that is primarily responsible for enforcing nondiscrimination prohibitions applicable to its recipients.

VOTING

- Despite requests from voters in a large Spanish-speaking community, election officials refuse to provide election materials, including registration forms and sample ballots, in Spanish or to allow Spanish speakers to bring translators into the voting booth.

- A polling official requires a dark-skinned voter, who speaks with a foreign accent and has an unfamiliar last name, to provide proof of American citizenship, but does not require proof of citizenship from white voters.

The election officials' conduct may violate the federal laws prohibiting voting discrimination. The Voting Rights Acts do not specifically prohibit national origin discrimination. However, provisions of the Acts make it illegal to limit or deny the right to vote of any citizen not only because of race or color, but also because of membership in a language minority group. In addition, the Acts also require in certain jurisdictions that election materials and assistance be provided in languages other than English.

Additionally, Section 208 of the Voting Rights Act, allows voters, who need help because of blindness, disability or because they cannot read or write, to bring someone (other than an employer or union representative) to help. This means that a voter who needs help reading the ballot in English can bring a friend or family member to translate. In some places, election officials must provide information, such as voter registration and the ballot, in certain language(s) other than English. This can include interpreters to help voters vote.

If you believe that you have been discriminated against in voting or denied assistance in casting your ballot, you may contact the Division's Voting Section at (800) 253-3931.

APPENDIX II
MAPS OF THE WORLD

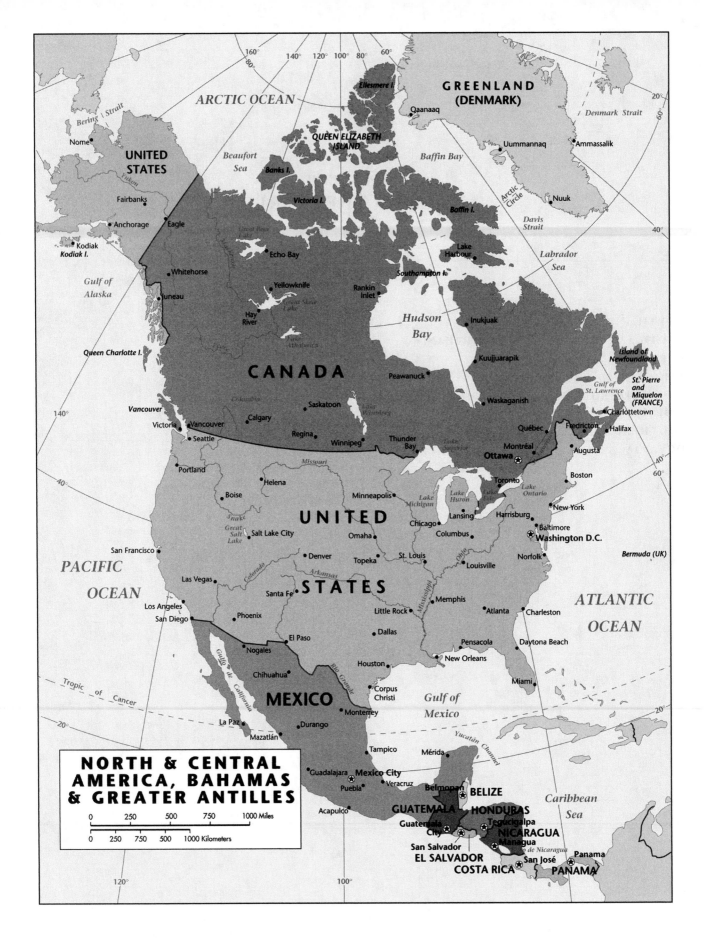

NORTH & CENTRAL AMERICA, BAHAMAS & GREATER ANTILLES

0   250   500   750   1000 Miles

0   250   500   750   1000 Kilometers

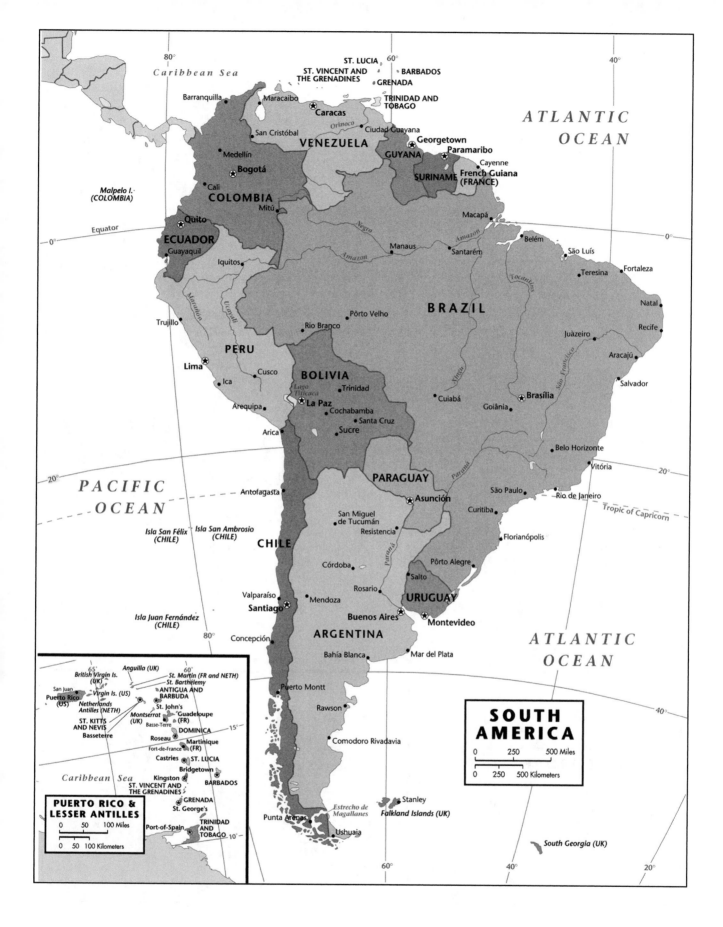

SOUTH AMERICA

0	250	500 Miles

0	250	500 Kilometers

PUERTO RICO & LESSER ANTILLES

0	50	100 Miles

0	50	100 Kilometers

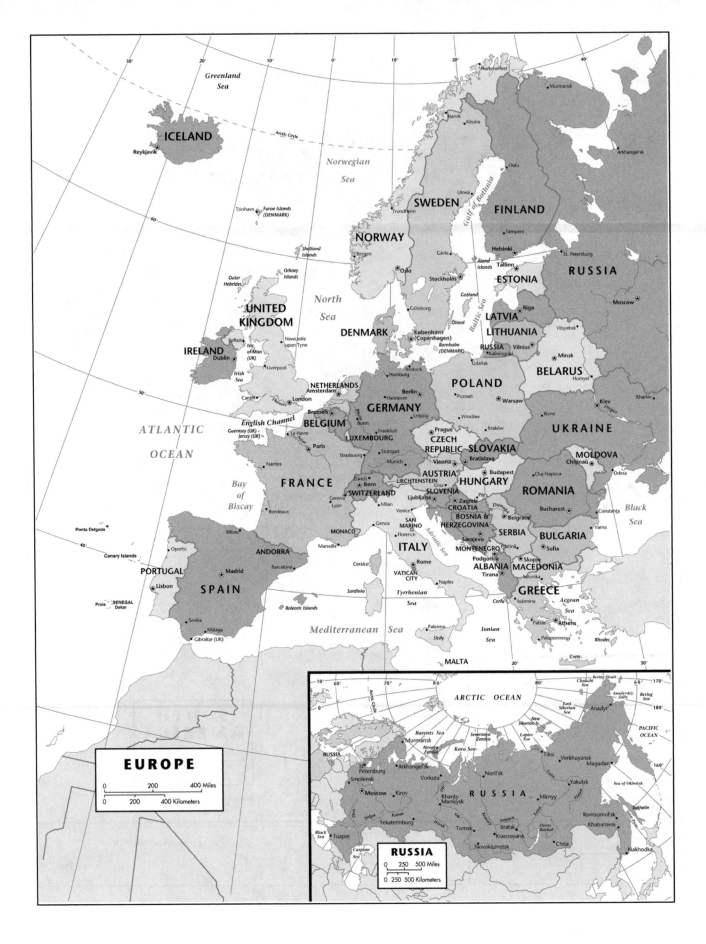

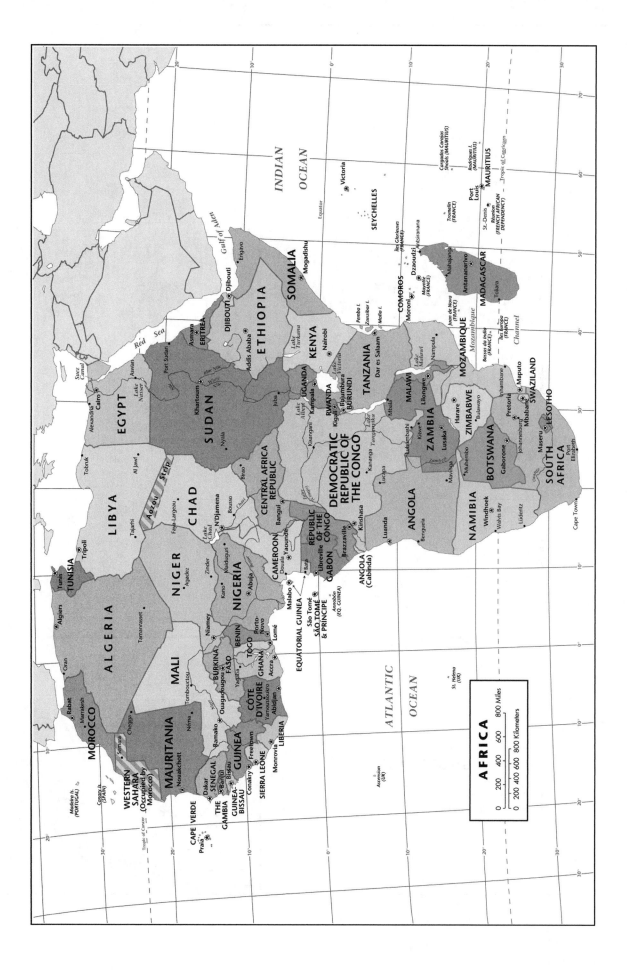

AFRICA

| 0 | 200 | 400 | 600 | 800 Miles |
| 0 | 200 400 | 600 | 800 Kilometers |

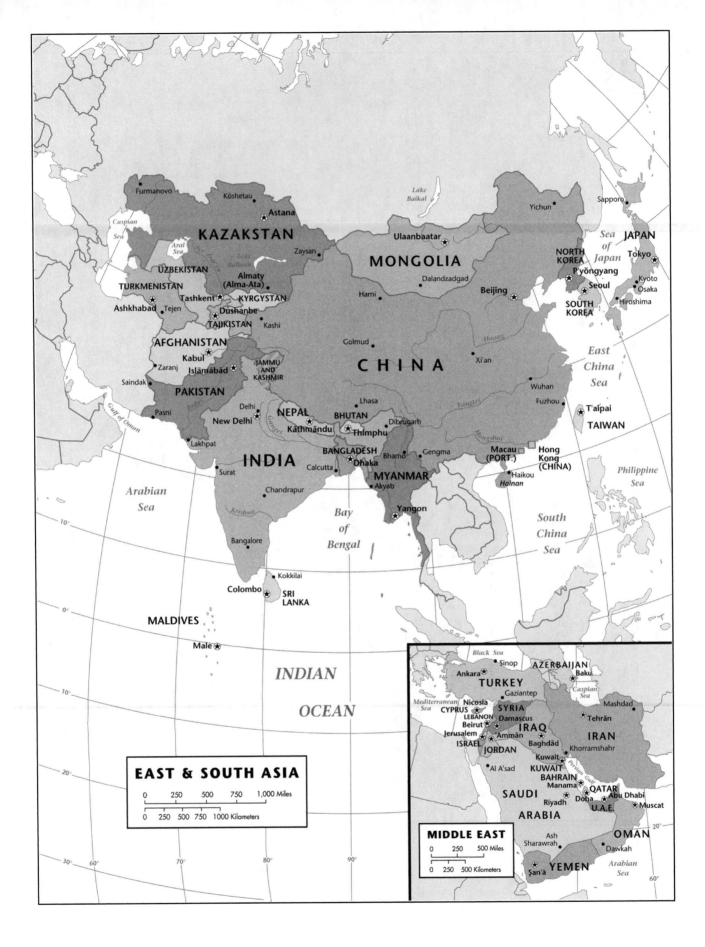

EAST & SOUTH ASIA

0   250   500   750   1,000 Miles

0   250   500   750   1000 Kilometers

MIDDLE EAST

0   250   500 Miles

0   250   500 Kilometers

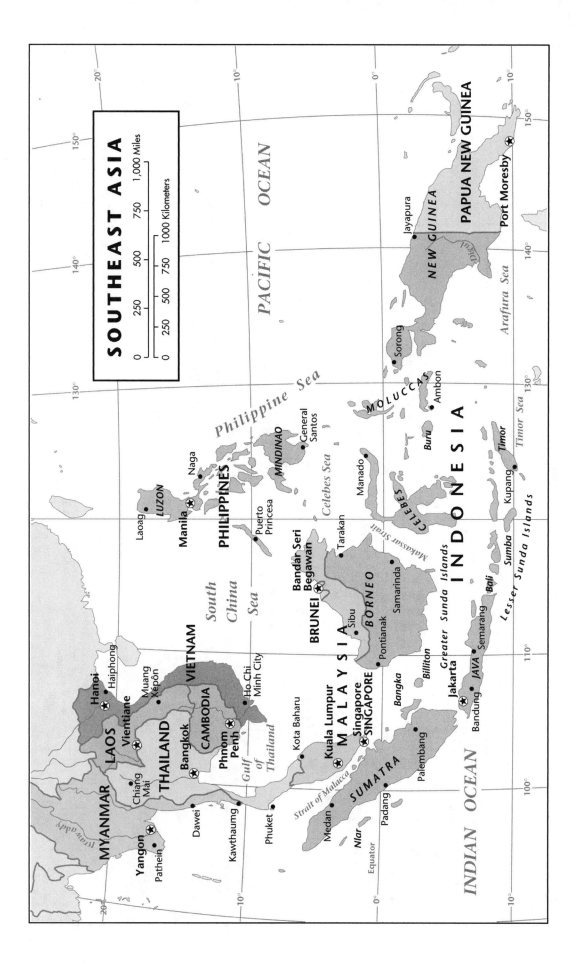

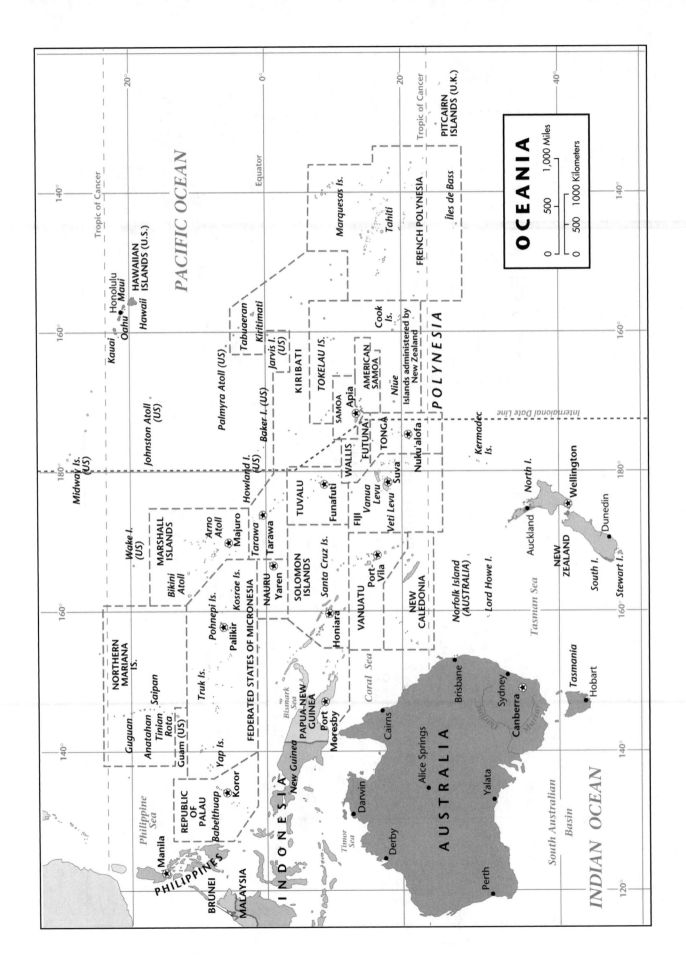

IMPORTANT NAMES
AND ADDRESSES

American Border Patrol
2160 E. Fry Blvd., Ste. 426
Sierra Vista, AZ 85635
1-800-600-8642
(520) 803-7703
E-mail: info@americanborderpatrol.com
URL: http://www.americanborderpatrol.com/

American Civil Liberties Union
125 Broad St., 18th Floor
New York, NY 10004
1-888-567-2258
URL: http://www.aclu.org/

Amnesty International USA
5 Penn Plaza
New York, NY 10001
(212) 807-8400
FAX: (212) 627-1451
E-mail: aimember@aiusa.org
URL: http://www.amnestyusa.org/

**Bureau of Population, Refugees, and
Migration**
U.S. Department of State
2201 C St. NW
Washington, DC 20520
(202) 647-4000
URL: http://www.state.gov/g/prm/

Cato Institute
1000 Massachusetts Ave. NW
Washington, DC 20001-5403
(202) 842-0200
FAX: (202) 842-3490
URL: http://www.cato.org/

Center for Immigration Studies
1522 K St. NW, Ste. 820
Washington, DC 20005-1202
(202) 466-8185
FAX: (202) 466-8076
E-mail: center@cis.org
URL: http://www.cis.org/

**Federation for American Immigration
Reform**
25 Massachusetts Ave. NW, Ste. 330
Washington, DC 20001
(202) 328-7004
FAX: (202) 387-3447
URL: http://www.fairus.org/

Human Rights Watch
350 Fifth Ave., 34th Floor
New York, NY 10118-3299
(212) 290-4700
FAX: (212) 736-1300
E-mail: hrwnyc@hrw.org
URL: http://www.hrw.org/

Immigration Works USA
1101 Pennsylvania Ave. SE, Ste. 204
Washington, DC 20003
(202) 506-4541
FAX: (202) 506-4642
E-mail: info@immigrationworksusa.org
URL: http://www.immigrationworksusa.org/

Institute of International Education
809 United Nations Plaza
New York, NY 10017-3580
(212) 883-8200
FAX: (212) 984-5452
URL: http://www.iie.org/

**Lutheran Immigration and Refugee
Service**
700 Light St.
Baltimore, MD 21230
(410) 230-2700
FAX: (410) 230-2890
E-mail: lirs@lirs.org
URL: http://www.lirs.org/

**Mexican American Legal Defense and
Education Fund**
634 S. Spring St., 11th Floor
Los Angeles, CA 90014
(213) 629-2512
FAX: (213) 629-0266
URL: http://www.maldef.org/

Migration Policy Institute
1400 16th St. NW, Ste. 300
Washington, DC 20036
(202) 266-1940
FAX: (202) 266-1900
E-mail: info@migrationpolicy.org
URL: http://www.migrationpolicy.org/

National Conference of State Legislatures
444 N. Capitol St. NW, Ste. 515
Washington, DC 20001
(202) 624-5400
FAX: (202) 737-1069
URL: http://www.ncsl.org/

National Council of La Raza
Raul Yzaguirre Bldg.
1126 16th St. NW
Washington, DC 20036
(202) 785-1670
FAX: (202) 776-1792
E-mail: comments@nclr.org
URL: http://www.nclr.org/

National Foundation for American Policy
2111 Wilson Blvd., Ste. 700
Arlington, VA 22201
(703) 351-5042
URL: http://www.nfap.net/

National Immigration Forum
50 F St. NW, Ste. 300
Washington, DC 20001
(202) 347-0040
FAX: (202) 347-0058
URL: http://www.immigrationforum.org/

**New York City Department of City
Planning**
22 Reade St.
New York, NY 10007-1216
(212) 720-3300
FAX: (212) 720-3219
URL: http://www.nyc.gov/html/dcp/

Office of Refugee Resettlement
Administration for Children and Families
370 L'Enfant Promenade SW
Washington, DC 20201
URL: http://www.acf.hhs.gov/programs/orr/

Pew Hispanic Center
1615 L St. NW, Ste. 700
Washington, DC 20036-5610
(202) 419-3600
FAX: (202) 419-3608
E-mail: info@pewhispanic.org
URL: http://www.pewhispanic.org/

ProLiteracy
1320 Jamesville Ave.
Syracuse, NY 13210
1-888-528-2224
FAX: (315) 422-6369
E-mail: info@proliteracy.org
URL: http://www.proliteracy.org/

Refugee Council USA
3211 Fourth St. NE
Washington, DC 20017-1194
(202) 541-5404
FAX: (202) 541-3468
E-mail: info@rcusa.org
URL: http://www.refugeecouncilusa.org/

United Nations High Commissioner for Refugees
Case Postale 2500
CH-1211 Genève 2 Dépôt, Switzerland
(011-41) 22-739-8111
URL: http://www.unhcr.org/cgi-bin/texis
/vtx/home

Urban Institute
2100 M St. NW
Washington, DC 20037
(202) 833-7200
URL: http://www.urban.org/

U.S. Census Bureau
4600 Silver Hill Rd.
Washington, DC 20233

(301) 763-2422
URL: http://www.census.gov/

U.S. Citizenship and Immigration Services
2675 Prosperity Ave.
Fairfax, VA 22031-4906
1-800-375-5283
URL: http://www.uscis.gov/

U.S. Committee for Refugees and Immigrants
2231 Crystal Dr., Ste. 350
Arlington, VA 22202-3711
(703) 310-1130
FAX: (703) 769-4241
URL: http://www.refugees.org/

U.S. Customs and Border Protection
1300 Pennsylvania Ave. NW
Washington, DC 20229
1-877-CBP-5511
URL: http://www.cbp.gov/xp/cgov/

U.S. Department of Health & Human Services
200 Independence Ave. SW
Washington, DC 20201
1-877-696-6775
(202) 619-0257
URL: http://www.hhs.gov/

U.S. Department of Homeland Security
Washington, DC 20528
(202) 282-8000
URL: http://www.dhs.gov/

U.S. Department of Justice
950 Pennsylvania Ave. NW
Washington, DC 20530-0001
(202) 514-2000
E-mail: AskDOJ@usdoj.gov
URL: http://www.usdoj.gov/

U.S. Department of Labor
Frances Perkins Bldg.
200 Constitution Ave. NW
Washington, DC 20210

1-866-4-USA-DOL
URL: http://www.dol.gov/

U.S. House of Representatives Committee on the Judiciary Subcommittee on Immigration, Citizenship, Refugees, Border Security, and International Law
2138 Rayburn House Office Bldg.
Washington, DC 20515
(202) 225-3951
URL: http://www.house.gov/judiciary/
immigration.htm

U.S. Immigration and Customs Enforcement
500 12th St. SW
Washington, DC 20536
1-866-DHS-2-ICE
URL: http://www.ice.gov/

US/Mexico Border Counties Coalition
310 N. Mesa, Ste. 824
El Paso, TX 79901
(915) 838-6860
FAX: (915) 838-6880
URL: http://www.bordercounties.org/

U.S. Senate Committee on the Judiciary Subcommittee on Immigration, Refugees, and Border Security
224 Dirksen Senate Office Bldg.
Washington, DC 20510
(202) 224-8352
FAX: (202) 228-2260
URL: http://judiciary.senate.gov/
subcommittees/immigration109.cfm

U.S. Social Security Administration
Windsor Park Bldg.
6401 Security Blvd.
Baltimore, MD 21235
1-800-772-1213
URL: http://www.ssa.gov/

RESOURCES

The U.S. government provides most of the statistical information concerning immigration and naturalization. Much of the information comes from branches of the U.S. Department of Homeland Security (DHS). The primary source is the annual *Yearbook of Immigration Statistics*, an online publication of the U.S. Citizenship and Immigration Services (USCIS). The USCIS quarterly report *Student and Exchange Visitor Information System, General Summary Quarterly Review* tracks the location and status of foreign students who attend U.S. schools. Another DHS report that provides valuable data is *Annual Flow Report: Refugees and Asylees, 2007* (July 2008).

Because immigration affects so many areas, information on this topic can also be found in reports issued by government agencies outside the DHS. For example, the U.S. Department of Agriculture oversees and provides information on the Food Stamp Program. The Social Security Administration controls the Earnings Suspense File and jointly conducts the E-Verify program with the DHS. The Social Security Administration's *Annual Statistical Supplement to the Social Security Bulletin, 2007* (April 2008) offers information on immigrant tax contributions and benefits. The Centers for Disease Control and Prevention monitors health issues in publications such as *Reported Tuberculosis in the United States, 2007* (September 2008). The U.S. Coast Guard reports attempted illegal immigrants intercepted in the oceans and seas in *Alien Migrant Interdiction* (October 2008). The U.S. Census Bureau collects and distributes the nation's statistics in *Statistical Abstract of the United States: 2009* (2008).

The U.S. Department of State details results of issued visas in *Report of the Visa Office 2007* (2008) and *Visa Bulletin for February 2009* (January 2009). Refugee admissions and future admission levels are provided in *Proposed Refugees Admissions for Fiscal Year 2009: Report to the Congress* (2008). The *Trafficking in Persons Report* (June 2008) offers data on U.S. efforts to combat human trafficking and assist victims.

The U.S. Department of Justice published *Attorney General's Annual Report to Congress and Assessment of the U.S. Government Activities to Combat Trafficking in Persons, Fiscal Year 2007* (May 2008). The U.S. Department of Labor provides information on jobs in *Foreign-born Workers: Labor Force Characteristics in 2007* (March 2008).

Information about schools, students, and staffing came from the U.S. Department of Education in *Schools and Staffing Survey* (2006), *Participation in Education* (2008), and *English Language Acquisition: Fiscal Year 2009 Budget Request* (2008).

The U.S. Government Accountability Office (GAO) studies many aspects of immigration. Among the reports used in this publication were *U.S. Asylum System: Significant Variation Existed in Asylum Outcomes across Immigration Courts and Judges* (September 2008), *Homeland Security: U.S. Visitor and Immigrant Status Indicator Technology Program Planning and Execution Improvements Needed* (December 2008), and *Immigration Enforcement: Weaknesses Hinder Employment Verification and Worksite Enforcement Efforts* (August 2005).

The Congressional Research Service (CRS) is a think tank that works exclusively for members and committees of Congress. The CRS publications used in this book include *Farm Labor: The Adverse Effect Wage Rate (AEWR)* (March 2008), *Border Security: Barriers along the U.S. International Border* (May 2008, Blas Nuñez-Neto and Yule Kim), and *U.S. International Borders: Brief Facts* (November 2006, Janice Cheryl Beaver). The National Conference of State Legislatures published *State Laws Related to Immigrants and Immigration in 2008, January 1–November 30, 2008* (December 2008).

Organizations that support and oppose immigration have published extensive information on various immigration issues. Reports used in this book include the Migration Policy Institute's *Adult English Language Instruction in the United States: Determining Need and Investing Wisely* (July

2007, Margie McHugh, Julia Gelatt, and Michael Fix). The Center for Immigration Studies published *Immigrants in the United States, 2007: A Profile of America's Foreign-Born Population* (November 2007, Steven A. Camarota), *Who Pays? Foreign Students Do Not Help with the Balance of Payments* (June 2008, David North), and *Homeward Bound: Recent Immigration Enforcement and the Decline in the Illegal Alien Population* (July 2008, Steven A. Camarota and Karen Jensenius). The Institute of International Education provided detailed information about foreign students in U.S. colleges and universities in *Open Doors 2008 "Fast Facts"* (November 2008). The Inter-American Development Bank studied the impact of money immigrants send to their home countries to support family members in *The Changing Pattern of Remittances: 2008 Survey of Remittances from the United States to Latin America* (April 2008) and *Survey of Latin American Immigrants in the United States* (April 2008). The Pew Research Center for the People and the Press published *American Mobility: Who Moves? Who Stays Put? Where's Home?* (October 2008, D'Vera Cohn and Rich Morin), *An Even More Partisan Agenda for 2008* (January 2008), and *Latino Settlement in the New Century* (October 2008, Richard Fry). The Pew Hispanic Center delivered results of its research in *Trends in Unauthorized Immigration: Undocumented Inflow Now Trails Legal Inflow* (October 2008, Jeffrey S. Passel and D'Vera Cohn), *Hispanics See Their Situation in U.S. Deteriorating; Oppose Key Immigration Enforcement Measures* (September 2008, Mark Hugo Lopez and Susan Minushkin), *Hispanics and the Economic Downturn: Housing Woes and Remittance Cuts* (January 2009, Mark Hugo Lopez, Gretchen Livingston, and Rakesh

Kochhar), and *Hispanics and the New Administration: Immigration Slips As a Priority* (January 2009, Mark Hugo Lopez and Gretchen Livingston). Western Washington University's Border Policy Research Institute provided *International Mobility and Trade Corridor (IMTC) Project Passenger Intercept Survey Final Report* (September 2008, Melissa Miller, Hugh Conroy, and David Davidson). An in-depth look at border issues was provided by the US/Mexico Border Counties Coalition in *At the Cross Roads: US/Mexico Border Counties in Transition* (March 2006, Dennis L. Soden et al.).

The Center for Public Priorities studied the plight of unaccompanied immigrant children and published *A Child Alone and without Papers* (September 2008, Amy Thompson). The National Opinion Research Center surveyed doctoral graduates of American universities for *Doctorate Recipients from United States Universities: Summary Report 2006* (2007, Thomas B. Hoffer et al.). Georgetown University's Center for Applied Research in the Apostolate provided information on foreign-born seminarians in *Catholic Ministry Formation Enrollments: Statistical Overview for 2007–2008* (April 2008, Mary L. Gautier). The Heritage Foundation published *The Fiscal Cost of Low-Skill Immigrants to the U.S. Taxpayer* (May 2007, Robert E. Rector and Christine Kim). The National Foundation for American Policy studied foreign-born athletes for *Coming to America: Immigrants, Baseball and the Contributions of Foreign-born Players to America's Pastime* (October 2006, Stuart Anderson and L. Brian Andrew). Gale, Cengage Learning thanks all these organizations for permission to reproduce their data and graphics.

INDEX

Page references in italics refer to photographs. References with the letter t following them indicate the presence of a table. The letter f indicates a figure. If more than one table or figure appears on a particular page, the exact item number for the table or figure being referenced is provided.

A

Abuse, domestic, 20
ACTC (Additional Child Tax Credit), 85–86, 86(t6.2)
Active-duty military, 38
Adams, John, 2
Additional Child Tax Credit (ACTC), 85–86, 86(t6.2)
Address change notification, 23
Adjustment of status, 35
Admissions classification. *See* Classification
Admissions wait time, 63
Adoption, 35–36, 35*f*, 36*f*, 36*t*
Adult immigrant population, 68*f*
Adult limited English proficiency immigrants, 94–96
Adverse effect wage rates, 48*t*
Affirmative asylum claims, 57, 58*f*, 58(t4.6)
Africa, 141*f*
Agricultural workers, 15, 42–45, 49*t*, 110
Agriprocessors Inc., 68–69
Airline travel, 74
Alfonso, José, 72
Alien and Sedition Acts, 2
Alien Registration Act, 11, 22
Alien Registration Receipt Card, 22
Al-Qaeda, 78
American Competitiveness in the 21st Century Act, 37
American Council on International Personnel, 125–127
American Party, 2
Amnesty, 129–131

Anti-immigration sentiment
    anti-Irish sentiment, 2
    Asian immigration, 7, 8
    white supremacists, 7
Antiterrorism measures. *See* Counter-terrorism measures
Antitrafficking measures, 59–60, 60(t4.11)
A-number system, 11
Application processing wait time, 63, 64(t5.2)
Arizona, 25, 70–71
Arkansas, 93(f6.6), 100
Armed forces, 38
Arrests, 81
Article 1, U.S. Constitution, 1–2
Asia, 142*f*, 143*f*
Asian immigrants
    Chinese Exclusion Act, 7–8
    Immigration Act of 1917, 9
    legal permanent residents, 37
    quotas, 10
Asylees
    claims filing, 57
    countries of nationality, 56, 58*t*
    court challenges, 57–58
    Cuban migrants, 75–76
    definition, 57
    expedited removal, 58–59
    flow, 58*f*
    parole authority, 12
    refugee as distinct from asylee, 54
Athletes, 45–46, 49*f*
Attorney general, 12

B

Balanced Budget Act, 21
Baseball players, 45–46
Basic Naturalization Act, 8
Basic Pilot Program, 16, 19
Battered brides, 20

Bechtolsheim, Andreas von, 105
Bersin, Alan, 74
Bilingual Education Act, 91
Biometric data, 22, 75, 127
Birth, countries of. *See* Countries of nativity
Bock, Laszlo, 108
Border issues
    apprehensions, 77*f*
    Canada, 77–78, 78*t*, 79*f*, 80*f*
    crossing card costs, 65
    crossing points, 66
    entrance/exit monitoring, 73–74
    Homeland Security Act, 23
    land, 76–77
    Mexico, 69–70, 70*f*, 71*t*, 76, 79–81
    National Security Entry-Exit Registration System, 75
    Save America Comprehensive Immigration Act, 129–130, 132
    water, 75–76
Border Patrol, U.S., 10, 73
    See also Customs and Border Protection
Boyda, Nancy, 129
Bracero Program, 12–13, 80
Budget of federal government immigration programs, 87–88
Bureau of Immigration, 8
Bury, David C., 25
Bush, George W.
    Homeland Security Act, 23
    Military Personnel Citizenship Processing Act, 38
    REAL ID Act, 23
    Secure Fence Act, 76
Business cycle, 98–100

C

California, 24–25, 76, 77*f*, 81
Canada, 77–78, 78*t*, 79*f*, 80*f*
Cascade Gateway, 78

income, 33*t*

marital status, 30(*f*3.4)

nineteenth century, 2

number of immigrants living in the U.S., 28*f*

poverty status, 34*f*

projections for native and foreign-born population, 28*t*

region of birth, 28*f*, 29*f*

Ports of entry, 132

Post–Civil War era, 7

Post–World War II era, 11

Potato famine, 2

Poverty

illegal aliens, 69, 69*t*

immigrants and their U.S. born children, by nativity, 85*t*

immigrants compared to natives, 84–85, 84*f*

by nativity, citizenship status, and arrival period, 34*f*

women, 119

working immigrants, 31

Preference categories, 36–37, 39*t*

Presidential proclamations, 46, 48

Priests, 102–103, 103*f*

Prison population, 81

Privacy issues, 24, 117–118

Professional athletes, 45–46, 49*f*

Prohibited countries list, 23

ProLiteracy, 94

Proposed Refugees Admissions, 55

Proposition 187 (California), 24

Proposition 200 (Arizona), 25

Public accommodations discrimination, 135

Public assistance. *See* Welfare benefits

Public opinion

federal government raids, 72

Hispanic priorities for Obama administration, 112*f*

importance of immigration as an issue, 111–112, 112(*t*7.10)

Latin American immigrants' opinion on discrimination, 98*f*

of Latinos on their situation in the U.S., 66*f*

travel documents, 79

workplace raids, 72, 73*f*

Q

Quotas, 8–12

R

Racial profiling, 72–73

Raids, workplace, 72–73, 73*f*

Reagan, Ronald, 11

REAL ID Act, 23, 37, 55

Reciprocal visa fees, 64

Recordkeeping, 126

Refugee Act of 1980, 12, 53, 54

Refugee Relief Act, 54

Refugees

admissions legislation, 53–54

admissions limits, 54–55, 55(*t*4.3)

admissions numbers, 54, 54*f*

arrivals, by admission category, 56(*t*4.5)

arrivals, by country of nationality, 55(*t*4.1)

assistance budget, 61*f*

demographics, 56(*t*4.4)

1950s, 11

post–World War II era, 12

priority admissions categories, 55–56

social services, 61

by state of residence, 55(*t*4.2)

Regents, Martinez v., 97

Region of birth

current statistics, 28, 29*f*

legal permanent residents, 37, 40*t*

naturalized citizens, 39, 42*f*, 43*f*

Regional responses to border issues, 69–70

Regions of last residence, 3*t*–6*t*

Registration

nonimmigrants, 22

World War II, 11

Remittances, 97–98, 99*t*, 100*f*

Repatriated Mexican children, 68*t*

Republican Party, 2

Requirements for naturalization, 37–38

Resettlement, refugee, 53–55, 61

Ressam, Ahmed, 78

Restaurants, immigrant workforce and, 71

Restitution, 11

Returns and removals, 48–51, 50*f*, 58–59, 121

Reyes, Silvestre, 132

Rights of immigrants, 100

Roosevelt, Franklin D., 8, 11

Roosevelt, Theodore, 8

S

San Diego, California, 76, 77*f*

Sanctions, employer, 16

Save America Comprehensive Immigration Act, 118–122, 129–132

Science and technology, employment issues, 109, 113–114

Seasonal agricultural workers, 42–45, 49*t*

Secret societies, 2, 7

Secure Electronic Employment Verification System, 126, 127

Secure Fence Act, 76–77

Select Commission on Immigration and Refugee Policy, 13

Seminary students, 103, 103*f*

September 11 attacks, 15, 22

Service workers, 110, 119

SEVIS (Student and Exchange Visitor Information System), 23, 108

Simpson, Alan K., 20

Small towns, 101–102

Social Security

costs, 89–90

E-Verify system, 115–118

New Employee Verification Act, 128–129

Save America Comprehensive Immigration Act, 131

totalization agreements, 91*t*

welfare reform, 21

Social services

costs, 83–84

discrimination, 135

illegal aliens, 69, 70

refugees, 61–62

Society for Human Resources Management, 125–127

Socioeconomic status, 86(*t*6.3)

South America, 139*f*

South Asia, 142*f*

Southeast Asia, 143*f*

Southwest border, 69–70, 70*f*

Spanish language, 101–103

Special agricultural workers, 15

Specialized Refugee Foster Care Program, 62

Specialty occupations, 40

Sports, 45–46, 49*f*

Spousal abuse, 20

SSI (Supplemental Security Income), 21

State Criminal Alien Assistance Program, 90

State Department. *See* Department of State, U.S.

State laws, 7, 24–25, 25*t*, 70–72, 126–127

State Legalization Impact Assistance Grant program, 16

States

college tuition denials, 97

costs of illegal aliens, 83–84

education costs, 90–91, 92–94

foreign-born population, 28, 29*t*

high-growth industries, 110

illegal aliens, 69–72

incarceration costs reimbursement, 90

limited English proficiency students, 93*f*, 95*t*

Medicare allocations, 88

REAL ID Act, 23–24

refugee arrivals, 54, 55(*t*4.2)

Save America Comprehensive Immigration Act, 130

Statistical information

admissions classifications, 34(*t*3.7)

adoptions, 35*f*, 36*f*, 36*t*

adult immigrant population, 68*f*

U

Underground economy, 116
Undocumented aliens. *See* Illegal aliens
Uninsured immigrants, 84f, 85
United Nations High Commissioner for
 Refugees, 53
University students. *See* International
 students
Urban areas, 9
US/Mexico Border Counties Coalition,
 69–70
US-VISIT, 73, 74

V

Vehicle barrier systems, 77
Venters, Darrell, 103
Vietnam War, 13
Violence against Women Act, 20
Violence victims, 59–60
Visa Waiver Program, 74–75
Visas
 athletes, 45–46
 Continued Presence visa applications,
  60(t4.10)
 costs, 64–65
 denials, categories of, 46, 48
 Diversity Visa program, 20
 foreign students, 23
 H class, 39–46, 46f
 H-1B, 108–109, 114–115
 Immigration and Nationality Act
  Amendments, 12
 ineligibilities, 50f
 legal permanent residents, 36–37
 processing fees, 45(t3.15)
 State Department processing, 39
 students, 108, 108f
 T visa applications, 60(t4.10)
 tourists and students, 39
 trafficking victims, 59
 Visa Waiver Program, 74–75
 wait time, 63, 64(t5.1, t5.2, t5.3)
Voting rights, 135–136
Voting Rights Acts, 136

W

Wages and earnings
 adverse effect wage rate compared to
  minimum wage, by state, 48t
 Save America Comprehensive
  Immigration Act, 121–122
 seasonal agricultural workers, 43
 Social Security, 89–90
 See also Income
Wait time
 application processing, 63, 64(t5.1, t5.2,
  t5.3)
 US-VISIT system, 74
Water borders, 75–76
Welfare benefits
 discrimination, 135
 fiscal deficit from low-skilled immigrant
  households, 90f
 for households headed by immigrants
  without a high school diploma, 89(f6.3)
 illegal aliens, 69
 immigrant use, 85–86, 86(t6.2)
 immigrant use of compared to native use
  of, 84, 84f
 Immigration Reform and Control
  Act, 16
 low-skilled immigrant households,
  88–89
 refugees, 61–62
 trafficking victims, 59
Welfare reform, 21
Western Hemisphere, 11
Western Hemisphere Travel Initiative, 78
White supremacists, 7
William Wilberforce Trafficking Victims
 Protection Reauthorization Act, 59
Wilson, Woodrow, 9
Women, 118–120
Workers
 agricultural, 15, 42–45, 49t, 110
 athletes, 49f
 domestic, 119
 H class visas issued, by region, 46f
 H-1 visa program, 40–42
 H-1B visas, 108–109
 highly skilled, 113–114, 123–124
 Indian, 111(t7.8)
 low-wage, 121–122
 Mexican, 112(t7.9)
 service workers, 110, 119
 undocumented workers' impact on the
  business cycle, 98–100
 visa classification, 39–40
Workplace raids, 72–73, 73f
Worksite enforcement
 E-Verify system, 115–118
 New Employee Verification Act,
  125–129
 Save America Comprehensive
  Immigration Act, 130–131
World War I, 9
World War II, 10–11, 22

Y

Yang, Jerry, 105